DIET FOR A
STRONG HEART_____

by the same authors:
The Cancer-Prevention Diet

DIET FOR A STRONG HEART

Michio Kushi's Macrobiotic
Dietary Guidelines
for the Prevention of
High Blood Pressure,
Heart Attack, and Stroke

By MICHIO KUSHI
with ALEX JACK

Foreword by H. Robert Silverstein, M.D., F.A.C.C.

ST. MARTIN'S PRESS
NEW YORK

Note to the reader:
It is advisable for the reader to seek the guidance of a physician
and an appropriate nutritionist before implementing the
approach to health suggested by this book. It is essential that
any reader who has any reason to suspect that he or she suffers
from cardiovascular disease contact a physician promptly.
Neither this nor any other book should be used as a substitute
for professional medical care or treatment.

Library of Congress Cataloging in Publication Data

Kushi, Michio.
    Diet for a strong heart.

    1. Hypertension—Diet therapy—Recipes.   2. Macrobiotic
diet—Recipes.   3. Heart—Diseases—Prevention.   I. Jack,
Alex, 1945-   .   II. Title.
RC685.H8K85   1985   616.1'320654   85-1751
ISBN 0-312-20998-3
ISBN 0-312-00120-7 (pbk.)

Design by Mina Greenstein

Contents

Illustrations

Tables

Foreword

The single best advice that I could give you the reader is to follow Michio Kushi's guidance and direction in this book. You may learn something from me, as a medical doctor specializing in cardiology, but you will learn an immense amount from him.

Basically, Michio Kushi and co-author Alex Jack are talking about doing things "right." It is a very simple position: Be optimistic, be diligent, and eat a macrobiotic diet, which is mostly vegetarian. Be reasonable about everything; do not go crashing into eccentric diets, faddish exercise regimens, or other such activities.

As a cardiologist fully grounded in standard Western medicine, I believe that Michio Kushi and Alex Jack are absolutely correct on diet, exercise, and attitude, and in their approach to smoking and drinking. Theirs is a thoughtful, commonsense program, one that refuses to "bet your life" on many of the assumptions and methods of modern medicine and science. They would have you stay well and avoid the need for taking medication for high blood pressure, avoid varicose vein stripping, and avoid heart bypass surgery—all through this deceptively simple dietary approach. That is also my position. I feel that this book offers a sound prescription for preventing diseases of the heart and circulatory system, and thereby for avoiding the need for a great deal of medication and surgery.

This is not to say that there aren't certain areas of interpretation, and perhaps even fact, where I might disagree with the authors. However, I believe the *substance* of their macrobiotic system to be correct and as acceptable an approach to the understanding of health and body function as there is. It is an approach founded on both intuition and the scientific method. Some may find fault with this reliance on intuition. But we should not discount intuition too quickly. At *my* very best, I function as an intuitive physician, rather than as a physician adhering only to "established fact." That course will lead one to mechanical diagnosis and treatment, and to a lack of insight. One must have the discipline to know and understand fact, and then the flexibility and confidence to rely on one's own intuition. My intuition and belief is that the authors are correct. This is my judgment after full training and board certification in internal medicine as well as in cardiovascular disease, and after having performed more than a thousand coronary angiograms, and after having cared for patients as a practicing cardiologist for twelve years.

Diet for a Strong Heart combines a wealth of scientific background and research with traditional Oriental medicine and philosophy. It explains thoroughly the way the heart and the circulatory system function and affect your life. And it demonstrates clearly how your life style and eating patterns affect the heart and the circulatory system. It describes each of the heart-related diseases—how they develop, what brings them about, and how they can be relieved through diet. It then goes on to advise us how to implement the macrobiotic, "long life," way in our daily lives. The knowledge and principles embodied in this book, and in the macrobiotic system in general, by this name or any other, could have a profound impact on your health and life span. The discussion of the psychological and emotional factors relating to health and sickness is especially informative. I encourage everyone who opens this book to be sure to read the section on the relation between stress and diet in Chapter 13.

In today's societies, which put such a premium on artifice and instant gratification, these principles and guidelines may seem to some to be rather strange and spartan. But I assure you that, with a little patience and thought, they will not seem odd or extreme at all. That appearance of strangeness only shows how far humanity has deviated from traditional, natural ways.

* * *

It may be helpful for the reader to know a little about my own background. As a child I was overweight, and I have been weight conscious since then. I had no idea what it was that made me heavy. I was never particularly unhealthy. My parents have high blood pressure and high cholesterol, and my father smokes. I smoked for a while and until relatively recently consumed the standard American diet. I am a *slow* learner, and it has taken me a very *long* time to come to a more holistic understanding of health, including my own.

In 1966 I started my internship and became acutely aware that obesity was a major problem for heart disease and diabetes. Even then I was not really sure why people were overweight, being overweight myself, again. The first "diet" that I became aligned with was the American Heart Association diet. It was somewhat lower in saturated fats, higher in polyunsaturated fat, and expressed a concern about salt, but it did not fundamentally address itself to the quality of food, nor did it really restrict sugar, animal products, synthesized and preserved foods, and canned and frozen products.

I then passed through various fad diets. Each of these was completely unsuccessful, and eating habits were not substantially changed. They were piecemeal, superficial "diets," which usually reduced appetite and focused on specific nutrients while ignoring the whole picture, and solved nothing in the long run. As I began to study biochemistry and understand its relevance in traditional medicine, and its role in heeart disease, diabetes, diseases of the bowels, osteoporosis, and others, it became apparent to me that there had to be an ideal "fuel" for the human "machine."

I also discovered that if you take the lips, teeth, tongue, throat, esophagus, stomach, small and large bowels, and attached digestive organs of a human to a comparative anatomist and a biochemist and ask, "What kind of food should this animal eat?" the answer will be *predominantly vegetarian food.* Not exclusively vegetarian, because there are four canine teeth for tearing flesh. Four out of thirty-two. Basically, and simply, the other twenty-eight teeth, as well as the organs and tissues, manifest that the human body will run most efficiently on cereal grain and vegetable foods that are relatively whole and unprocessed, and unchemicalized. This is the ideal. The human body is designed to run optimally on a very high whole complex carbohydrate diet. And the macrobiotic diet is the closest that I can find to that ideal. On the macrobiotic diet my own cholesterol count has come down from 280 to 130, and I have experienced many other physical, mental, and emotional benefits.

The diet that I now recommend in my practice is essentially the macrobiotic diet. I have found that patients who follow a macrobiotic approach seldom need my services or those of my colleagues. It is gratifying to see them once a year as their blood pressure significantly drops down to normal levels, as their cholesterol falls to normal, as their weight improves, as their diabetes recedes, and in general, as they avoid illness and continue to stay well. The macrobiotic approach really works. I do not say this with scientific certitude, but there are numerous scientific studies that support these conclusions, and many are summarized in this book.

Read *Diet for a Strong Heart* for both its information and its philosophy. Absorb what you can, and begin to implement a macrobiotic dietary approach. If you are not seriously ill, I would only recommend moderation in the beginning. If your current diet is radically different from the macrobiotic, a *gradual* transition is definitely called for. If you are ill, you should seek help from a qualified macrobiotics teacher to guide you, and of course you should keep your physician informed of changes in your diet. In this way, most cardiovascular conditions can be prevented without the need for any of the excellent emergency surgery and other seeming miracles that modern medicine can offer.

Finally, I would urge you to feel free to adapt the macrobiotic guidelines to your own personal needs. A spirit of flexibility and a respect for nature are essential aspects of the macrobiotic philosophy. So you should not dogmatically or rigidly adhere to rules or adopt exercises you are not comfortable with. But rather you should feel your own way, and learn for yourself, at your own pace. For example, in my own case, I prefer downhill skiing to yoga or other Oriental exercises; my cardiovascular system is stimulated more by disco music than by the bamboo flute or classical music. My advice would be that you follow the macrobiotic approach 95 percent of the time, and save the extra five percent to do as you wish.

Diet for a Strong Heart points the way to health and beauty, longevity and personal success. Do it. Join me. Be kind, keep a positive attitude, make "proper" commitments, and give yourself the best. If you become macrobiotic, then we might meet as friends rather than as doctor and patient, and enjoy a long, healthy life together.

—H. ROBERT SILVERSTEIN, M.D.
Hartford, Connecticut
October 15, 1984

Fellow of the American College of Cardiologists
Clinical Assistant Professor, University of
    Connecticut School of Medicine
Member, Section of Cardiology, St. Francis Hospital
Courtesy Staffs, Mt. Sinai Hospital and Hartford Hospital

Preface

When I was nineteen years old, my political science and law studies at Tokyo University were interrupted by my being drafted into the army. The Second World War was ending, and with the end came the turmoil of destruction. Besides the death of many millions of people, the war brought poverty, misery, and grief without solace to many parts of the world. But life never dies so long as nature continues its cycle, distributing its grace and benefits upon the Earth. A new world began gradually to be constructed, the social order recovered, economic development stabilized, and the dream and hope of humanity for a world of peace and international order began to grow.

What we learned from the war, however, soon seemed to have been forgotten as a new sense of prosperity swept the planet. Instead of modesty and humility, selfishness and greed again predominated. Instead of love and compassion, prejudice and discrimination again began to guide. Philosophy and science did not reflect deeply enough on the origin and real causes of the misery and destruction that we had created upon the Earth. Thinking remained self-centered. Monetary and material satisfaction governed the use of nature and the environment. Blue skies, clear water, and green fields became contaminated. Countless wild and domesticated animals were killed, as well as microbes and bacteria that are also part of the natural order. Heavy chemicalized and artificially produced products replaced the natural, organic quality of food as traditional cooking methods declined. A sensitivity and respect for basic human values and the priceless biological, cultural, and spiritual traditions of the human race all but vanished.

During the last generation, faulty nutritional theories, combined with the increased consumption of animal food and refined foods, have conquered modern Western and Far Eastern society and many areas of the developing world. Human civilization is now facing an unprecedented crisis of biological degeneration, characterized by heart disease, cancer, mental illness, loss of reproductive ability, and other physical and psychological disorders, that may lead to the possible extinction of our species from this Earth regardless of whether or not we can prevent nuclear war.

To prevent this catastrophe—the loss of our human quality and spirit—it is essential to recover the macrobiotic perspective that has guided humanity in both East and West for thousands of years. Macrobiotics—which combines a spirit of reverence toward the universe, nature, and other people with the practice of a more natural way of life, including proper daily dietary practice—was once taught and observed in ancient Greece, the Far East, the biblical Holy Land, and other traditional cultures up until the present. To recover our true humanity and respect for God and the order of the universe, we need to return to a more simple, practical life, follow a traditional way of eating, and cultivate a spirit of modesty, humility, compassion, and love.

Together with several million people who practice macrobiotics and a more natural way of living, we deeply appreciate the recent efforts of the many individuals and organizations working to reorient social awareness and build a more peaceful world. These efforts include the development of environmental guidelines, the preservation of natural resources, and the promotion of dietary goals by governments, public agencies, research institutions, social organizations, scholars, farmers, businesspeople, homemakers, students, and others, as well as by medical, nutritional, psychiatric, and other health professionals.

This book addresses itself to the origin, prevention, and relief of heart and circulatory diseases, which are the leading cause of death in modern society. Its aim is to prevent cardiovascular disease and develop healthier and more peaceful individuals and families. We know, however, that many parts of this book may need further study, evaluation, and scientific verification. We are grateful to all those working in this direction, seeking not only for relief of the symptoms of any particular form of illness but also, totally and comprehensively, for ways to turn humanity from a physical, psychological, and spiritual degeneration far beyond what we are able to suggest in this small volume.

My co-author, Alex Jack, is a person of sincere, honest, and profound understanding. He has traveled extensively throughout the world, studying the relation between humanity and the environment. He has dedicated his life to the improvement of society and the creation of a world of lasting peace. After working as an author and journalist, most recently as editor of *East West Journal,* he joined me in writing *The Cancer-Prevention Diet,* to which this book is a companion. For these projects, he gathered the necessary historical and scientific material and has been able to express in a literary way what I wish to convey to society. Without his collaboration and assistance, these books would not have been completed. I wish to extend my gratitude to Alex from the bottom of my heart for his dedication and perseverance.

For this book, we owe thanks to so many people, especially George and Lima Ohsawa, modern founders of macrobiotics, who have inspired and guided countless individuals and families to greater health and happiness. We are grateful to Dr. Edward Kass and Dr. Frank Sacks; the other medical associates at Harvard Medical School; and to Dr. William Castelli, director of the Framingham Heart Study, all of whom have undertaken pioneer studies of the macrobiotic dietary approach. We are also grateful to H. Robert Silverstein, M.D., of St. Francis Hospital in Hartford; to Dr. Kenneth Greenspan of Columbia Presbyterian Hospital in New York City; to George Barasch of the New York Cardiac Center; to J. P. Deslypere, M.D., and colleagues at the Academic Hospital in Ghent; to Mark Mead of Reed College in Oregon; and to other medical friends who are investigating or treating heart patients with a macrobiotic approach. Our thanks also to Senator George McGovern, former chairman of the Senate Select Committee on Nutrition and Human Needs and author of *Dietary Goals for the United States;* and to the many nutritionists, physicians, nurses, and other health professionals who have participated in the East West Foundation's annual conferences on diet and degenerative disease.

We are grateful to the people whose case histories are told in this book for sharing their experience with others. We are deeply indebted to our associates at the Kushi Foundation, and the Kushi Institute, and at Macrobiotics International Centers around the world, for their hard work in the day-to-day activity of providing macrobiotic dietary counseling and cooking instruction. I am very thankful for the constant companionship and devotion of my wife Aveline, who oversaw the preparation of the recipes and menus in this book. My son Lawrence, who has a doctorate in nutrition from the Harvard School of Public Health and is an epidemiologist in the field of heart disease and cancer, assisted me in reviewing some of the scientific areas of current heart disease research. We are also thankful for the support, encouragement, and advice of other family members and friends. Esther Jack, Alex's mother, proofread the galleys and made some editorial suggestions for which we are grateful. We would also like to thank Donna Cowan, Ed Esko, Karin Stephan, Elaine and Chuck Altman, Flo Nakamura, Evelyne Harboun, and Mary Brower for their assistance and counsel. To Julie Coopersmith, our literary agent; Barbara Anderson, our editor; Victor Guerra, our production editor; and our other friends at St. Martin's Press we extend our thanks for their help in seeing this book into its final form. Most of the illustrations were drawn by Melissa Sweet, and we thank her for her valuable contribution.

With this work, we would especially like to honor the memories of Alexander Jack and Rev. David Rhys Williams, Alex's grandfathers, who both died of heart disease. We would like further to dedicate this book to the realization of one healthy, peaceful world and the joyful union of all human hearts.

—MICHIO KUSHI
Brookline, Massachusetts
January 21, 1985

DIET FOR A
STRONG HEART_____

PART I
Preventing Heart Disease Naturally

1

The Heart Disease Epidemic

In the Middle Ages, the Black Death earned its reputation by killing about one-third of the population of Europe. Today, cardiovascular disease claims the lives of over 50 percent of the people in the United States and in many other advanced industrial societies (see Figure 1). We do not ordinarily think of high blood pressure, stroke, and heart attack as plagues because the conditions leading to them can take decades to develop and because they can to some extent be controlled medically. But actually heart disease is more deadly than all other modern scourges combined, including cancer and loss of life from car accidents, crime, and war.

One out of every five men in this country will have a heart attack by age sixty. If stroke, peripheral vascular disease, and other circulatory disorders are also considered, then one out of three men will suffer a major heart or blood vessel ailment in their forties or fifties. The rate among women is considerably less, about one in six.[1]

This year, according to the American Heart Association, 1.5 million Americans will have a heart attack, and 550,000 of them will die.[2] Another half-million will suffer a stroke, 165,000 of which will prove fatal. Those who survive these two afflictions will join the 6.5 million people who have had a heart attack or stroke and are still living. Thirty-seven million adults in this country have hypertension or high blood pressure, and this group forms the pool from which one of these potentially lethal conditions usually de-

3

velops. Other cardiovascular diseases, such as pulmonary heart disease, aneurysm, arterial embolism, arterial thrombosis, and phlebitis, will account for about 225,000 deaths this year. Another 7,700 deaths result from rheumatic fever or rheumatic heart disease. With respect to medical treatment, 1.6 million cardiovascular operations and procedures are currently performed each year in the United States, including 159,000 coronary artery bypass grafts, 177,000 pacemaker operations, and 414,000 cardiac catheterizations. At life's other end, in the next twelve months 25,000 babies will be born with congenital heart defects. About one-quarter of these infants will die, and the survivors will join the nearly half-million persons with heart defects still living.

Over the last fifteen years, the death rate from heart disease in the United States has begun to decline, among both sexes, in all age groups, and among all races and ethnic backgrounds. This decline is apparently due to a combination of factors that include dietary changes, reduced smoking, and increased exercise. While mortality is down, according to one medical journal, "at present there is practically no information on what is happening to the incidence of new coronary heart disease events."[3] For example, heart disease appears to be on the rise among young people.

In a 1981 California study, researchers measured the serum cholesterol levels of six-year-old children drawn from a representative group of white, black, Asian, Hispanic, and other families.[4] Cholesterol levels ranged from 113 to 260 mg, with a mean of 190. Twenty-nine percent of the children had values of 200 or more. The researchers correlated these high levels primarily with the consumption of eggs and red meat. In contrast, children in traditional societies, where heart disease is uncommon, have cholesterol levels generally below 150 and often around 100. A level of 190 among California first-graders corresponds with the high-risk category for coronary heart disease in less industrially developed countries such as China, where the rate of heart disease is low.[5]

During the Vietnam War, doctors examined the bodies of American soldiers killed in combat to determine the cardiovascular condition of relatively healthy and active young males.[6] Autopsies showed that 45 percent had some evidence of coronary atherosclerosis (hardening of the arteries) and 26 percent showed hardening in more than one heart vessel. The average age of the

Figure 1. The Rise of Degenerative Disease

U.S. death rates per 100,000 for selected causes, 1970–1975.

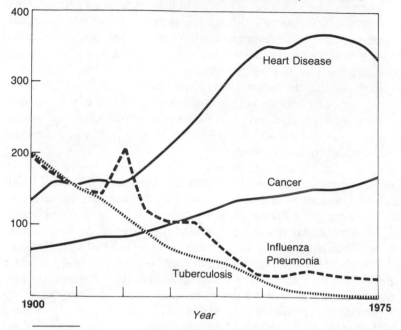

Source: National Center for Health Statistics, 1974.

young men was twenty-two. These rates had actually fallen since the Korean War, when a similar study was performed. However, the rates were considerably higher than those determined by a long-term Chicago study conducted from 1920 to 1953, which found that only 7.3 percent of patients under fifty years of age had atherosclerosis.[7]

At New York University Medical Center, Mildred S. Seelig, M.D., has been investigating atherosclerosis and other heart conditions in thousands of children and infants under two-and-a-half years of age. In a recent report to her medical colleagues, she concluded:

> The cardiovascular diseases of infancy and childhood that are common enough to require specialty medical care and surgical correction are a development of the past 30 to 40 years, as is the epidemic of sudden death of men under fifty

from ischemic [degenerative] heart disease. Less widely recognized is the evidence that sudden death from IHD [ischemic heart disease] has also occurred in infancy and childhood, with increasing frequency during the same period of time, as has generalized arteriosclerosis in very young infants, and atherosclerosis, hyperlipemia, and hypertension in older infants and children. The initiating cardiovascular lesion can begin very early in life (in some individuals during gestation; in many during early infancy). The years during which cardiovascular diseases of all ages have increased in incidence correlates with the years during which major dietary changes were made in the industrialized countries.[8]

Dr. Seelig goes on to cite decreased breastfeeding since the 1920s and the processing of cow's milk as possible primary factors contributing to this increase of heart disorders in the very young.

Cardiovascular disease is the leading cause of death in many other societies than the United States (see Table 1). In Finland, which has the world's highest milk consumption, the rate of heart disease is even higher than in the United States, which rates second per capita. In Great Britain, coronary heart disease mortality increased fifteen times from 1921 to 1946 and 80 percent in young men from 1950 to 1973.[9] In Sweden, heart attacks rose fivefold between 1950 and 1964. In the Soviet Union, mortality from coronary heart disease went up about 18 percent between 1964 and 1975.[10] In Japan, where overall heart disease is still less common than in Western countries, degenerative heart ailments rose 45 percent from 1970 to 1980. Interestingly, during this decade, Japanese consumption of fat from animal sources of food exceeded that from vegetable sources for the first time.[11]

Once rare or unknown, coronary heart disease is emerging in the developing world. In middle- and upper-class districts in Buenos Aires, New Delhi, Cairo, and Johannesburg, heart disease rates are soaring as the rich diet and life-style of the more affluent nations take hold. For example, in Zimbabwe in central Africa, physician Michael Gilford recalls: "Twenty-five or thirty years ago, we were aware that we were not noticing cases of myocardial infarction or angina pectoris, conditions that are associated with atherosclerosis. . . . In 1958 I met a Zimbabwe woman, employed as a nanny in a European household in Salisbury, with a typical

Table 1. CORONARY HEART DISEASE AROUND THE WORLD
Deaths per 100,000 people

Country	Men	Women
Finland	872	262
United States	793	318
New Zealand	740	311
Ireland	672	288
Australia	787	311
United Kingdom	702	254
Canada	663	247
Norway	581	173
Netherlands	502	168
Israel	625	352
Denmark	606	225
Belgium	463	163
West Germany	457	150
Sweden	588	214
Austria	435	164
Venezuela	323	189
Switzerland	279	90
Italy	309	127
France	205	72
Japan	115	61

Source: Robert Levy, et al., eds., *Nutrition, Lipids, and Coronary Heart Disease* (New York: Raven Press, 1979).

history of anginal pain."[12] Only in the late 1960s and 1970s, Dr. Gilford notes, following the increased popularity of the refined modern diet, did coronary heart disease begin to be encountered with regularity.

THE HISTORY OF HEART DISEASE

In Genesis, when the angels of the Lord appeared before Abraham, he welcomed them into his tent, saying, "I will fetch a morsel of bread and comfort ye your hearts." With his wife, Sarah, Abraham prepared a meal centered on whole cereal grains. The angels foretold that in a year Sarah would bear a son, from whom would spring a mighty nation. Later, when the divine emissaries went to destroy Sodom and Gomorrah, Abraham and Sarah's nephew Lot won the angels' protection by offering them a dish made from unleavened grain.[13]

Traditional societies in the Middle East, Europe, Asia, and elsewhere intuitively understood the relationship between personal and social health and a balanced daily diet. In the Yellow Emperor's Classic of Internal Medicine, the medical book of ancient China, the heart is likened to the monarch of the body who governs the other principal officials or organs: "When the monarch is bright, the officials below him will feel secure, and when this principle is applied to nourish life, one will enjoy longevity without health hazards; when the same principle is applied to rule the world, the world will be in great prosperity."[14] For strengthening the heart, the world's oldest medical text recommends consumption of millet and warns that "an excessive consumption of salted foods [e.g., meat and fish] will cause the blood vessels to become stiffened. . . ."[15]

The world's scriptures, legends, and myths enshrine the ways in which different cultures have provided nourishment, harmonized with their environment, and either advanced or declined. In Hebrew, the word covenant originally meant to eat together.[16] In the Old Testament, God promised Moses that the Children of Israel would be happy and prosper so long as they observed the dietary laws and observed Passover by eating unleavened bread. In the New Testament, Jesus offered his followers wholemeal bread made from barley at the Sermon on the Mount, the Last Supper, and on the road to Emmaus. Among early Christians, whole grain bread symbolized eternal life.

Bread, or the staff of life—whole cereal grains, including brown rice, whole wheat, barley, millet, oats, rye, and corn—was the cornerstone of all civilizations previous to our own. Supplemented with fresh garden vegetables, beans, sea vegetables, fermented foods, and small amounts of seasonal fruit, seeds, and nuts, grains were eaten daily and formed the center of every meal. Animal food was consumed very sparingly and eaten with substantial quantities of grain and vegetables.

Until modern times, when this way of eating changed, heart disease, cancer, and other degenerative illnesses were almost unknown. Still, there were periods of imbalance and excess when ancient peoples forgot their dietary codes and abused their health. In the Old Testament, for instance, plague is associated with worship of the Golden Calf, a symbol of idolatry and of putting personal desires and appetites above divine and natural order. At the biological level, we may view the Golden Calf as symbolizing a rejection of the grains, vegetables, and other herb-bearing seeds that the Lord, the sages, and the prophets upheld as the proper foods for human consumption. "Oh, for a few bites of meat," the wayward Israelites lamented in the wilderness, recalling the familiar comforts of bondage. "Oh, that we had some of the delicious fish we enjoyed so much in Egypt. . . ."[17]

The Emergence of Heart Disease

World food patterns remained relatively constant from the time of the Neolithic revolution to the Middle Ages. Following the Crusades to the East, the Mongol incursions to the West, and the discovery of the New World, foods, spices, and stimulants crossed hemispheres and natural climatic zones, lowering natural immunity to disease and precipitating epidemics. With the advent of the Industrial Revolution in the seventeenth century, traditional ways of eating that had existed for thousands of years entered their final decline. The introduction of farm machinery, crop rotation, and rock fertilizers (mineral compounds from the earth) in the eighteenth century increased agricultural yields and reduced rural populations. Enclosure laws transformed farmland into pasture, and cattle, traditionally used for plowing and turning millstones for grinding grain, were bred selectively for their meat and milk. Improvements in milling made white flour widely available. By 1800, white bread, once limited only to the aristocracy, was eaten in England by nearly all members of the lower classes.[18] In medieval times, sugar had been locked away in apothecary shops as a dangerous and prohibitively expensive drug. By 1815, the international slave trade turned sugar from a luxury into a staple, and annual per capita consumption rose to 15 pounds.[19] Foreign trade also stimulated coffee, tea, and chocolate consumption as well as alcohol intake.

As traditional food patterns declined, a host of infectious diseases developed and became the leading causes of death in the manufacturing countries and their foreign colonies. Individual cases of heart disease, cancer, and other degenerative disorders began to surface in the upper classes, which were most prone to dietary excess. In 1768, for example, Heberdeen, a British physician, described the first clinical case of angina pectoris, a degenerative heart ailment characterized by acute pains in the chest and shortness of breath.

Yet a century later, heart disease continued to present little menace to public health. In 1876, *Scientific American* published a survey of mortality rates in New York, the nation's largest city. Among adults and older children, the principal causes of death were tuberculosis, 26.6 percent; other lung disorders, 19.2 percent; diarrheal diseases, 18.7 percent; diphtheria, 15.6 percent; croup, 6.3 percent; typhoid fever, 4.2 percent; smallpox, 3.4 percent; whooping cough, 2.7 percent; puerperal diseases, 1.4 percent; scarlatina, 1.3 percent; measles, 0.3 percent; and typhus fever, 0.3 percent. The diseases that are epidemic today—heart disease, cancer, and diabetes—are not even listed.[20]

In 1896, Sir William Osler, the father of modern medical education, noted in lectures on the heart: "During the ten years in which I lived in Montreal, I did not see a case of the disease [angina pectoris] either in private practice or at the Montreal General Hospital. At Blockley (Philadelphia Hospital), too, it was an exceedingly rare affection. I do not remember to have had a case under my personal care. . . ."[21]

By World War I, heart disease emerged as a major ailment, accounting for about 9 percent of fatalities in the United States.[22] Various factors contributed to its rise, including the reduction of infectious diseases, longer life-spans, and better medical diagnosis. The primary causes, however, appear to be dietary, and they may be traced back to the change in patterns of food consumption begun during the latter part of the nineteenth century.

After the Civil War, with the coming of the railroad, the establishment of cattle drives to rail depots, and the building of commercial stockyards, meat consumption rose substantially and America's romance with beefsteak began. Fat consumption also increased with the introduction of commercial vegetable oils and the development of margarines. The introduction of steel rollers into the milling process—introduced first in Minnesota in 1880 and later in the rest of the Grain Belt—completely stripped the germ and bran from wheat, making available an even finer white flour. In 1890, pasteurized milk became available, and the invention of the cream separator, the milking machine, and advances in commercial refrigeration launched the modern dairy industry. Between 1875 and 1915, annual sugar consumption doubled from about 40 pounds per capita to 80 pounds.[23] By the turn of the century, Coca-Cola and other soft drinks had become widely available, and their popularity increased with each new decade.

The medicine of this era favored drugs and surgery, as it does to an even greater extent today. Yet the connection between diet and disease did not go entirely unobserved. In his lectures on heart ailments, Dr. Osler advised, "Diet is in many cases the central point in the treatment. The subjects of angina are often men with large appetites, accustomed to eat freely of rich and strong foods. First, limit the amount taken, which in most persons above forty years of age is far too great; second, see that the quality is suitable by excluding from the dietary rich, highly seasoned foods. . . . There is 'death in the pot' for angina victims, and a surfeit may be as fatal as poison."[24]

In 1904, the word *atherosclerosis* was coined to describe the hardening of the arteries. In 1912, several decades of coronary research culminated in the first clinical description of myocardial infarction in a medical journal. In the 1920s, *heart attack,* the common term for this condition, became a household word.

Biological Degeneration

Following World War I, the pace of scientific and technological change accelerated, and eating patterns changed even more fundamentally. In agriculture, chemical fertilizers and pesticides, developed in the nineteenth century, displaced organic farming. The creation of mammoth incubators after the war led to the mass production of poultry. In the 1920s, home refrigeration came into vogue, and prepackaged frozen foods reduced the consumption of fresh garden produce. Refined, canned, and dehydrated foods also took an increasing share of the market. In the 1930s, the vitamin industry was developed to sell back to the consumer the nutrients removed by refining grain. Artificial colors, preservatives, and

Table 2. FOOD CHANGES, 1910–1976

(Per capita annual consumption in pounds unless otherwise noted.)

Food	1910	1976	Change
Eggs	305 whole	276 whole	−10%
Meat	136.2	165.2	+21%
Beef	55.5	95.4	+72%
Poultry	18.0	52.9	+194%
Fish	11.4	13.7	+20%
Canned Tuna	.2	3.1 (1974)	+1,300%
Grains	294.0	144.0	−51%
Wheat	214.0	112.0	−48%
Corn	51.1	7.7	−85%
Rice	7.2	7.2	none
Rye	3.6	0.8	−78%
Barley	3.5	1.2	−66%
Oats	3.5	3.5	none
Buckwheat	2.1	0.05	−98%
Beans, Peas	13.0	7.0	−46%
Fresh Vegetables	188.0	144.5	−23%
Fresh Cabbage	23.2 (1920)	8.3 (1965)	−64%
Sweet Potato	22.5	4.4	−80%
Fresh Potato	80.4	48.3	−40%
Frozen Potato	6.6 (1960)	36.8	+457%
Tomato Products	5.0 (1920)	22.4	+348%
Canned Vegetables	12.6 (1920)	53.0	+320%
Frozen Vegetables	.57 (1940)	9.9	+1,650%
Fresh Fruit	123.0	82.0	−33%
Processed Fruit	20.5	134.6	+556%
Grapefruit	1.0	9.0	+800%
Frozen Citrus	1.0 (1948)	117.0	+11,600%
Frozen Foods	3.1 (1940)	88.8	+2,764%
Dairy	320.2	354.3	+11%
Whole Milk	29.3 gal.	21.5 gal.	−27%
Low Fat Milk	6.8 gal.	10.6 gal.	+56%
Cheese	4.9	20.7	+322%
Ice Cream	1.9	18.1	+852%
Frozen Dairy	3.4	50.2	+1,376%
Yogurt	.5 (1967)	2.0	+300%
Margarine	1.5	12.5	+733%

Table 2 *(continued)*

Food	1910	1976	Change
Sweeteners	89.0	134.6	+51%
Corn Syrup	3.8	32.7	+761%
Sugar	73.7 (1909)	94.8	+29%
Soft Drinks	1.1 gal.	30.8 gal.	+2,638%
Saccharine	2.0 (1960)	8.0	+300%
Tea	1.0	0.8	−20%
Coffee	9.2	12.8	+39%
Alcohol	2.69 gal.	2.69 gal.	none
Food Colors	.03 oz. (1940)	.34 oz. (1977)	+995%
Total Food	4.4 per day	4.1 per day	−9%
Calories	3,490″ ″	3,380″ ″	−3%
Protein	102 gms.	103 gms.	+1%
Fat	124 gms.	159 gms.	+28%
Carbohydrate	495 gms.	390 gms.	−21%

Source: U.S. Department of Agriculture statistics summarized in *The Changing American Diet,* published by the Center for Science in the Public Interest and adapted for this chart. Figures do not measure quality, whether organically grown, or naturally processed. For example, the USDA makes no distinction between whole wheat or white refined bread (included in Grain and Wheat categories).

other additives found their way into daily food as new synthetic flavors, cosmetic appearance, and extended shelf life replaced wholesomeness and nutrition as primary concerns.

Between the two world wars, the death rate from heart disease in the United States recorded its greatest single jump, rising from about 11 percent in 1920 to 45 percent in 1940.[25] Table 2 summarizes some of the changes in our way of eating over the last half-century. These changes have laid the foundation for heart disease, cancer, and other modern ills. Increased cigarette smoking and industrial pollution, and a more sedentary way of life resulting from the spread of the automobile and other modern conveniences, all contributed to this rise.

Following World War II, beef, milk, cheese, ice cream, and other dairy products replaced whole grains, bread, noodles, and pasta as the staples in most of the industrialized world. Through breeding, artificial insemination, and growth hormones, the cattle population of the nation doubled. Today there is one cow for every two Americans.[26] In the 1950s and 1960s, fast food became a way of life. The temples of these Golden Calves—McDonald's, Burger King, Dairy Queen—dotted the landscape. Eighty-five percent of American women gave up breastfeeding for infant formula.[27] In addition to heart disease, other chronic illnesses and signs of social disharmony continued to soar (see Table 3). Cancer, which affected about one American in twenty-five at the beginning of the century, now affects nearly one in three. A generation ago the rate of mental illness was about one in twenty people. It has now more than doubled to over one in ten. In the last few years, herpes and other sexually transmitted diseases (STD) have assumed epidemic proportions. Infertility is on the increase. According to medical tests, the average sperm count in American males has dropped 39 percent since the 1920s, and 45 percent of the nation's nearly 27.5 million couples have been unable to have children or have had difficulty in conceiving.[28] About 800,000 American women, many of childbearing age, currently have their ovaries or uteruses surgically removed each year, mostly as a preventive measure against cancer.

Several new diseases have appeared to further challenge public health. These include Legionnaire's disease, toxic shock syndrome, and AIDS, for which no medical solutions are in sight. At the same time, old diseases are returning in more virulent form that include new strains of pneumonia and other infectious diseases for which antibiotics are ineffectual. Few if any diseases can really be cured by modern medical methods such as surgery, radiation therapy, or drugs. In some cases symptoms of illness can temporarily be suppressed and pain and other discomfort eased. Fundamentally, however, disease cannot be cured and sooner or later reappears, even though diagnosed by a different specialist and given a new name. Patients are increasingly finding that they must heal themselves of the effects of the medical treatment as well as of the original disease.

Effects on Society

The effects of heart disease on national life and international security are profound and far-reaching. The smooth functioning of

Table 3. RECENT HEALTH AND SOCIAL STATISTICS—
U.S.A.

Illness or Condition	Americans Currently Affected
Heart disease	42,330,000
High blood pressure	37,000,000
Allergies	35,400,000
Arthritis	31,600,000
Alcoholism	14,272,000
Diabetes	11,000,000
Mental retardation	5,654,000
Cancer	4,640,000
Epilepsy	2,135,000
Strokes	1,830,000
Abortions	1,500,000 per year
Cerebral palsy	750,000
Birth defects	12,750,000
Parkinson's disease	1,500,000
Multiple sclerosis	500,000
Syphillis, gonorrhea, and older sexually transmitted diseases	1,064,000
Herpes and newer sexually transmitted diseases	20–30,000,000
Divorce	1 in 2 marriages
Crime	1 crime index offense every 2 seconds
	1 violent crime every 24 seconds
	1 property crime every 3 seconds
Drug use	160,000,000 prescriptions per year
Mental illness	22–56,500,000
Infertility	1 out of 5 couples
Sperm count	30–40 percent decline since 1920
Sterility	20 percent sexually active males
Hysterectomies	800,000 per year

Source: Conservative estimates based on 1980 U.S. population of 226,504,825 from most recent national health statistics compiled by groups including American Cancer Society, American Diabetes Association, American Heart Association, American Parkinson's Disease Association, Arthritis Foundation, Center for Disease Control, Epilepsy Foundation of America, Federal Census Department, Massachusetts Department of Mental Health, National Institute on Drug Abuse, Multiple Sclerosis Society, Planned Parenthood, and United Cerebral Palsy Association.

Table 4. THE HEALTH OF THE PRESIDENTS

Name	Cause of Death
Washington	Throat infection
J. Adams	Hardening of the arteries
Jefferson	Old age, exhaustion
Madison	Hardening of the arteries
Monroe	Tuberculosis
J. Q. Adams	Stroke
Jackson	Pulmonary disease
Van Buren	Pulmonary heart disease
W. H. Harrison	Pneumonia
Tyler	Stroke
Polk	Cholera
Taylor	Cholera
Fillmore	Stroke
Pierce	Cirrhosis of the liver
Buchanan	Heart failure
Lincoln	Assassination
A. Johnson	Stroke
Grant	Throat cancer
Hayes	Heart attack
Garfield	Assassination
Arthur	Stroke
Cleveland	Heart attack
B. Harrison	Pneumonia
McKinley	Assassination
T. Roosevelt	Heart disease
Taft	Heart disease
Wilson	Stroke
Harding	Heart attack
Coolidge	Heart attack
F. D. Roosevelt	Stroke
Hoover	Hemorrhage and cancer
Truman	Cardiovascular disease
Eisenhower	Heart failure
Kennedy	Assassination
L. B. Johnson	Heart attack

Source: Rudolph Mark, M.D., *The Health of the Presidents* (New York: G. P. Putnam's Sons, 1960). The cause of death of early presidents is based on modern medical diagnosis of recorded symptoms. Information on presidents who have died since 1960 updated by Kushi and Jack.

government has been impaired, and in some cases the government itself suddenly changed, with the incapacitation, death, or lingering disability of a leader. The American presidency has been particularly hard hit. Woodrow Wilson's stroke immobilized the executive branch of the government and may have had an adverse effect on the critical postwar period. In *The Health of the Presidents*, Rudolph Marx, M.D., describes the effects of Wilson's stroke on foreign policy:

> The progressive degeneration of the central nervous system induced a rigidity of mind. The less sympathetic features of the old schoolmaster came to the surface—an air of authority and superiority, no longer censored by the weakened superego. His apparent arrogance embittered Wilson's antagonists and estranged some of his lukewarm supporters in the Senate.[29]

Dwight D. Eisenhower's and Lyndon Johnson's heart attacks and Richard Nixon's phlebitis all may have adversely affected their performance in office. Interestingly, in the twentieth century, nearly every chief executive in Washington, except for those felled by assassins' bullets, died from some form of heart or circulatory disorder. Although heart disorders were not well understood in previous centuries, modern medical historians have concluded that many of America's earlier presidents also died from some form of heart disease (see Table 4).

The effects of heart disease on the economy are also extensive. In 1984, the medical costs, home nursing expenses, and lost output due to disability for this form of illness were estimated by the American Heart Association at $64.4 billion.[30] The indirect costs in lowered productivity, increased insurance premiums, and family turmoil have not been calculated and can only be inferred. Medical costs are a primary cause of inflation, rising at a rate about twice as fast as the rest of the economy.

There are also social consequences that are much less perceptible. For example, the socioeconomic composition of juries has changed significantly as more and more middle-aged and elderly people have been excused from jury duty for medical reasons. In an article on a murder and armored car robbery trial, the *New York Times* recently reported:

Medical problems and doctors' notes abounded. There was a litany of heart trouble, hypertension, diabetes, deafness and stories of helping ailing, homebound parents in their 80's and 90's. Two men flapped bags of pills at the judge. "If I get too nervous, I just pass right out," said another. One woman who said she had chronic heart trouble told the judge that if she served, "The risk would be yours."[31]

Heart disease, directly or indirectly, touches nearly every aspect of modern life. Thus, strengthening our hearts will make for a more healthy, peaceful, and responsible society.

The Road Ahead

On the basis of the trends discussed in this chapter, we can see that modern civilization as a whole is suffering from deep-seated biological degeneration. This trend affects the populations of the United States, Canada, the Soviet Union, Western and Eastern Europe, Japan, China, Australia, and developing regions of Asia, Africa, and Latin America. As with the nuclear arms race, the time left for us to reverse it is short.

Like the generation of Abraham, Sarah, and Lot, we find ourselves in a world beset by catastrophe. As a civilization, we have lost our vision and judgment. We prefer illness to health. We mistake war for peace. We confuse our own limited will with that of nature and the infinite universe. At the simplest level, many of us can no longer distinguish between a grain and a bean, a seed and a fruit, and food for health and food for enjoyment.

An angel of the Lord appearing in our midst today would very likely be offered a hamburger, a slice of pizza, or an ice cream cone. Like Lot's wife, who was turned into a pillar of salt, our lives will be crippled by atherosclerosis, arthritis, and a rigid mentality if we look back and follow the unnatural and chaotic way of life, especially the day-to-day eating patterns, with which we grew up. We must wean ourselves from the Golden Calf and its products.

The task before us is no less than the complete regeneration of the human race, beginning with ourselves and extending, with love and understanding, to our family, friends, and community. The infinite universe has chosen each of us to come to this Earth to be healthy, happy, and together realize our endless dream of one peaceful world. Let us joyfully rediscover the natural way of life that unites us with those who have come before and those who will follow. Let us return to whole cereal grains—the traditional staff of life—and once again, in the words of the psalmist, nourish each other with "the bread which strengtheneth humanity's heart."[32]

2

The Macrobiotic Approach to Heart Disease

Following World War II, I completed my studies in international law at Tokyo University and decided to devote my life to helping solve the problems of modern society. Outside the capital city, in a little school, I met a remarkable man named Yukikazu Sakurazawa, or George Ohsawa as he came to be known in later life. He introduced me to macrobiotics.

As a young man, Ohsawa had grown up on a diet high in beef, pork, white rice, white flour, milk, and sugar. The modern way of eating had swept into Japan following the Meiji Restoration and the colonization of Taiwan, site of vast sugar plantations, at the end of the nineteenth century. This change in diet included the influx of tropical foods into Japan's temperate climate in violation of ecological principles. The infectious diseases of modern civilization followed. In 1909, young Ohsawa contracted tuberculosis, from which his mother had died several years previously. Japanese doctors, trained in the modern scientific method, examined his diseased lungs and gave him medication to relieve the symptoms. He was told there was no cure for his illness and was sent home to die.

One day while awaiting his fate, the ailing sixteen-year-old came across a small book in a second-hand bookstore in Kyoto entitled *The Curative Method by Diet*. The author, Sagen Ishizuka, M.D., had been educated in modern methods but remained firmly convinced of the value of the long traditional nutritional practices of healthy families in his own country and in other parts of the Far East. He believed that nearly all modern diseases could be healed by avoiding meat, sugar, and refined foods and by adhering to a simple balanced diet consisting chiefly of brown rice and vegetables.

Ishizuka had originally developed his method in 1884 while serving as a military doctor on the battlefield in the Sino-Japanese War. There was a defiant horse in his unit that refused to be mounted, and the company commander offered to give the spirited animal to anyone who could ride it. After three days of carefully observing the horse's habits, Ishizuka appeared before the assembled regiment astride the majestic charger. To everyone's amazement, the once wild stallion had become obedient and gentle. "It is not the technique of horsemanship which counts for being able to mount the horse," Ishizuka explained to his astonished fellow officers. "The secret is the food." When left to itself in the fields, the horse ate only small quantities of wild grasses and herbs. In the stables, it had been fed excessive amounts of processed grain by the trainers. By adjusting both the quality and quantity of the nourishment, Ishizuka completely modified the horse's disposition.

After the war, Ishizuka went on to study the effects of food on human health. He was one of the first researchers to investigate the acid/alkaline ratio of nutrients and conclude that the modern diet, which contains extremes of both sodium and potassium—two major antagonistic and complementary mineral elements—was dangerously imbalanced. In Tokyo, Dr. Ishizuka opened a clinic and introduced his methods to thousands of people, many with serious or terminal illnesses. The success rate was high, and he was fondly known as Dr. Vegetable or Dr. Radish on account of the long white radish he recommended to detoxify the body following the consumption of animal food.[1]

After discovering Ishizuka's little book, George Ohsawa changed his diet and began to eat brown rice, miso soup, land and sea vegetables, and other traditionally prepared foods and beverages. In a short time, the tuberculosis disappeared. "It cured me completely," he later recalled. "For forty-eight years since, I have not been sick except for one occasion when I deliberately contracted the terrible (and usually incurable) disease named tropical ulcers. This was at Dr. Schweitzer's hospital in Lambarene, Africa, and was part of my quest for the biggest medical difficulties in the world. Through macrobiotic medicine, I overcame this disease in a few days."[2]

During these five decades, Ohsawa expanded Ishizuka's method for treating personal illness to solving the problems of modern society. He studied the teachings of Confucius, Lao Tzu, Buddha, and the Vedic sages as well as the Bible, Shakespeare, and contemporary Western authors such as Lewis Carroll, Samuel Butler, and Arnold Toynbee. From 1929 to 1935 he lived in Paris teaching Oriental medicine and philosophy, as well as judo, haiku, and flower arrangement.

Like Benjamin Franklin and Thomas Jefferson, whom he admired, Ohsawa taught that agricultural self-sufficiency was the foundation of civilization and that the industrial nations of the world, including Japan, the United States, France, Germany, and the Soviet Union, would decline because of biological degeneration following the spread of modern chemical agriculture and the rise of heart disease, cancer, and mental illness. During World War II, Ohsawa was jailed in Japan for publishing antimilitarist material and setting off alone on a peace march to Manchuria. He was arrested, tortured, and sentenced to death. However, before he could be executed, the war ended and he was freed.

After the war, Ohsawa traveled to India, Africa, Vietnam, Europe, and North America, introducing his methods and insights to thousands of people. Over the years he wrote three hundred books, including a history of China, a biography of Gandhi, a study of cancer and diet, and a new theory of atomic transmutation. "I would have to write a large book to explain the mechanism and the therapeutics of heart disease," he observed at the end of his life in 1965. "It is a very interesting subject but at my age I do not have the time. You will have to learn through study and write the book yourselves."[3] A year later, in his mid-seventies, after an active and adventurous life, George Ohsawa's own heart stopped beating.

MACROBIOTICS IN ANTIQUITY

Ohsawa called his teachings, which synthesize the wisdom of East and West, *macrobiotics* after the old Greek term for "long life" or "great life." The expression was first used by Hippocrates in the fifth century B.C. The Father of Western medicine taught a natural healing method emphasizing environmental and dietary factors. His philosophy was summed up in the aphorism, "Let food be thy medicine and medicine thy food." The Hippocratic Oath, still taken by doctors, states in part: "I will apply dietetic measures for the benefit of the sick according to my ability and judgment; I will keep them from harm and injustice. I will neither give a deadly drug to anybody if asked for it, nor will I make a suggestion to this effect. . . . I will not use the knife [surgery]. . . ."[4]

In Hippocrates' view, food nourished the humors in the blood, and an imbalance or excess of these vital forces led to disease. By regulating the daily food intake, the quality of blood could be brought back into equilibrium and health restored. To strengthen the blood and vital organs, he particularly recommended a broth made from whole grain barley, the chief staple of the Hellenistic world. In a memorable passage on the functioning of the heart, Hippocrates anticipated William Harvey's famous discovery of blood circulation nearly two thousand years later:

> The vessels communicate with one another and the blood flows from one to another. I do not know where the commencement is to be found, for in a circle you can find neither commencement nor end, but from the heart the arteries take their origin and through the vessel, the blood is distributed to all the body, to which it gives warmth and life; they are the sources of human nature and are like rivers that purl through the body and supply the body with life; the heart and the vessels are perpetually moving, and we may compare the movement of the blood with courses of rivers returning to their sources after a passage through numerous channels.[5]

Other classical authors, including Herodotus, Aristotle, Galen, and Lucian, also used the word *macrobiotics* in discussing health and longevity. In early Western literature, the term became synonymous with a simple grain and vegetable diet and a natural way of life. The ancient Ethiopians, the Thessalians, Biblical patriarchs such as Abraham, and other long-lived people were described respectfully as macrobiotic, and the term entered the common vocabulary. During the Renaissance, for example, macrobiotics was popularized by Rabelais, the French humanist, in *Gurgantua and Pantagruel,* his satire on the foibles and follies of modern civilization.

In more recent times, macrobiotics found a champion in Christoph Hufeland, M.D., an eighteenth-century philosopher, professor of medicine, and physician to Goethe. At a time when the leaders of the age were fighting to establish republics and nation-states, Hufeland proclaimed himself "a citizen of the world." Bucking the scientific tide, he devoted his life to extolling the virtues of a simple grain and vegetable diet, warned of the health hazards of meat and sugar, and promoted breastfeeding, exercise, and self-healing. In his most famous book, *Macrobiotics or the Art of Prolonging Life,* published in 1797 and translated into many foreign languages, he explained:

> The more a man follows Nature, and is obedient to her laws, the longer he will live; the further he deviates from these, the shorter will be his existence. . . . The healing power of nature must, above all things, be supported from the beginning, because it is the principal means which lies in ourselves for rendering the causes of disease ineffectual. This may be done chiefly by not accustoming the body at first too much to artificial assistance; otherwise Nature will be so used that she will depend on foreign aid, and at length lose altogether the power of assisting herself.[6]

In this book, Hufeland goes on to note that about 1.2 percent of the European population then living would die from apoplexy (stroke). In addition to proper diet, he stressed the importance of regular exercise to strengthen the heart and vascular system along with other vital organs. He was probably the first person to recommend jogging for cardiovascular conditions, as a careful reading of the following passage shows:

> A foundation may be laid for good lungs, by pure open air; and afterwards, by speaking, singing, running; for a sound stomach by wholesome food, easy of digestion; but neither too strong and stimulating, nor too highly seasoned; for a sound skin by cleanliness, washing, bathing, pure air, a temperature neither too hot nor too cold, and, afterwards, by exercise; and for a strong heart and vessels, by all the above means; in par-

ticular by wholesome nourishment, and afterwards by bodily motion.[7]

MODERN MACROBIOTICS

After studying macrobiotics with George Ohsawa, I left Japan for New York, home of the newly formed United Nations, to devote myself to world peace and world federal government. When I arrived in America in 1949, the relation between diet and disease was poorly understood. The nation had just gone through the Great Depression and a world war. In the immediate postwar period, the United States sought to put this era of deprivation and sacrifice behind it and, through developing the economy, attain new levels of material prosperity. Cheap fuel, synthetic materials, and converted wartime technology transformed daily life at all levels. Urban areas encroached upon once productive farmland and untouched seashore. New methods of transportation and communication contracted distances, and inexpensive mass-produced goods replaced durable consumer items and handcrafted wares.

In the area of agriculture and food, the modern supermarket was born. Thanks to heavy machinery and chemical fertilizers, crop yields soared, transcontinental markets opened, and advances in freezing, canning, and preserving made it possible to further increase production, stretch quality, and stimulate demand. The new wave of food technology made it possible to override the seasons and provide a cornucopia of tropical foods year round. Sugarcane and dairy milk replaced rice and wheat as the world's number one and two crops, and the declining cereal grain produced was almost completely refined and then fortified with artificial ingredients. The majority of grain, moreover, went to fattening livestock rather than feeding people. As the economy grew, higher incomes put beef and dairy products on the table nearly every day. Families could also afford to eat out more often. Hamburgers, hot dogs, pizza, French fries, soft drinks, candy bars, ice cream, potato chips, and other fast foods became a way of life. When preparing food at home, families ate together less frequently and desired quick, convenient foods in order to have more time to watch the newly developed medium of television.

In the area of health, wartime advances in antibiotics, surgery, and radiotherapy contributed to a new era of emergency medical intervention. Success in lowering infant mortality, controlling infectious diseases, and suppressing the symptoms of polio contributed to the expectation that there was a technological or biochemical solution to every ill. It was only a question of time, resources, and scientific detective work until that solution was discovered.

In this atmosphere of unbounded optimism in modern society's ability to control, conquer, and even improve upon nature, the food of the past—whole grains, fresh vegetables, and local, seasonal fruit—appeared as plain and primitive as our grandparents' jalopies, wireless radios, and pocket watches. The new, enriched food of the future would usher in a taller, stronger, and more intelligent generation. As with the peaceful use of atomic energy, almost no one seriously questioned the value of this new food at the time. When President Eisenhower launched Atoms for Peace, he codenamed the project Operation Wheaties. The nation's program for the domestic use of nuclear energy was formulated at a series of White House breakfasts.[8]

Against this background, macrobiotics largely went unheeded in the 1950s and early 1960s. Its emphasis on organic foods, locally grown and seasonal produce, home-cooked meals, and simple home remedies made it seem like a throwback to a more austere and less scientific era. Its claims to prevent and relieve serious illnesses through diet, exercise, self-reflection, and a more natural way of life were generally ignored or criticized in medical, academic, and government circles.

America's and Europe's young people, however, were more receptive to macrobiotics. Some of them were looking for a safe, natural way to grow and develop as a healthful alternative to the mind-altering drugs that became widely available in the 1960s. Others were concerned about the relationship between world hunger and the use of grain reserves for cattle feed rather than human consumption. Still others were concerned about environmental pollution and the toxic effects of the chemicals used to grow or preserve foods and beverages. By the late 1960s, awareness of the value of healthy food had developed into a national and international movement. Those of us in the movement went beyond the existing health food industry, which was focused primarily on vitamins and other supplements to the diet, and selected the name *natural foods* to encompass the concern for returning to a more balanced daily way of eating. Spearheaded by Erewhon Trading Company, the East West Foundation, the *East West Journal*, and many other macrobiotic enterprises and educational centers, this movement raised the public's consciousness of soil and food quality and reintroduced into contemporary life the concept of daily food as preventive medicine.

In January 1977, the premises and goals of the natural foods movement, which had grown to embrace many different food and agricultural organizations, received support in *Dietary Goals for the United States*, a report issued by the Senate Select Committee on Nutrition and Human Needs. Headed by former presidential candidate George McGovern and vice-presidential nominee Robert Dole, the committee took testimony and held hearings on the nation's health. The final document concluded:

> During this century, the composition of the average diet in the United States has changed radically. Complex carbohydrates—fruit, vegetables, and grain products—which were the mainstay of the diet, now play a minority role. At the same time, fat and sugar consumption have risen to the point where these two dietary elements alone now comprise at least 60 percent of total calorie intake, up from 50 percent in the early 1900s.
>
> In the view of doctors and nutritionists consulted by the Select Committee, these and other changes in the diet amount to a wave of malnutrition—of both over- and under-consumption—that may be as profoundly damaging to the Nation's health as the widespread contagious diseases of the early part of this century.
>
> The over-consumption of fat, generally, and saturated fat in particular, as well as cholesterol, sugar, salt, and alcohol have been related to six of the leading causes of death: Heart disease, cancer, cerebrovascular diseases, diabetes, arteriosclerosis, and cirrhosis of the liver.[9]

After more than a generation of neglect, the Senate report opened the door to nutritional common sense in this country. There had been earlier studies linking diet and degenerative disease, but these had made little impact on the medical profession and rarely received publicity. Through the mid-1970s, many physicians continued to ignore dietary considerations, and heart patients in coronary care units were routinely served meals including steak, fried potatoes, ice cream, and other foods high in fat or sugar.

Despite organized opposition from the meat and dairy food lobbies, *Dietary Goals* was well received by a great number of readers, nutritionists, and educational and consumer organizations and sent shock waves through the food industry, the medical profession, public school lunch programs, and other segments of society responsible for providing basic nutrition. The Report's call for increased consumption of whole grains, vegetables, and fresh fruit and for decreased consumption of fat, cholesterol, sugar, and refined foods was echoed by many medical associations and bodies. During the last fifteen years, at least thirty-seven international health organizations and task forces on cardiovascular disease have issued similar recommendations. These organizations include the International Association of Cardiology, the Intersociety Commission on Heart Disease Resources, the World Health Organization, the Canadian Department of National Health and Welfare, the American Heart Association, the Royal College of Physicians and the British Cardiac Society, the Australian National Heart Foundation, the West German Federal Health Office, and the Netherlands Nutritional Council.

In 1979, the U.S. Surgeon General issued a report, *Health Promotion and Disease Prevention*, that went even further than *Dietary Goals* in suggesting that already existing heart disease could be relieved by dietary measures:

> Direct evidence from animal studies supports the linkage of atherosclerosis with high levels of fats (particularly saturated) and cholesterol in the diet . . . [and] that Americans who habitually eat less fat-rich diets (vegetarians and Seventh Day Adventists, for example) have less heart disease than other Americans; and that atherosclerotic plaques in certain arteries may be reversed by cholesterol-lowering diets.[10]

Some of the studies that the Surgeon General referred to took place at Harvard Medical School and involved comparing the dietary practices and cholesterol and blood pressure levels of people in the Boston area eating macrobiotically with people enrolled in the Framingham Heart Study eating the Standard American Diet. The Framingham Heart Study, the longest and most influential heart disease study, is an ongoing research project in Framingham, Massachusetts, that has followed five thousand men and women for over three decades, assessing dietary and other lifestyle factors. It was this study that introduced into public consciousness the identification of high serum cholesterol, high blood pressure, and cigarette smoking as the three primary risk factors of cardiovascular disease.

Beginning in the early 1970s, Drs. Edward Kass and Frank Sacks at Harvard Medical School and their colleagues at greater Boston medical centers, later including William Castelli, M.D., current director of the Framingham Heart Study, undertook a series of experiments to evaluate the possible health benefits of the macrobiotic dietary approach. The results of these ongoing studies have been published in professional journals, including the *American Journal of Epidemiology,* the *New England Journal of Medicine,* and the *Journal of the American Medical Association.* Scientific studies of the macrobiotic diet have been published by other researchers in the *Journal of the American Dietetic Association* and *Atherosclerosis.*

Among many interesting findings, the researchers discovered that the macrobiotic community had the lowest serum cholesterol values ever reported for a group living in modern society. The values were similar to those of people living in traditional societies in North America, South America, Asia, and Africa where heart disease is almost unknown (see Table 5). During the last decade, these research studies at Harvard on macrobiotics have contributed significantly to the current change in thinking about diet and heart disease within the medical community. In a later chapter, we shall look at this research in detail.

Meanwhile, investigators at other institutions are looking at the value of macrobiotics in preventing and relieving other serious illnesses and providing a secure foundation for daily health. Researchers at Tulane University School of Public Health and Tropical Medicine, under the direction of James Carter, M.D., chairman of the Department of Nutrition, are developing a long-term medical study to evaluate the relationship between macrobiotics and

Table 5. CHOLESTEROL AND HEART DISEASE

Type of Diet	Average Cholesterol Range	Countries	Incidence of Coronary Heart Disease
High-cholesterol, high-fat, high-sugar	220–280	U.S., Australia, New Zealand, Northern and Central Europe	High
Low-fat, low-cholesterol, polyunsaturated oils	180–190	Greece, Yugoslavia, Italy, Puerto Rico, urban Japan	Moderate
Low-fat, high-fiber, seafood and fish	150–160	Rural Latin America, Mediterranean Islands, rural Japan	Low
Grains, vegetables	100–140	Traditional societies	Rare or nonexistent

Source: Data adapted from *American Heart Association Handbook* (New York: E. P. Dutton, 1980).

recovery from cancer among patients in the New Orleans area. In another study, a team of investigators from Boston University, the University of Minnesota School of Public Health, Harvard School of Public Health, and New England Baptist Hospital, headed up by Robert Lerman, M.D., Director of Clinical Nutrition at University Hospital in Boston, is evaluating the progress of an estimated seven hundred cancer patients who have sought macrobiotic guidance from me in the last few years. These persons will be matched with controls from the Eastern Cooperative Oncology Group tumor registry at the Dana-Farber Cancer Institute in Boston.

For studies on selected individual forms of cancer, physicians in Philadelphia are collecting medical records of cancer patients who have implemented macrobiotics, beginning with the pancreas. In Washington, D.C., a Congressional House Subcommittee on Health and Long-Term Care, chaired by Congressman Claude Pepper, concluded in 1984 that the "macrobiotic diet appears to be nutritionally adequate. . . . The diet would also be consistent with the recently released dietary guidelines of the National Academy of Sciences and the American Cancer Society in regard to possible reduction of cancer risks."[11] In New York, a macrobiotic project to wipe out AIDS has been started. Dozens of members of the gay community with AIDS and Kaposi's sarcoma, a form of skin cancer associated with this disorder, have sought dietary counseling. Generally their condition is stabilizing or improving on the new diet, and immunologists from some of the medical schools are collecting their blood samples and monitoring their progress for future documentation.

At the Shattuck Hospital in Boston, results of a double-blind study of the macrobiotic diet on a ward of long-term psychiatric and geriatric patients are being prepared for publication. Macrobiotic food was also served in Shattuck's cafeteria for two years, and about half of the five hundred doctors, nurses, and other staff took advantage of this service. In Chesapeake, Virginia, the Tidewater Detention Center is initiating a macrobiotic food program for juvenile offenders. A preliminary study showed that instances of aggressive behavior and other infractions declined 45 percent following removal of sugar from the inmates' food and snacks.[12]

Internationally, a United Nations Macrobiotics Society has been established in New York. Its guiding force, Katsuhide Kitatani, U.N. Development Director for Southeast Asia, overcame stomach cancer on the macrobiotic diet. The group already has a hundred and fifty members from the U.N. secretariat and member delegations and meets regularly to discuss problems of world health and world peace. In Geneva, Switzerland, I have been invited to lecture at the World Health Organization, and a macrobiotic society is being organized at UNESCO headquarters. Meanwhile, friends from some of our centers in Western Europe have been invited to teach in Rumania, Czechoslovakia, and other Eastern European countries and bring in macrobiotic literature for the first time. Articles on macrobiotics have begun to appear in Russian and Arabic magazines.

Nearer to home, at our international headquarters here in Boston, we have installed a national toll-free telephone number with information on macrobiotic literature, seminars and workshops on heart disease and cancer, cooking classes, and other activities across the country; referrals to recommended counselors, physicians, and other dietary and health care professionals; and local and mail-order sources for whole foods and products. This number, as well as a directory of Macrobiotics International Centers, is included in the resource section at the end of the book. A new macrobiotic educational facility, Mt. Kushi Seminary, has been opened in the lovely Berkshire Mountains at a former Franciscan retreat. Throughout the year, the center will host a variety of programs sponsored by the Kushi Institute and Kushi Foundation, including orientation, cooking classes, and dietary and way-of-life counseling sessions for visitors and their families. There are also special summer camps in the Pocono Mountains of Pennsylvania and in the Swiss Alps. Macrobiotic congresses meet annually in North America, the Caribbean, the Middle East, and Europe to discuss regional, continental, and global issues of health and peace.

Though still small and evolving, modern macrobiotics is the seed from which a mighty tree can grow, to nourish, shelter, and secure the future health and happiness of the human family for endless generations.

3

How the
Heart Beats

"The blood cannot but flow continuously like the currents of a river, or the sun and the moon in their orbits," the sages of ancient China observed in the Yellow Emperor's Classic of Internal Medicine.[1] The view of the body as a microcosm prevailed in both East and West until the beginning of modern times. "The heart is the beginning of life, even as the sun may be called the heart of the world," William Harvey noted on the eve of the Industrial Revolution. "The heart is the foundation of life, the source of all actions."[2] In the Vedas of ancient India, the heart is described as "a lotus with nine gates."[3] Dante likened the heart to a rose.

In modern medical texts, this natural imagery is largely missing. The heart is usually described as a four-chambered pump, and its relationship with the rest of the body is explained through metaphors drawn from hydraulics, engineering, auto mechanics, and most recently computer science. There are many reasons why modern science has developed such a fragmented view of life and health. One reason is that modern anatomy has measured the size and location of the heart and other organs but has not yet discovered the overall dynamic function of these organs in relationship to each other and to the cosmos. This is because that present-day anatomy draws most of its knowledge from autopsies rather than living organisms. Of course, when the body is dead, there isn't much going on inside besides decay. However, during a person's life, all our organs are working in concert with one another. Thus, to strengthen the heart, we need to strengthen the kidneys, liver, spleen, pancreas, and lungs since the healthy functioning of the heart depends on the healthy functioning of our entire system.

UNDERSTANDING YIN AND YANG

Everything in the universe is eternally changing, and this change proceeds according to the infinite order of the universe. The order of the universe was discovered, understood, and expressed at different times and different places throughout human history, forming the universal and common basis for all great religious, spiritual, philosophical, scientific, medical, and social traditions. The way to practice this universal and eternal order in daily life was taught by the Yellow Emperor, Hippocrates, Confucius, Lao Tzu, Buddha, Abraham, Jesus, and other great teachers in ancient times and has been rediscovered, reapplied, and taught under many names and forms over the past two thousand years.

From observing nature and our day-to-day thought and activity, we can see that everything is in motion. Everything changes: Electrons spin around a central nucleus in the atom; the Earth rotates on its axis while orbiting the sun; the solar system is revolving around the galaxy; and galaxies are moving away from one another with enormous velocity as the universe continues to cycle and expand. Opposites attract each other to achieve harmony, the similar repel each other to avoid disharmony. One tendency changes into its opposite, which shall return to the previous state.

In the Far East, the two interrelated universal tendencies that govern all phenomena were known as yin and yang. On the Earth, we experience yang as centripetal energy coming from the sun, the planets, the stars, distant galaxies, and finally cosmic space. This incoming, downward force pushes everything toward the surface of the Earth and causes the planet to spin and to orbit around the sun. In traditional cultures, this energy was known as Heaven's force. Modern science calls it gravity.

At the same time, the Earth generates an opposite centrifugal, yin, force because of the rotation on its axis. The outgoing, upward energy from the core of the planet was known as Earth's force.

The interplay between these two forces creates all manifestations on our planet, and likewise throughout the universe (see Table 6). Each movement creates respective physical tendencies. Yang force creates contraction, density, heaviness, rapid motion, and high temperature. Yin force creates expansion, diffusion, lightness, slower motion, and lower temperature. At their extremes each force changes into its opposite. For example, high temperature causes expansion and low temperature causes contraction.

Yin and yang are not static conditions but rather tendencies that cycle continuously, each changing into the other. At the biological level, yang is identified with masculine energy, while yin is associated with feminine energy. However, nothing is completely one or the other, and the ratio between the two forces is subject to constant fluctuation. Originating from God, or the infinite universe, yin and yang are manifested in myriad forms, ultimately merging and returning to their source. Yin and yang are the eternal laws governing all phenomena, from the movements of subatomic particles to the composition of blood and tissue to the formation of galaxies. By knowing how to balance these forces in our own lives, we can turn sickness into health, conflict into harmony, and sorrow into joy.

The rhythmic beating of the human heart is one of nature's most beautiful expressions of yin and yang, expanding and contracting more than 100,000 times a day, three billion times in a lifetime. The heartbeat is a perfect model of the universal laws of change. Blood flows in and out, the gates, or valves, open and close. The river of nourishment cycles continuously through the body, and the heart, like a majestic waterwheel, gently regulates its flow.

Our health and judgment depend on the smooth functioning of the heart and other vascular organs. Without proper nourishment and oxygen, the cells of the body, including our brain cells, degenerate and we lose our physical vitality and mental clarity and ultimately die. In the Gospel According to Thomas, Jesus says, "If they ask you, 'What is the sign of your Father in you?', say to them: 'It is movement and repose.' "[4] The heart is a perfect metaphor for the expression of God—the infinite order of the universe —within each of us. To preserve the health of this organ, we must preserve a balance between yin and yang, between expansion and contraction.

Table 6. EXAMPLES OF YIN AND YANG

Attribute	*YIN* ▽* *Centrifugal force*	*YANG* △* *Centripetal force*
Tendency	Expansion	Contraction
Function	Diffusion	Fusion
	Dispersion	Assimilation
	Separation	Gathering
	Decomposition	Organization
Movement	More inactive, slower	More active, faster
Vibration	Shorter wave and higher frequency	Longer wave and lower frequency
Direction	Ascent and vertical	Descent and horizontal
Position	More outward and peripheral	More inward and central
Weight	Lighter	Heavier
Temperature	Colder	Hotter
Light	Darker	Brighter
Humidity	Wetter	Drier
Density	Thinner	Thicker
Size	Larger	Smaller
Shape	More expansive and fragile	More contractive and harder
Form	Longer	Shorter
Texture	Softer	Harder
Atomic particle	Electron	Proton
Elements	N, O, P, Ca, etc.	H, C, Na, As, Mg., etc.
Environment	Vibration. . . . . .Air. . . . . . .Water. . . . . .Earth	
Climatic effects	Tropical climate	Colder climate
Biological	More vegetable quality	More animal quality
Sex	Female	Male
Organ structure	More hollow and expansive	More compacted and condensed
Nerves	More peripheral, orthosympathetic	More central, parasympathetic
Attitude, emotion	More gentle, negative, defensive	More active, positive, aggressive
Work	More psychological and mental	More physical and social
Consciousness	More universal	More specific
Mental function	Dealing more with the future	Dealing more with the past
Culture	More spiritually oriented	More materially oriented
Dimension	Space	Time

*For convenience, the symbols ▽, for Yin, and △, for Yang, are used.

36

OUR SPIRAL DEVELOPMENT

In the womb, the embryo continuously receives Heaven's force, entering the mother spirally through the upper magnetic pole, the center of the hair spiral on the head. The embryo also receives, from the rotating Earth, forces generated in an expanding direction, going upward through the lower magnetic pole, the mother's uterus. Both forces charge the embryo from above and below, generating vital forces of electromagnetic energy. In the Far East, this energy was traditionally known as *ki, chi,* or *prana.* We call this charged state of the embryo "being alive."

These two charging forces, together with the rotational movement of the embryo, produce expanding energy radiating out from the inside of the embryo toward the surrounding space, forming an invisible electromagnetic layer of energy around the fetus. Between the electromagnetic layer around the embryo and the center of the embryo, an electromagnetic charge is exchanged in the form of invisible currents that spiral in from the layer toward the inner part of the embryo as it rotates in twelve different ways. When these invisible currents reach the central part of the embryo, they each form a spiral. Some form inward-moving spirals due to their slow speed, and others form outward-moving spirals due to their faster speed. These spirals, inward and outward, grow continuously during the embryonic period, developing into various major organs and functions. The inward spirals form more compacted organs that are slower in movement, and the outward spirals create more expanded organs that are faster in movement. Among these organs, those having yang compacted structure and yin slow movement balance with those having yin expanded structure and yang active movement, as if forming pairs. The six pairs of balancing organs and functions are listed in Table 7.

In the embryo, the primitive heart starts to beat in response to the rhythmic pulsations of Heaven's and Earth's forces on about the twenty-fourth day, causing blood to circulate throughout the embryonic disc and primitive placenta. At maturity, the circulatory system approximates an infinite spiral. The blood pulsating through the arteries and veins forms a figure eight, or inverted infinity sign in three dimensions. At the center of the spiral, the heart propels blood into orbit throughout the body, delivering nourishment and oxygen to the cells through a network of increas-

Table 7. THE SIX PAIRS OF ORGANS
AND FUNCTIONS

Compacted Organs; Slow Movement	Expanded Organs; Active Movement
Lungs	Large intestine
Spleen and pancreas	Stomach
Heart	Small intestine
Kidneys	Bladder
Heart governor	Triple heater
Liver	Gallbladder

ingly finer vessels. Carbon dioxide and waste material from the cells are picked up and returned through the veins to the right side of the heart. Here the blood orbits to the lungs to exchange carbon dioxide for a fresh supply of oxygen. From the left side of the body, the blood once again starts a new orbit through the body.

Altogether there are seven separate branches of the body's spirallic system, distributing blood to the seven different regions. The seven circuits of the circulatory system are (1) the heart or coronary area itself, (2) the upper extremities (shoulders and arms), (3) the neck, head, and brain, (4) the lungs, (5) the abdominal area and digestive organs, (6) the renal circuit (the kidneys and bladder), and (7) the pelvis and lower extremities, including the legs. The pathways that link these major circuits to the heart are called the Great Vessels and include the inferior vena cava, the superior vena cava, the pulmonary artery, the pulmonary vein, the aorta, and the coronary arteries.

The circulatory system can be compared to a tree. Each of its major circuits fork into numerous smaller branches that in turn divide into millions of peripheral arterioles and capillaries. Ultimately, the capillaries differentiate into the trillions of cells within the body. The central regions of the circulatory system can be likened to the bough and stem of a tree, while the peripheral regions correspond to the branches and leaves. The body's cells comprise the most peripheral part of the circulatory system and correspond to the tree's fruit.

After forming the heart and other major organs and functions, electromagnetic energy begins to discharge in both upward and downward directions. Energy discharged upward has been charged more at the peripheral parts of both sides of the embryo, and energy discharged downward has been charged more at the central part of the embryo. These discharged energies also form outer spirals that later develop as arms and legs. Electromagnetic currents running through the arms and legs in the form of channels, or meridians, terminate in the formation of fingers and toes.

The meridians running throughout the body are somewhat like the meridians running on the surface of the Earth (see Figure 2). Electromagnetic currents running along the surface layer of the Earth form mountain ranges, aligned mainly in a north–south direction. There are some mountain ranges running east–west or northeast–southwest that have arisen in the past before or during axis shifts of the earth, which have changed the magnetic poles. On the mountain ranges there are springs, waterfalls, and streams, as well as volcanoes, valleys, forests, and plains. Each of these places has certain characteristics, produced by atmospheric pressure and other surface conditions together with underground forces and movement. Similarly, along the body meridians there are points analogous to various natural phenomena arising on mountain ranges. Some points on the meridians are more watery in nature—the electromagnetic current is streaming, pooling, falling, and bubbling up. Other points are characterized more by the energy of fire, the energy of metal, the energy of trees, or the energy of soil, or of other characteristics. These points are traditionally named according to their character, although in modern Oriental medicine a series of numbers has been fixed to identify them. These points exist mainly along the meridians, particularly around the joints of the arms and legs, and between these points, balancing points are further produced. In this way, more than 360 points are produced throughout our body along the twelve major meridians and more than 2,000 points are produced along the surface of the entire body.

The heart meridian, for example, branches into three directions (see Figure 3). One extends from the heart region downward to the small intestine, the heart's complementary and antagonistic organ. The second runs from the heart up through the side of the throat to the eye. The third passes through the lungs, descends, comes out at the underarm, runs down the middle of the inside of the upper arm, runs down the forearm, crosses the wrist and

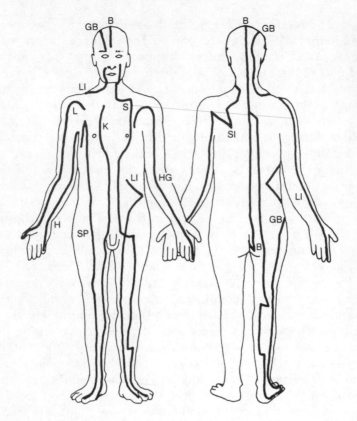

Figure 2. Electromagnetic Energy Circulation through the Meridians

H	= Heart	B	= Bladder
L	= Lung	S	= Stomach
SP	= Spleen	HG	= Heart governor
K	= Kidney	SI	= Small intestine
GB	= Gallbladder	LI	= Large intestine

palm, and ends at the inside end of the little finger on each hand, where it meets the small intestine meridian.

Among the twelve basic meridians, the heart governor meridian and the triple heater meridian have no specific organs to and from which energy enters and leaves. Their currents have more comprehensive functions. In the case of the heart governor meridian, energy generated by the movement of the heart region administers the circulation of blood and body fluids throughout the

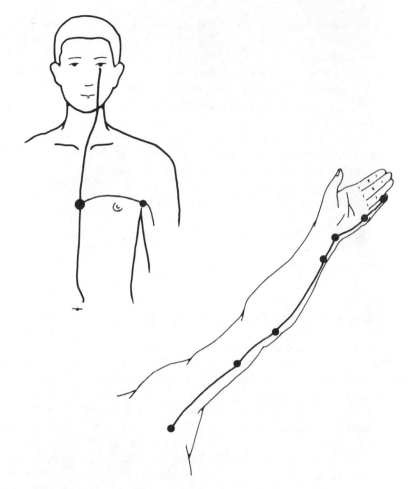

Figure 3. The Heart Meridian

body. In the case of the triple heater meridian, vibrations discharged from the metabolic movement of the upper heart region, middle stomach region, and lower abdominal region are constantly adjusting and controlling heat metabolism throughout the body. These two meridians influence and are reciprocally affected by the other ten meridians. At every moment, electromagnetic energy flows from one meridian to another as a continuous current, which is constantly receiving charges from the external environment through various points and constantly discharging through various other points as the current continues to flow.

Oriental medicine traditionally devised treatments using these meridians and the points along them to harmonize electromagnetic currents throughout the body. When the energy flow along certain meridians is lower than normal, stimulation is applied to supply energy or activate energy flow. When certain meridians have excessive energy, stimulation is applied to disperse energy in order to achieve a harmonious relation among the meridians. The arts for supplying or dispersing energy have been developed and applied in traditional European, African, and American Indian societies as well as in the Far East for many thousands of years. The arts of harmonizing energy include acupuncture, moxibustion, shiatsu or meridian massage, palm healing, and yoga and other physical exercises.

FUNCTIONING OF THE HEART

In the Far East, the heart is identified with the self, or innermost soul. It is the place where Heaven's and Earth's forces collide and meet, giving rise to the rhythmic expansion and contraction of the heartbeat. The heart is divided into four petals, or chambers (see Figure 4). The two upper regions are called the atria and the two lower regions the ventricles. The atria are smaller in size than the ventricles, have thinner walls, and serve to collect blood returning from the body or lungs. The ventricles are larger in size than the atria, have thicker walls, and pump the blood to the rest of the body and the lungs. A septum, or wall, divides the two sides of the heart, preventing blood or other fluids from entering or exiting except through the arteries and veins. The right atrium and ventricle are often referred to as the right heart and the left atrium and ventricle as the left heart.

When the atria expand with returning blood, the ventricles contract. When the atria contract, the ventricles expand and refill. The scientific terms for these movements are *systole* and *diastole*. *Systole* means "squeezing together" or contraction and is the yang phase of the cycle. *Diastole* means expansion or refilling and is the yin phase of the cycle. The two phases of the cycle occur almost

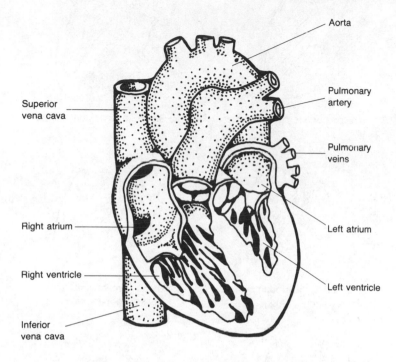

Figure 4. The Chambers of the Heart and Great Vessels

simultaneously and last less than a second (see Figures 5 and 6). Deoxygenated blood from the body enters the right atrium and flows to the right ventricle, which sends it to the lungs through the pulmonary artery. In the lungs, oxygen and carbon dioxide are

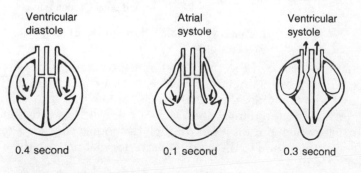

Figure 5. The Heart's Pumping Cycle

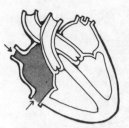

A. Blood enters right atrium.

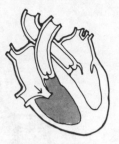

B. Blood flows to right ventricle.

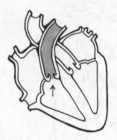

C. Blood flows through pulmonary artery to lungs.

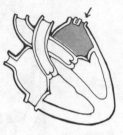

D. Blood enters left atrium from pulmonary vein.

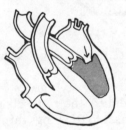

E. Blood flows to left ventricle.

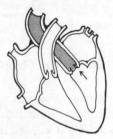

F. Blood is pumped to head and body through aorta.

Figure 6. Blood Circulation through the Heart

exchanged between the the blood and the atmosphere across a moist membrane connecting the alveoli, or air sacs, and the capillaries. From the lungs, the freshly oxygenated blood enters the left atrium via the pulmonary vein. From there it passes to the left ventricle, which pumps it out through the connecting aorta to the rest of the body and to the coronary arteries that nourish the heart itself.

Each minute, about six quarts of blood pass through the heart to the extremities of the body and back again. With each beat, the left ventricle of the heart pumps exactly the same amount of blood to the aorta as the right ventricle pumps to the lungs. Four valves open and close simultaneously to allow equal amounts of blood to flow into each chamber and prevent fluid from rushing backward while refilling.

The heartbeat itself is activated by the sinoatrial node, a small bundle of nerve tissue in the right atrium, which further branches and divides into scores of minute nerve endings (see Figure 7). A wave of electricity moves downward from the sinoatrial node to the atrioventricular node and the ventricles, causing the muscular walls of each large chamber to contract and pump out blood. The wall of the heart is composed of four sheaths of tissue: (1) the *endocardium,* a smooth membrane covering the valves and chambers of the heart, (2) the *epicardium,* a shiny membrane on the surface of the heart, (3) the *myocardium,* a thick layer of cardiac muscle that extends up to an inch in thickness around the hard-working left ventricle, and (4) the *pericardium,* the outermost sac, which contains a lubricating fluid allowing the heart to beat with a minimum of friction.

The vascular system consists of a variety of blood vessels. These vessels distribute blood to the organs and extremities of the body; facilitate the exchange of gases, nutrients, and other substances

Figure 7. The Heart's Electrical System

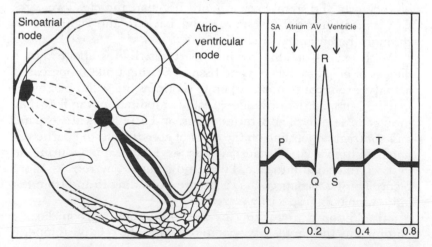

between the blood, lymph, and cells; and transport the blood back to the heart. The size and thickness of the blood vessels vary, as does the blood pressure. The arteries, which carry blood away from the heart, are the largest and thickest of the vessels. Because of their proximity to the heart, they also have the highest pressure, and the blood rushes through them with the greatest velocity. From the heart, the aorta branches into major arteries servicing the seven major circuits of the body.

In the course of their journey, the arteries divide into smaller arterioles and finally into capillaries. In these tiny vessels, the exchange of oxygen and nourishment between the cells and blood takes place. Only .01 mm in diameter, the capillaries are so minute that only one cell at a time can pass through their membrane. This makes for a highly effective distribution of oxygen and nutrients and utilization of energy. The capillaries, whose combined surface area is larger than a football field and extends altogether tens of thousands of miles, accounts for most of the vascular system.

From the capillaries, the blood begins its return journey to the heart through tiny connecting vessels called *venules.* The venules in turn join larger vessels, or veins, and the veins empty into the inferior or superior vena cavae, the two great vessels returning blood to the right atrium. The blood pressure in the veins is lower than in the arteries, and the walls of the veins are thinner than their arterial counterparts.

The heart nourishes itself by two coronary arteries that branch off the aorta and spiral back around the heart muscle. Two coronary veins return the venous blood back to the right atrium through the coronary sinus.

With each beat, the resting heart distributes about 2 to 3 ounces of blood to the cells and tissues. During times of increased activity, excitement, or stress, up to six times the volume of blood may be pumped. During sleep, rest, or meditation, the flow may drop considerably. The arteries, veins, and capillaries also expand and contract depending on the level of activity and the particular needs of the varying organs and tissues. For example, during digestion, the small intestine, liver, and spleen may require more blood. During urination, the renal circuit leading to and from the kidneys may be especially activated.

In addition to regulating oxygen intake and carbon dioxide elimination, the circulatory system regulates the relative temperature of the body and facilitates the removal of other waste products. A variety of sensors and other monitoring devices are used to activate these processes or convey information to other systems, such as the brain, which also help the body as a whole adapt to its environment. Blood pressure, for example, must remain steady or be compensated for by corresponding adjustments in other regions if it suddenly rises or falls in one specific area. Nervous impulses to and from the brain stem constantly monitor blood pressure. Imbalances arising from internal or external stimuli may trigger the release of hormones into the bloodstream, resulting in changes in arterial diameters, venous capacity, heart rate, or stroke volume (the amount of blood pumped out of the heart during each contraction) in an effort to modify the blood pressure. Similarly, the heartbeat may be modified by hormones that stimulate the sinoatrial node, either slowing down or stepping up electrical activity in response to a variety of stimuli.

The brain also houses a cardiac-inhibiting center that slows the heart through impulses in the vagus nerves connected to the sinoatrial node. Specialized cells, called *stretch receptors,* within the walls of the aorta and the carotid arteries to the brain monitor minute fluctuations in pressure and relay this data to the brain centers. Stretch receptors in the heart and lungs transmit information on the volume of blood within these regions and can result in short-term adjustments via the sympathetic nerves. Hormones from the brain also modify long-term blood volume by regulating fluid retention in the kidneys.

Another set of monitors called *chemoreceptors* monitors the chemical composition of the arterial blood. Also located in the aorta and carotid arteries, these cells observe fluctuations in oxygen and carbon monoxide levels and can modify the respiration rate. Further sensors in the skeletal muscles are activated by vigorous physical activity and help the body adapt to hard work or exercise. There are also thermosensitive cells that monitor minute changes in temperature and can transmit impulses resulting in the raising or lowering of body temperature.

The adrenal glands secrete two major hormones, norepinephrine and epinephrine, that can also affect the heartbeat and the activity of the heart muscle and blood vessels. These hormones, part of a group of strong substances called *catecholamines,* are often activated during emotional stress or other periods of intense activity. Another substance, angiotension II, produced in the blood vessel walls of the kidneys, regulates the balance of sodium and water in the bloodstream and thus affects blood pressure.

THE HEART AND LOVE

The relation of the heart to physical functioning is fairly well understood by most people. The emotional and spiritual function of this organ is less understood. The heart, as we all intuitively know, is associated with love. But why is this so? Why don't we associate feelings of affection, sympathy, and attraction with other bodily organs or glands? As Jonathan Swift satirically signed his correspondence, "With all of my heart and a piece of my liver."

The answer is simple. The human heart is centrally situated in the body, midway between Heaven and Earth. Physically, the heart is slightly to the left side of the chest cavity. The left ventricle, the largest chamber of the heart, which pumps blood to the rest of the body, shows the predominant influence of Heaven's force. It is a primary channel for the development of judgment, strength, perseverance, intuition, and other yang qualities. However, the heartbeat itself is initiated in the right side of the heart in the atrium. This channel governs wisdom, gentleness, devotion, reason, and other predominantly yin qualities. Thus, we see once again nature's wondrous complemental and antagonistic relationship. The upper right sinoatrial node regulating the heartbeat is balanced by the lower left ventricle regulating blood circulation to head and body.

Love is the perfect union of male and female—or yin and yang forces. In the East, we say that the Tao or Order of the Universe is yin and yang. In the West, we say God is Love. Upon reflection, we find that these two ways of looking at ultimate reality are the same. In the human heart, the forces of contraction and expansion —yang and yin—are perfectly balanced. A healthy heart is truly the gateway of love.

4

Diet, Ecology, and the Heart

Traditional cultures may not have mapped and classified every branch of the circulatory system. However, they respected the flow of blood through the heart and connected it with the orbits of the sun and moon, the passage of the seasons, and the cycles of planting and harvest. A very simple principle guided their understanding and practice: Food creates blood and blood creates life.

From ancient times, each civilization developed a way of eating that was in harmony with its local environment. Bound together by common food, mythology, and language, primitive societies learned to adjust to their unique surroundings and to maintain a balance with nature. Degenerative disease was almost unknown, and these early cultures often lasted for a hundred generations or more.

The belief that primitive hunting societies lived chiefly on mountain lion, antelope, boar, and other game has been shown to be in error. Paleolithic tribes hunted primarily wild cereals and grasses and foraged for plants, berries, roots, and tubers. In an article on the origin of the human diet in its science section, the *New York Times* reported:

> Recent investigations into the dietary habits of prehistoric peoples and their primate predecessors suggest that heavy meat-eating by modern affluent societies may be exceeding the biological capacities evolution built into the human body. The result may be a host of diet-related health problems, such as

Figure 8. World Climates

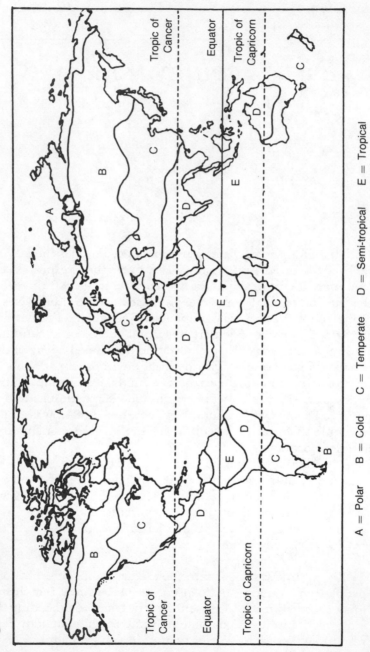

A = Polar   B = Cold   C = Temperate   D = Semi-tropical   E = Tropical

diabetes, obesity, high blood pressure, coronary heart disease, and some cancers.

The studies challenge the notion that human beings evolved as aggressive hunting animals who depended primarily upon meat for survival. The new view—coming from findings in such fields as archaeology, anthropology, primatology, and comparative anatomy—instead portrays early humans and their forebears more as herbivores than carnivores. According to these studies, the prehistoric table for at least the last million and a half years was probably set with three times more plant than animal foods, the reverse of what the average American currently eats.[1]

The few Stone Age cultures remaining today continue to consume primarily vegetable-quality food. Scientists who studied fifty-eight contemporary hunter–gatherer societies found that their diets contained from 50 to 70 percent complex carbohydrates from plant sources. Animal food comprised 25 to 35 percent of the total volume, and none of the tribes consumed milk, sugar, alcohol, or salt added at the meal.[2]

With the introduction of farming in Neolithic times, domesticated grains replaced wild strains as the principal fare. The staff of life, celebrated in ancient teachings, differed with each culture according to geography and climate. In the Orient it was largely rice and millet. In the Middle East it was mostly barley and wheat. In Europe it was mostly oats and rye, in Russia buckwheat, in Africa sorghum, and in the Americas Indian corn. This staple was supplemented with beans and legumes, seeds and nuts, garden vegetables, sea vegetables, seasonal fruits, and small, condiment-size amounts of fish, poultry, meat, or other animal products.

Even today, cooked whole grains and beans continue to form the basic nourishment in regions into which the modern way of life has not fully penetrated. Thus, corn tortillas and black beans form the daily diet in rural and low-income urban areas of Mexico and some parts of Central America. Rice and soybean products make up the staple fare outside the major cities in China, Southeast Asia, and Indonesia. Whole wheat chapati bread and lentils provide sustenance in India, Pakistan, and Afghanistan. Bulghur, tahini, hummus, and falafel—made from wheat and various beans and seeds—are eaten throughout North Africa and the Middle East.

The two exceptions to this pattern of eating, which extends across the temperate zones of the world, are in the polar regions and in the tropics. In the northern latitudes, where the growing season is short, a balanced diet higher in animal food and seafood evolved over the millennia. In cold regions, while this animal food was often consumed fresh and raw, vegetable-quality food was cooked longer than in warm climates, and salt was used more in cooking and in preserving foods for use throughout the year. In the southern latitudes, where animal food rapidly spoils, people tended to adopt a more completely vegetarian diet higher in fruits, spices, and liquids. Cooking was lighter and raw foods were consumed more frequently in these hotter regions.

The different ways of eating in the polar and cold regions, the temperate zones, and the tropical and semitropical regions are a good illustration of the dynamic balance of yin and yang (see Figure 8, page 50). At the poles, the Earth's features are stiller. There are barren stretches of snow and ice, long periods of intense cold, and abundant darkness. We may classify the polar and cold environment as yin. In the tropics, the landscape teems with life, the weather is hot and humid, and the days are bright and sunny. We may classify the more active tropical and semitropical environment as yang. In between these two extremes, our four-season temperature climate displays moderate fertility, medium temperature, and a more balanced cycle of days and nights.

COMPARING APPLES AND ORANGES

As we saw in the last chapter, yin and yang never exist in isolation. They are always found together in different proportions, and at their extremes they produce their opposites. As we go farther north into a cold yin environment, the forms of life become more yang—smaller, harder, and stronger. As we go farther south into a hot yang environment, the flora and fauna become more yin—larger, softer, and more delicate. In the temperate zones, the size and shape of plants and animals are more balanced. Thus, cranberries and currants grow naturally in colder climates, apples and pears grow in temperate climates, and mangoes and coconuts grow in hot climates (see Table 8).

Table 8. YIN AND YANG IN THE ANIMAL AND VEGETABLE KINGDOMS

Yin and Yang in the Animal Kingdom

	Yin (▽) Centrifugal	Yang (△) Centripetal
Environment	Warmer and more tropical; also in warm current	Colder and more polar; also in cold current.
Air humidity	More humid	More dry
Species	Generally more ancient	Generally more modern
Size	Larger, more expanded	Smaller, more compacted
Activity	Slower moving and more inactive	Faster moving and more active
Body temperature	Colder	Warmer
Texture	Softer, more watery and oily	Harder and drier
Color of flesh	Transparent–white–brown–pink–red–black	
Odor	More odor	Less odor
Taste	Putrid—sour—sweet—salty—bitter	
Chemical components	Less sodium (Na) and other yang elements	More sodium (Na) and other yang elements
Nutritional components	Fat . . . . . Protein . . . . . Minerals	
Cooking time	Shorter	Longer

Of course, these climatic divisions are the most basic, and there are many subdivisions. Within the same division, people who live in the high mountains naturally eat differently from people who live in the lower plains. People who live far inland naturally differ in their way of eating from those living along coastal regions or by major waterways. Even within the same local environment, varying soil conditions, temperatures, and levels of precipitation can give rise to unique strains and varieties of life.

There is a wonderful order and harmony to nature. Through the innumerable species, as well as natural formations such as valleys and mountains, deserts and lakes, and continents and

Table 8 *(continued)*

Yin and Yang in the Vegetable Kingdom

	Yin (▽) Centrifugal	Yang (△) Centripetal
Environment	Warmer, more tropical	Colder, more polar
Season	Grows more in spring and summer	Grows more in autumn and winter
Soil	More watery and sedimentary	More dry and volcanic
Growing direction	Vertically growing upwards; expanding horizontally underground	Vertically growing downward expanding horizontally above the ground
Growing speed	Growing faster	Growing slower
Size	Larger, more expanded	Smaller, more compacted
Height	Taller	Shorter
Texture	Softer	Harder
Water content	More juicy and watery	More dry
Color	Purple–blue–green–yellow–brown–orange–red	
Odor	Stronger smell	Less smell
Taste	Spicy—sour—sweet—salty—bitter	
Chemical components	More K and other yin elements	Less K and other yin elements
Nutritional components	Fat—protein—carbohydrate—mineral	
Cooking time	Faster cooking	Slower cooking

oceans, we can observe the rhythmic melody of yin and yang. On the basis of shape, size, color, aroma, taste, and other qualities, we can classify the entire scope of foods according to the relative balance of these two forces. The substances that we ingest fall into three broad categories: strong yang, balanced, and strong yin. Within each category, there are gradations among the various items as well as differences of quality within each item according to its manner of cultivation, season of growth, way of preparation, manner of storage, and other considerations.

Table 9 is compiled for the world's temperate zones, including most of the United States and Canada, Europe, the Soviet Union, China, Japan, and parts of Africa and Latin America. Items in each column are arranged in order of relative strength, e.g., eggs are more contracted, or yang, than meat; whole grains are more centered, or balanced, than beans; and sugar is more expansive, or yin, than coffee and tea.

A number of interesting relationships emerge from studying this order. The foods in the strong yang column are primarily animal foods and are naturally eaten in higher proportions in the colder regions of the world. The foods in the strong yin column are mostly vegetable-quality and are usually native to the tropics. Those in the middle column are common to temperate zones. In addition, we find that the balanced foods are chiefly whole foods and that they are prepared and eaten in whole form. In contrast, both the strong yang and the strong yin foods are primarily processed foods and are prepared and consumed in fragments rather than as wholes.

From this table, we see that the modern diet combines foods mostly from the strong yang category and the strong yin category. Historically, most of these foods originated in either colder northern climates or hotter southern climates, even though they are now produced in temperate zones owing to transplanting, hybridization, refrigeration, and artificial methods of preservation. In their original habitats, some of these foods are part of a balanced natural diet, for example, curry and spices in southern India, coconuts in the Pacific Islands, and meat and dairy food in Siberia and Alaska. However, when consumed on a daily basis in a four-season climate, strong yin and strong yang foods are unnatural. Sooner or later they lead to serious imbalance and a biological degeneration of the human beings who eat them.

THE EFFECTS OF MEAT AND DAIRY FOOD

Meat, poultry, fish, and seafood give the body an immediate burst of energy and strength. In the colder regions of the world, animal

Table 9. A YIN/YANG CLASSIFICATION OF FOOD, BEVERAGES, AND OTHER SUBSTANCES

Strong Yang

Refined salt
Eggs
Meat
Hard cheese
Poultry
Fish
Seafood

Balanced

Whole grains
Beans and bean products
Vegetables
Sea vegetables
Sea salt
Spring or well water
Nonaromatic, nonstimulant teas
Seeds and nuts
Locally grown, seasonal fruit
Unrefined vegetable oils

Strong Yin

Medications (with a few exceptions)
Drugs (marijuana, LSD, etc.)
Most foods containing chemicals, preservatives, dyes, or pesticides
Most vitamin pills (with a few exceptions)
Alcohol
Sugar, molasses, honey, and refined sweeteners
Aromatic and stimulant beverages (coffee, black tea, mint tea, etc.)
Spices (curry, cumin, pepper, nutmeg, dill, etc.)
Saturated and refined vegetable oils
Milk, butter, soft cheese, yogurt, ice cream
Tropical fruits and vegetables
White rice, white flour

food serves to warm the body quickly and thus helps balance the extremely low outside temperature. Among native peoples of the arctic, animal food comprises about 30 to 40 percent of the traditional diet. The remainder consists of vegetable materials taken from the intestines of slaughtered caribou, plants, roots, berries, and seaweed scraped from coastal cliffs at low tide. Similarly, reindeer milk was traditionally eaten in small volume to increase vitality. In less frigid but still cool regions, yogurt made from fermented goat, sheep, or horse's milk was consumed to aid digestion. For the most part, the people who consumed these meat and dairy products were hardworking farmers or seafarers, and any excess toxins from animal food consumption could be discharged from their bodies through their normally strenuous activity. As we shall see, physical activity is an important factor in maintaining our health and is complementary to our way of eating.

In temperate latitudes, animal foods naturally make up a much smaller part of the daily diet than in cold or polar regions. Three out of the four seasons are warm, hot, and cool, with winters that are less cold than in arctic regions. About 10 percent animal food consumption is the upper limit for our temperate zone. This proportion is confirmed anatomically by the ratio of human teeth suitable for consumption of vegetable-quality food (8 incisors and 20 molars and pre-molars) and animal-quality food (4 canines). However, the modern diet in four-season latitudes commonly averages from 50 to 75 percent meat, dairy, and other animal products.

Taken on a daily basis in this excessive volume, animal food has an adverse effect on personal health, especially on sedentary modern urban populations. For example, it takes twice as long to digest meat as it does to digest grains and vegetables. Meat thus begins to putrefy in the stomach, producing toxins and amines, destroying bacterial culture in the small intestine, and causing degeneration of the villi where metabolized food is absorbed into the blood. Saturated fat and cholesterol from meat accumulate around active organs, such as the heart and liver, and can lead to hardening of the arteries and coronary disease. In the large intestine, protein wastes from meat tend to clog the transverse colon, hampering proper elimination and leading to further retention of toxic by-products in the body. To compensate for eating meat, our system requires more oxygen in the bloodstream. The breath rate rises, making it difficult to maintain a calm and peaceful mind. Thinking in general becomes defensive, suspicious, rigid and sometimes aggressive—all negative expressions of yang energy.

Dairy food, which often accompanies meat consumption in our society, contributes a soothing, stabilizing, and overall calming influence on a digestive, nervous, and circulatory system subjected to volatile red meat elements. However, dairy food can produce illnesses of its own or in combination with other factors. Casein, the protein in cheese, milk, cream, and butter, cannot be assimilated by most people and begins to accumulate in the undigested state in the upper intestine and putrefy, producing mucus and toxins and leading to a weakening of the gastric, intestinal, pancreatic, and bile systems. Since more oxygen is needed to carry hemoglobin to cells enveloped with mucus, regular dairy intake also contributes to uneven thinking, dulled reactions, and emotional dependency.

BALANCING EXTREMES

Whenever we eat from one extreme, we are automatically attracted to food from the other extreme in an effort to maintain equilibrium. Thus at breakfast, to offset our customary pair of eggs, we take orange juice, several slices of white bread fortified with additives, and a cup of coffee with cream and sugar. At lunch our hamburger is bathed in mustard, catsup, relish, and other spices, and we eat it with French fries and soda. At dinner our fried chicken is served with mashed potato and gravy, a tomato salad, and for dessert a fruit cup with pineapples and bananas.

Although we are not aware of it, we are balancing yin and yang all the time regardless of how we eat. The problem with the modern diet is that we are trying to balance foods that are not natural to our own local environment or grown under similar climatic conditions. Many of the everyday foods we take for granted originally derive from tropical or semitropical regions or are shipped into our area from places thousands of miles away. Orange juice and frozen citrus foods, for example, come from Florida and Brazil, coffee from El Salvador and Uganda, sugar from Hawaii, spices from India, and pineapples and bananas from Hawaii and Guatemala. Though now grown in northern climates, potatoes and tomatoes are native to Latin America, and it may take thousands of years before they adapt evolutionarily to our environment. The syrup in soft drinks comes from kola nuts originating in tropical parts of Africa.

The more meat, eggs, cheese, and fish we eat, the more tropical food we must consume to counter their effects. The rise of yang animal food consumption in modern civilization has been accompanied by successively stronger influxes of yin food. First, in the seventeenth and eighteenth centuries, rising animal food intake was balanced by an increased intake of sugar, coffee, and tea. In the nineteenth and early twentieth centuries, the rise of the beef industry in the American West, Argentina, and Australia laid the foundation for a surge in alcohol and soft drink consumption. Finally, in the mid- and late twentieth century, the spiral has widened, and modern society's craving for excessive yin energy to balance hamburgers, steaks, and increased meat consumption has taken the form of an explosion of marijuana, opium, and other drug and pill intake. The effects of these addictions, especially on family life, have been heavy, and society has usually moved to limit or prohibit the stronger forms of yin. However, these efforts to legislate biology have not succeeded. Only if the underlying cause— excess meat, poultry, dairy food, refined salt, and other strong yang consumption—is alleviated will the demand for stimulants, sweets, alcohol, drugs, and other strong yin consumption diminish.

Modern medicine operates on this same principle, though it has not recognized the underlying mechanism at work. Many of the pharmaceuticals used to counterbalance heart disease, cancer, and other degenerative disorders are tropical in origin. For example, Capoten, a synthetic drug used to control high blood pressure, is derived from a substance in the venom of the South American pit viper.

Though meat and sugar, cheese and wine, and quiche and cocaine form a rough sort of natural balance, the human body is unable to withstand such extreme efforts at homeostasis. The natural, smooth contraction and expansion of the intestinal tract, or peristalsis, becomes irregular and begins to deteriorate through successive shocks of extreme yin or yang substances. Absorbed into the bloodstream and the vital organs, these materials create imbalance, eventually leading to abnormal discharges, chronic disease, and degeneration of the organism.

In the case of the heart and circulatory system, hard fats and cholesterol may accumulate around the major vessels, eventually penetrating to the tissues of the heart walls and immobilizing the heart. The aorta, pulmonary artery, and other vessels often become clogged with plaque from this source, giving rise to atherosclerosis. Blood clots may form and cause thrombosis or embolism in the brain, legs, and other organs and extremities, as well as the coronary arteries.

Sugar, honey, and other sweeteners also lead to the formation of fatty acids and buildup of plaque in the circulatory system. These strong yin substances, along with excessive liquid, fruits, juices, foods of tropical origin, stimulants, alcohol, drugs, and medication, loosen the elasticity of heart tissues. General enlargement of the heart caused by the loosening of tissues may lead to abnormal blood pressure. Inharmonious coordination between right atrium and left atrium due to the expansion and loosening or contraction and hardening of a part of the heart may cause heart murmur and irregular breathing. Imbalanced food intake can lead to congenital heart defects in the next generation.

Today we eat more meat than the Inuit (Eskimos) and more sugar than the Cubans, and get less exercise than either. The unnatural marriage of a semipolar and semitropical diet is the underlying biological foundation for many of the social, political, and environmental problems of our era. In geopolitical terms, the strong, aggressive yang northern societies whose diet is more carnivorous have historically dominated the weak, gentle yin southern cultures who have been nourished on primarily vegetable-quality foods. Today dietary lines have blurred, and the north is importing tomatoes, oranges, bananas, pineapples, avocados, sugar, spices for cola, marijuana, and cocaine from the south in return for infant formula, cheese, ice cream, hamburgers, hot dogs, and pizza. Both sides ultimately lose out in this exchange, as does the environment of which they are a part. With the spread of heart disease and cancer, modern society's 400-year-old dietary experiment in violating ecological principles of balance—the order of the universe—is coming to an abrupt and tragic end.

5

Making Balance Naturally

By selecting food that was in harmony with the local environment, our ancestors retained their immediate responsiveness to the natural world. Their reactions were intuitive and appropriate to the geography and climate of which they were an integral part. As complex civilizations developed in which food was transported over vast distances from areas with completely different climates and soil conditions, we grew increasingly out of touch with the natural world around us. The more that intuition decayed, the more we established institutions, including law and morality, science and nutrition, to restrain and guide us through our increasingly chaotic feelings.

Over the last four centuries, modern civilization entirely forgot about whole foods, neglected proper cooking techniques, and lost meaningful contact with the heavens, the seasons, the weather, the soil, and most growing things. With the development of air transportation, refrigerated cargo container shipping, and television advertising, natural climatic boundaries between cultures have completely dissolved, leading to confusion about what is natural and what is unnatural.

The infectious, chronic, and acute diseases of modern civilization have accompanied the spread of modern agriculture and the modern way of eating around the world. In the Third World, degenerative disorders that took four centuries to develop in Europe and North America are emerging within a generation or less. Despite this international trend, there are a few cultures and subcultures that have preserved their traditional way of eating and thus preserved their hearts.

ASIA

In areas of Asia where the traditional diet is still observed and modern life has made little impact, heart disease remains almost nonexistent. These regions include Siberia, Mongolia, the Armenian and Azerbaijan republics of Soviet Central Asia, and tropical New Guinea. According to Soviet cardiologists, the inhabitants of colder northern regions or mountainous central areas who consume a diet high in mutton, fermented milk or yogurt, and other animal products remain largely free from heart disease, while in the temperate regions ordinary Soviet citizens who eat high volumes of meat and dairy food suffer an epidemic of coronary disease.[1]

In remote parts of New Guinea that did not come in contact with modern civilization until after World War II, doctors report no signs of high blood pressure, diabetes, peripheral vascular disease, stroke, or heart attack. The staple food in this region is sweet potatoes, and the diet consists of 94 percent complex carbohydrates, 3 percent protein, and 3 percent fat.[2]

In China, heart disease was also virtually unknown until the twentieth century. In 1941, a medical researcher noted the rarity of arteriosclerosis, angina, and coronary thrombosis and connected their absence with the Chinese diet, which was low in cholesterol and in saturated fats and oils.[3] In the 1980s, the Chinese government embarked on a campaign to modernize the nation's diet after surveys revealed that the typical family spent three to four hours a day buying fresh produce at the market and preparing it at home.[4] The government is now introducing mass-produced baked goods and fast foods to channel the labor put into cooking into what it sees as more productive outlets. To this end, the Ministry of Light Industry (in charge of baked goods) has arranged with the U.S. Department of Agriculture to open several modern American-style bakeries in Peking. The goal of the new automated plants is to produce enough white bread, as well as doughnuts, shortcake, and other products, to feed the capital's seven million inhabitants. Ready-made sandwiches and other fast foods would eventually eliminate hot breakfasts and lunches. In southern China, parboiled white rice is being encouraged to save time and energy. Inexpensive soft drinks, popsicles, ice cream, and other snack and party foods are increasingly available throughout the country. Although overall heart disease rates in China remain well below Western levels, their incidence is increasing. A recent sampling in a Shanghai hospital indicated that from 8 to 16 percent of patients suffered from coronary disease.[5]

In Taiwan, cardiovascular disease has also risen over the last generation as refined rice displaced millet, taro potatoes, and sweet potatoes as the island's staples. Stroke rose 52 percent between 1952 and 1975 and is now the leading cause of death.[6]

In Japan, coronary heart disease is on the increase as well, though still only about 10 percent of American, Soviet, and European levels.[7] Stroke is the leading cause of death in Japan and appears to be associated with the now nearly universal consumption of refined white rice, as well as the rising consumption of sugar, monosodium glutamate, artificially prepared soy sauce, soft drinks, milk and other dairy foods, alcohol, and meat and other animal products.

In India, coronary disease is seven times higher in the south, where white rice is the staple, than in the north.[8] In the north, where whole grain chapati bread is the main food, degenerative diseases are less prevalent. Spices and raw foods are also consumed more in the more tropical south. While this is to a certain degree natural to balance the extreme heat (spices are activating and raw foods are cooling), current levels of consumption may be excessive. In an article on diet and heart disease, the *Journal of the Indian Medical Association* quoted an ancient Vedic physician named Sushruta who noted that excessive intake of hot spices and half-cooked food could interfere with the smooth functioning of the heart.[9]

AUSTRALIA AND OCEANIA

Australia and New Zealand rank among the top five nations in deaths from heart disease. Cardiovascular ailments, however, are unknown among native peoples of these regions, who follow a traditional diet of wild plants, roots, berries, sea vegetables, fresh game, insects, and fish and seafood. Beginning in the 1960s, acculturated aborigines who started eating white flour, beef, mutton, and other modern foods showed signs of high blood pressure and hardening of the arteries.[10]

In Oceania, heart disease is rare in traditional societies where coconut, taro potatoes, breadfruit, fish, and other products of the sea still form the foundation of the daily diet. For example, in the Cook Islands, 1,600 miles northeast of New Zealand, researchers found that the inhabitants of Atuiu and Mitiaro, who get 93 percent of their fat from coconut and other plant sources, have 2.5 times less hypertension than the Westernized inhabitants of nearby Rarotonga Island, who get 86 percent of their fat from animal sources.[11] Health also appeared to be related to different levels of activity and exercise. People on Atuiu and Mitiaro followed the traditional pattern of farming and fishing, while the Rarotongans tended to hold down civil service jobs and lead a more sedentary way of life.

AFRICA

In sub-Saharan Africa, heart disease was unknown until very recently.[12] In East Africa, doctors reported that they had never seen a case of high blood pressure before 1941 or heart attack before 1948. By 1963, the rate of high blood pressure among assimilated Ugandans rose to European levels. In South Africa, rates of coronary disease of blacks are 98 to 99 percent less than those of whites. The traditional Bantu diet consists of maize, millet, wheat, fermented cereal products, dried peas and beans, ground nuts, pumpkins, wild greens, tomatoes, onions, and small amounts of meat about twice a week. In Johannesburg and other metropolitan areas, lightly refined grains are now eaten regularly along with increasing amounts of sugar, tea, coffee, soft drinks, condensed milk, margarine, and canned fish. Stroke now accounts for about 10 percent of deaths among urban black South Africans, and high blood pressure is common. In rural areas, where processed foods, stimulants, and animal food are still scarce, cardiovascular disease is rare.

MIDDLE EAST

Heart disease is the leading cause of death in Israel and in other countries where the modern diet has taken root. Medical studies on the migration of Jews from Yemen to Israel have identified the specific foods responsible for part of this increase. Yemeni Jews born in Israel or who have lived there for over twenty-five years have substantially higher rates of hypertension and coronary disease than native-born Yemenis who have entered the country within the past ten years.[13] In Israel, the Yemenis continue to follow their traditional way of eating, except for a slight increase in oil consumption, especially margarine; and the addition of sugar (in Yemen, sugar consumption is negligible). In another study, only 2 percent of Israeli vegetarians had high blood pressure compared with 26 percent of nonvegetarians.[14]

EUROPE

Although heart disease is rampant throughout Europe, there is a striking difference in rates according to geography and climate. In Scandinavia, coronary disease rates are especially high, and this has been correlated to heavy consumption of saturated fat and cholesterol from meat and dairy foods. Rising consumption of tropical foodstuffs is probably also another major factor, though this has not been as widely studied. For example, after World War II, coconut oil became a staple for cooking in Sweden, and by the 1960s 50,000 tons were imported annually.

Heart disease is also epidemic in the Soviet Union west of the Ural mountains, Poland, East Germany, Great Britain, Ireland, Netherlands, Belgium, West Germany, and Austria. Coronary disease is about 50 percent less common in southern Europe, where more fiber from whole grains, fresh vegetables, and fruit is eaten and where olive oil and other vegetable-quality cooking oils are traditionally used. This includes France, Switzerland, Italy, Spain, Portugal, Greece, and the Mediterranean islands.

Interestingly, heart disease dropped sharply in northern Europe during both world wars as meat, eggs, cheese, milk, sugar, and other luxury items became scarce. In 1924, German pathologist Ludwig Aschoff first connected the decline in atherosclerosis with reduced intake of cholesterol and other fatlike substances.[15] During World War II, heart disease in Norway and many other countries occupied by the Germans declined by roughly 30 percent as processed foods and animal products became scarce and the consumption of cereals, vegetables, and skimmed milk rose.[16] When the war ended and the former diet high in fat and sugar resumed, mortality rates from heart disease returned to previous levels. Similar drops were noted in cancer and other degenerative disorders during this period. In the early 1950s, these unexpected findings alerted some Western doctors to the relation between diet and chronic illness and in the 1960s and 1970s contributed to the study of fat and cholesterol as primary causal factors in heart disease and some forms of cancer.

ARCTIC REGIONS

Hardening of the arteries and other heart and circulatory ailments were unknown among the native Inuit (Eskimos) prior to their contact with modern civilization. Traditional Inuit eat a diet high in animal products but not high in fat. Most of their animal intake comes from fish, whale, and other marine sources whose fat is mostly unsaturated. Native peoples also eat substantial amounts of plants, roots, and seaweeds. Over the last half-century, following the influx of sugar, stimulants, soft drinks, white flour, and other foods not common to the region, high blood pressure and heart attack have emerged.[17] Sugar consumption among native Alaskans, for example, rose four times between 1959 and 1967, and high blood pressure reached the levels of other Americans.

NORTH AMERICA

Among North American cultures and subcultures at low risk for heart disease, the Tarahumara are the most notable. The Tarahumaras live in the Sierra Madre Occidental Mountains in north central Mexico and eat a traditional diet of corn, beans, and squash. Meat is seldom eaten, and eggs are taken only occasionally. The 50,000 Tarahumaras use no mechanical energy in farming, travel only by foot, and engage in marathon kickball competitions sometimes ranging across 200 miles. Researchers who have studied this native culture report that high blood pressure and obesity are absent and death from cardiac and circulatory complications is unknown.[18]

In contrast, heart disease has begun to emerge in native people who have assimilated aspects of modern life. Among the Navajo, for example, diabetes, coronary disease, and cancer are emerging, and 5 percent of tribal members have high blood pressure. The Navajo's traditional diet has been largely displaced by mutton, bread, potatoes cooked in lard, and coffee with sugar. Compared with other Americans, their rate of heart disease is still low, and researchers attribute this to the Navajo's practice of "singing" together to achieve tribal harmony, to horseback riding and other vigorous exercise, and to smoking less.[19]

Among North Americans of primarily European descent, Seventh Day Adventists stand out for their low rates of heart disease.[20] About half the members of this Christian community are ovo-lacto vegetarians, meaning that they eat eggs and dairy food but not meat, poultry, or fish. Both vegetarian and nonvegetarian Seventh Day Adventists avoid pork, coffee, spices, highly refined foods, alcohol, and tobacco. According to a recent study of 25,000 church members in California, middle-aged men who were vegetarians suffered four times fewer fatal heart attacks than those who ate meat.[21] Among older men, the rate was six times fewer. Older vegetarian women were also at substantially less risk than those who consumed meat. The rate among younger women was low and about the same in both groups, which was attributed to the protective effects of ovulation and menstruation.

Among Asian Americans, studies show that immigrants who adopt the standard American diet soon acquire heart disease at the rate of other Americans even though incidence of the disease is low in their native homelands.[22] For example, Japanese who settle in Hawaii and adopt a partially Western diet have about twice the coronary disease rate as Japanese living in Japan. When they move to California and assimilate more completely, the coronary disease rate among those of ethnic Japanese background rises to that of other Americans. About twenty years ago, the studies of food habits among migrating populations first convinced doctors that genetics was not a primary factor in susceptibility to heart disease. Since then, a multitude of epidemiological studies from all around the world have shown that the different rates of heart disease are explained largely by diet and other environmental factors, not by heredity.

SOUTH AMERICA

Although modern medicine synthesizes many medications from plants and animals in the Amazon, heart disease itself is unknown among the native peoples living there. A medical study in Upper Xingu conducted from 1965 to 1979 showed no sign of stroke, angina, heart attack, or peripheral vascular disease among the Indian population.[23] Their diet consisted principally of manioc supplemented by corn, sweet potatoes, peanuts, bananas, pineapples, and fish. The Indians occasionally ate monkey and bird but otherwise not much game. Scientists reported that decision making among the community was equally divided among all members and that there was little competition or strife. As in most traditional societies, blood pressure was low and did not naturally rise with age. In contrast, heart disease is widespread in developed areas of Brazil as well as in metropolitan regions of Argentina, Venezuela, and other areas of South America.

In Washington, Moscow, Peking, New Delhi, Nairobi, and Rio, the Pepsi and McDonald's generation have abandoned their parents' and ancestors' way of eating for a diet high in saturated fat, dietary cholesterol, refined carbohydrates, and synthetic food. Before the onslaught of artificial flavors and chemical additives, the wonderful richness and variety of the world's cuisines are rapidly disappearing. A modern-day Noah's Flood of heart disease, cancer, mental illness, and diminished reproductive capacity caused by the foods, beverages, and medications we ingest threatens to destroy us internally. The conflagration is worldwide and affects nearly every family, every class, every ethnic group, and every nation (see Table 10). There is no escape through medicine, science, education, religion, or art. The only way out is for each individual to resolve from this day forward to select food in har-

Table 10. SPREAD OF CARDIOVASCULAR DISEASE IN TRADITIONAL SOCIETIES EXPOSED TO MODERN DIET

Society	High Blood Pressure	CHD*	Varicose Veins
Hunter–Gatherers			
Inuit (Eskimos)	+	+	+
Australian aborigines	+	+	
North American Indians		+	
Agriculturalists			
Uganda	+	+	+
Zimbabwe	0	+	
South Africa (Bantu)	+	+	+
Papua New Guinea	+	+	+
Pacific Islands	+	+	
Sub-Saharan Africa	+	+	+
Polynesia	+		+
Migrants			
Maoris	+	+	+
South African Indians	+	+	
Israelis	?	+	
Far East			
Japan		+	
Taiwan	+	+	P
Hawaiian groups		+	0

*Coronary Heart Disease
Increase = + / No change = 0 / Doubtful increase = ? / Already prevalent = P / No data = *Blank*
Source: H.C. Trowell and D.P. Burkitt, *Western Diseases* (Cambridge, Mass.: Harvard University Press, 1981).

mony with the local environment, to learn proper cooking techniques, and to reestablish contact with the soil and with the stars. How to grow proper food and how to balance our daily diet are essential to the continued survival and development of humanity for thousands of years to come.

6

The Standard
Macrobiotic Diet

The Standard Macrobiotic Diet has been practiced widely throughout history by all major cultures. In modern times, the diet has often been misunderstood because of a lack of information and basic understanding. The actual diet is very broad. It has been exercised by hundreds of thousands of people, especially in the last fifteen years by many individuals and families who have sought to attain better health and create a more healthy and peaceful society.

In comparison with current dietary habits, the Standard Macrobiotic Diet has the following nutritional characteristics: (1) more complex carbohydrates, less simple sugars; (2) more vegetable-quality protein, less animal food protein; (3) less overall consumption of fat, greater consumption of unsaturated fat and less saturated fat; (4) more consideration of balancing various vitamins, minerals, and other nutritional factors; (5) use of organically grown, natural-quality food utilizing more traditional food processing techniques and less artificial and chemically processed foods; and (7) consumption of more food rich in natural fiber and less food that has been devitalized.

The Standard Macrobiotic Diet is not designed for any particular person nor for any particular disease. It is designed for the general maintenance of physical and psychological health and the well-being of society as a whole. It further serves, in many instances, to prevent degenerative diseases and may be modified to

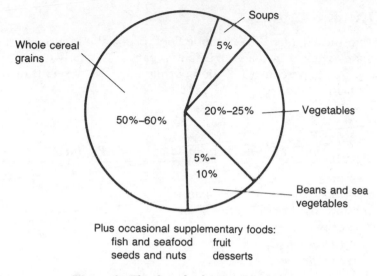

Plus occasional supplementary foods:
fish and seafood   fruit
seeds and nuts   desserts

Figure 9. The Standard Macrobiotic Diet

help relieve specific disorders. We usually speak of a macrobiotic dietary approach, rather than a macrobiotic diet, since everyone's selection of food and way of eating will differ slightly according to personal condition, level of activity, sex, age, climate, season, and individual needs and enjoyment. However, the Standard Macrobiotic Diet offers broad general guidelines regarding the overall percentages and types of foods to be consumed, as well as a balance of different cooking methods.

The accompanying chart (Figure 9) illustrates the four main categories of daily foods to be eaten, as well as the kinds of supplemental foods that may be consumed occasionally by those in good health. Persons with existing cardiovascular conditions or other illness may need to modify the diet further and avoid certain supplemental foods, especially animal food, fruit, desserts, raw food, and so forth until their condition improves. Complete dietary guidelines for heart and circulatory disease are provided in Part II of this book. For those in generally good health, the following guidelines are appropriate. In general, foods are listed according to yin/yang characteristics, beginning with the most centered items. In other cases, such as vegetables, alphabetization is used for convenience.

WHOLE GRAINS

Within the Standard Macrobiotic Diet, especially in a temperate climate, whole grains are an essential part of the daily diet. They comprise 40 percent to 60 percent (average 50 percent) of the daily food intake.

Kinds of Whole Grains and Grain Products

BROWN RICE

Brown rice—short, medium, and long grain
Genuine brown rice cream
Puffed brown rice
Brown rice flour products
Brown rice flakes

SWEET BROWN RICE

Sweet brown rice grain
Mochi (pounded sweet brown rice)
Sweet brown rice flour products

WILD RICE

Wild rice grain

WHOLE WHEAT

Whole wheat berries
Whole wheat bread
Whole wheat chapatis
Whole wheat noodles and pasta
Whole wheat flakes
Whole wheat flour products such as crackers, muffins, and
   others
Couscous
Bulghur
Fu (puffed wheat gluten)
Seitan (wheat gluten)

BARLEY
Barley grain
Pearl barley
Pearled barley
Puffed barley
Barley flour products

RYE
Rye grain
Rye bread
Rye flakes
Rye flour products

MILLET
Millet grain
Millet flour products
Puffed millet

OATS
Whole oats
Oatmeal
Oak flakes
Oat flour products and puffed oats

CORN
Corn on the cob
Corn grits
Corn meal
Whole corn dough products such as arepas, tortillas, etc.
Corn flour products such as corn bread, muffins, etc.
Puffed corn
Popped corn

BUCKWHEAT
Buckwheat groats
Buckwheat noodles and pasta
Buckwheat flour products such as pancakes, etc.

Cooking Styles for Whole Grains

Pressure cooking
Boiling

Cooking Styles for Whole Grains (cont.)

Steaming
Baking
Frying such as fried rice, fried noodles
Roasting
Other traditionally practiced and commonly used cooking
   styles

Cooking Varieties for Whole Grains

Cook with a pinch of sea salt
Occasionally cook with vegetables
Occasionally cook with beans
Occasionally cook with other grains
Occasionally cook with seaweed
Occasionally cook with fish or seafood (paella)
Occasionally cook in soup with vegetables and seaweeds
Cook as breakfast porridge
Other traditionally practiced and commonly used cooking
   varieties

Seasonings to Be Used When Cooking Whole Grains

Season with or without a pinch of sea salt
Season with or without a touch of tamari soy sauce (fermented
   soybean and grain soy sauce)
Season with or without miso (fermented soybean and grain
   paste)
Other traditionally practiced and commonly used seasonings

SOUP

The Standard Macrobiotic Diet recommends, under normal circumstances, a daily average consumption of two cups or bowls of soup.

Kinds of Soup

Light broth for noodles or pasta
Vegetable soup
Vegetable and seaweed (usually wakame or kombu seaweed) soup
Bean and vegetable soup
Grain and vegetable soup
Fish and vegetable soup
Fish, vegetable, and seaweed soup
Noodle vegetable soup
Mochi (pounded sweet brown rice) and vegetable soup
Bread and vegetable soup
Dumpling and vegetable soup
Stew with grains, vegetables, beans, seaweed, and/or fish and seafood
Other traditionally used and commonly consumed soups

Kinds of Vegetables Usually Used in Soup

Acorn squash	Escarole
Bok choy	Green beans
Broccoli	Hokkaido pumpkin
Brussels sprouts	Hubbard squash
Burdock	Jinenjo
Buttercup squash	Kale
Butternut squash	Lambsquarters
Cabbage	Leeks
Carrots	Lotus root
Carrot tops	Mushrooms
Celery	Mustard greens
Cauliflower	Onion
Chinese cabbage	Patty pan squash
Chives	Radish
Coltsfoot	Red Cabbage
Daikon	Rutabaga
Daikon greens	Scallions
Dandelion leaves	Shiitake mushrooms
Dandelion roots	Snap beans
Endive	Snow peas

Kinds of Vegetables Usually Used in Soup (cont.)

Sprouts
Summer squash
Turnips
Turnip greens
Watercress

Wax beans
Other traditionally used and
    commonly consumed
    vegetables

Kinds of Grains Usually Used in Soup

Brown rice
Corn
Millet
Barley
Oats
Buckwheat
Whole wheat noodles and
    pasta

Whole wheat dumplings
Buckwheat noodles and pasta
Couscous
Mochi (pounded sweet brown
    rice)
Other traditionally used and
    commonly consumed grains

Kinds of Beans Usually Used in Soup

Aduki beans
Black beans
Chick-peas (garbanzo beans)

Lentils
Split peas
Other beans

Kinds of Seaweeds Most Popularly Used in Soup

Nori seaweed
Wakame seaweed
Kombu seaweed

Dulse seaweed
Other seaweeds

Fish Occasionally Used in Soup

Carp
Cod
Dried Fish
Flounder
Haddock
Herring

Iriko (small dried fish)
Scrod
Snapper
Sole
Trout
Others

Seafood Occasionally Used in Soup

Cherrystone clams	Lobster
Clams	Octopus
Crab	Oysters

Seasonings for Soup

Miso (fermented soybean and grain paste)
Tamari soy sauce (fermented soybean and grain soy sauce)
Sea salt
Sesame or corn oil (occasionally)
Other traditionally used and commonly consumed condiments

Garnishes for Soup

Grated gingerroot (occasional use)	Parsley
	Scallions
Nori seaweed	Others

VEGETABLES

A variety of vegetable dishes prepared in a variety of cooking styles should comprise approximately 30 percent of the daily food intake.

Kinds of Vegetables

Acorn squash	Chinese cabbage
Bok choy	Chives
Broccoli	Coltsfoot
Burdock root	Cucumber
Buttercup squash	Daikon
Butternut squash	Daikon greens
Cabbage	Dandelion leaves
Celery	Dandelion roots
Carrots	Endive
Carrot tops	Escarole
Cauliflower	Green beans

Kinds of Vegetables (cont.)

Green peas
Hubbard squash
Hokkaido pumpkin
Iceberg lettuce
Jinenjo
Jerusalem artichoke
Kale
Leeks
Lotus root
Lambsquarters
Mushrooms
Mustard greens
Onion
Parsnip
Pumpkin
Patty pan squash
Radish

Red cabbage
Romaine lettuce
Scallions
Shiitake mushrooms
Snap beans
Summer squash
Turnip
Turnip greens
Watercress
Wax beans
Winter melon
Wild grasses which have been
   used widely for centuries
Other vegetables which have
   been traditionally used and
   commonly consumed

Cooking Styles for Vegetables

Raw salad
Pressed salad (salt and pressure added for a few hours to a few
   days)
Boiled salad (adding vegetables to boiling water and cooking
   for one to three minutes)
Boiling
Steaming
Baking
Broiling
Water sautéing
Oil sautéing (using a small volume of vegetable-quality oil)
Waterless cooking (cooking with a small volume of water until
   the water evaporates)
Deep frying (usually with a batter made of whole wheat
   unrefined flour)
Pickling
Other traditionally used and commonly practiced cooking
   styles

Seasonings for Vegetable Dishes

Miso (fermented soybean and grain paste)
Tamari soy sauce (fermented soybean and grain soy sauce)
Sea salt
Mirin (fermented sweetener made of sweet brown rice)
Brown rice vinegar
Umeboshi plum (pickled plum) vinegar
Oil (sesame, corn, mustard seed, safflower, or olive oil)

Cooking Varieties for Vegetables

A side dish
Cooked in soup
Cooked with grains
Cooked with beans
Cooked with seaweeds
An ingredient in sushi
Served with noodle or pasta dishes
Cooked and served with fish or seafood
An ingredient in dessert dishes

BEANS

The Standard Macrobiotic Diet recommends almost daily consumption of beans and bean products. Beans should comprise 5 percent to 10 percent of the daily food intake.

Kinds of Beans

Azuki beans	Navy beans
Black-eyed peas	Pinto beans
Black soybeans	Soybeans
Black turtle beans	Split peas
Chick-peas (garbanzo beans)	Whole dried peas
Great northern beans	Bean sprouts
Kidney beans	Other beans that have been
Lentils	traditionally used and
Mung beans	commonly consumed

Kinds of Bean Products

Dried tofu (soybean curd that has been dried)
Fresh tofu (soybean curd)
Okara (residue in making tofu)
Natto (fermented soybeans)
Tempeh (fermented soybeans)

Cooking Styles for Beans

Pressure cooking
Boiling
Roasting
Baking
Fermenting
Steaming
Other traditionally used and commonly practiced cooking
   styles

Cooking Varieties for Beans

Cook with a pinch of sea salt or miso
Cook with seaweed, usually kombu seaweed
Cook with carrots or onions
Cook with acorn or buttercup squash
Cook with chestnuts
Cook with vegetables
Cook as dessert
Other traditionally used and commonly practiced cooking styles

Seasonings Generally Used for Beans

Sea salt
Miso (fermented soybean and grain paste)
Tamari soy sauce (fermented soybean and grain soy sauce)
Mirin (fermented sweetener made from sweet brown rice)
Barley malt

Rice malt
Oil (vegetable quality)

Garnishes Generally Used with Beans
(will depend on the particular dish)

Grated gingerroot
Grated fresh daikon
Grated fresh radish
Grated fresh horseradish
Chopped fresh scallions
Chopped fresh onions
Other traditionally used and commonly consumed garnishes

SEAWEEDS

The macrobiotic diet recommends a small percentage of seaweeds
to be consumed daily or frequently as a seaweed dish or in various
food preparations.

Kinds of Seaweeds

Agar-agar
Arame
Dulse
Hiziki
Irish moss
Kombu
Mekabu

Nekabu
Nori
Wakame
Other seaweeds that have
    been traditionally used and
    commonly consumed

Cooking Styles for Seaweeds

Boiling
Steaming
Deep frying
Roasting
Toasting

Pickling
In waterless cooking
Drying
Soaked and raw

Cooking Varieties for Seaweeds

Cook seaweeds alone	Cook in sauces
Cook with beans	Cook with fish or seafood
Cook with grains	Cook in soup
Cook in vegetable dishes	Other
Cook as gelatin	

FISH AND SEAFOOD

For those in generally good health, the Standard Macrobiotic Diet allows fish and seafood as an occasional supplement to the previously discussed food categories—grains, soups, vegetables, beans, seaweeds, and beverages. The amount of fish or seafood varies according to personal needs and can range from once in a while to several times a week. The average, however, is twice a week. The kinds of fish and seafood recommended are those with less saturated fat and those that are most easily digested. Individuals with existing heart or circulatory ailments may need to avoid fish and seafood, depending on the circumstances, until the condition improves.

Kinds of Fish and Seafood

Carp	Scrod
Cod	Smelt
Dried fish	Snapper
Flounder	Sole
Haddock	Trout
Herring	Other white-meat fish
Iriko (small dried fish)	

Occasional-Use Seafood

Cherrystone clams	Lobsters
Clams	Scallops
Crab	Shrimp
Octopus	Other
Oysters	

Infrequent-Use Fish

Bluefish	Tuna
Salmon	Other blue-skinned and
Sardines	red-meat fish
Swordfish	

Garnishes Used to Balance Fish and Seafood Dishes

Chopped scallions	Raw fresh salad
Grated daikon	Lemon
Grated radish	Orange
Grated gingerroot	Fresh beefsteak plant leaves
Green mustard paste	Other traditionally used and
Grated horseradish	commonly consumed
Shredded daikon	garnishes

Seasonings for Fish and Seafood

Sea salt
Tamari soy sauce (fermented soybean and grain soy sauce)
Miso (fermented soybean and grain paste)
Black pepper corns
Red pepper
Rice vinegar
Sesame oil, corn oil, safflower oil, mustard seed oil, olive oil
Mirin (fermented sweet rice sweetener)
Umeboshi vinegar
Tofu sauce seasoned with some of the above ingredients
Kuzu sauce seasoned with some of the above ingredients
Oil sauce seasoned with some of the above ingredients
Other traditionally used and commonly consumed seasonings

FRUIT

The Standard Macrobiotic Diet includes the occasional consumption of fruit depending upon climate, season, personal needs, and circumstances. All traditionally used and commonly consumed fruits growing in a temperate climate are included. The regular use of tropical fruits in a temperate climate is discouraged.

Kinds of Fruit

Apples	Pears
Apricots	Persimmon
Blackberries	Plums
Blueberries	Raisins
Cantaloupe	Raspberries
Grapes	Strawberries
Honeydew melon	Tangerines
Lemons	Watermelon
Mulberries	Wild berries
Nectarines	Other fruit traditionally
Oranges	grown in a
Peaches	temperate climate

Variety of Serving Styles for Fruit

Fresh and raw
Fresh, raw, and soaked in lightly salted water
Grated
Boiled
Baked
Steamed
Juice as a beverage or flavoring
Preserves
Spread on bread or other baked flour products
As an ingredient in stuffing
As a dessert
As an ingredient and flavoring in kuzu or agar-agar gelatin
Baked in bread
Dried fruit as a snack, garnish, or dessert
Pickled fruit
Deep fried fruit (in a batter)
Served as a garnish
Fermented beverages
Other traditionally used and commonly consumed serving
  styles

PICKLES

The Standard Macrobiotic Diet recommends frequent use of pickles as a supplement to various main dishes and for the purpose of stimulating appetite and encouraging digestion. Some pickles are available in a natural food store, while many of them can be prepared at home. Some pickles are ready in a few hours, others require more pickling time—from a few days to a few seasons.

Kinds of Foods Often Used in Making Pickles

Burdock root	Red cabbage
Broccoli	Scallions
Cabbage	Squash
Carrots	Turnips
Cauliflower	Apricots
Chinese cabbage	Plums
Cucumbers	Anchovies
Daikon	Caviar
Leeks	Herring
Lotus roots	Salmon
Mustard greens	Sardines
Olives	Other traditionally used and
Onions	commonly selected foods
Pumpkin	for making pickles
Radishes, red and white	

Types of Pickling

Salt pickles
Salt and water pickles
Bran pickles
Brine pickles
Miso pickles (fermented soybean and grain paste)
Pressed pickles
Sauerkraut
Tamari soy sauce pickles (fermented soybean and grain soy sauce)

Types of Pickling (cont.)

Takuan pickles
Umeboshi pickles
Other traditionally used and commonly practiced pickling
methods

NUTS

The Standard Macrobiotic Diet includes occasional consumption
of various kinds of nuts in the form of snacks, garnishes, or as an
ingredient in desserts.

Kinds of Nuts

Almonds	Pinenuts
Chestnuts	Small Spanish nuts
Filberts	Walnuts
Peanuts	

Less-Frequent-Use Nuts (in a temperate climate)

Brazil nuts
Cashews
Hazel nuts
Macadamia nuts
Other traditionally used and commonly consumed nuts

Variety of Serving Styles for Nuts

Roasted with sea salt
Roasted without salt
Roasted and sweetened with barley malt
Roasted and sweetened with rice malt
Roasted and seasoned with tamari soy sauce (fermented
  soybean and grain soy sauce)
Ground into nut butter

Shaved and served as a topping, garnish, or ingredient in other
dishes
Cooked in grain flour products such as cookies, cakes, muffins,
pastries, pies, and other desserts and breads
Served with dried fruits as a snack
Other traditionally used and commonly practiced serving
methods

SEEDS

The Standard Macrobiotic Diet includes the occasional consumption of various seeds in various methods of preparation.

Kinds of Seeds

Black sesame seeds	Apricot seeds
White sesame seeds	Plum seeds
Pumpkin seeds	Umeboshi plum seeds
Squash seeds	Alfalfa seeds
Sunflower seeds	Other traditionally used and
Poppy seeds	commonly consumed seeds

Variety of Serving Styles for Seeds

AS CONDIMENTS
Dried and ground
Roasted and ground
Roasted and ground with sea salt
With umeboshi powder and sea salt
With miso (fermented soybean and grain paste)

AS GARNISHES
Sprinkled on various dishes such as grains, soups, vegetable dishes,
beans, fish and seafood, fruit, and desserts

AS SNACKS
Dried and served alone
Roasted and served alone

Variety of Serving Styles for Seeds (cont.)

Baked with flour products such as cookies, crackers, breads,
cakes, and other baked flour products
As an ingredient in candies
Other traditionally used and commonly consumed snacks

Seasonings Commonly Used with Seeds

Sea salt
Tamari soy sauce (fermented soybean and grain soy sauce)
Miso (fermented soybean and grain paste)
Barley malt
Rice malt
Other traditionally used and commonly consumed seasonings

SNACKS

The Standard Macrobiotic Diet includes daily or occasional use of
snacks of various kinds to be consumed in reasonable and moderate amount.

Kinds of Snacks

GRAIN-BASED SNACKS
Cookies, crackers, wafers, pancakes, muffins, bread
Puffed brown rice, barley, oats, millet, corn
Popcorn
Mochi (pounded sweet brown rice)
Noodles and pasta
Rice balls
Rice cakes
Homemade sushi
Roasted grains
Other traditionally used and commonly consumed natural
snacks

BEAN-BASED SNACKS
Roasted beans
Boiled beans

NUT-BASED SNACKS
Nuts roasted and seasoned with sea salt
Nuts roasted and seasoned with tamari soy sauce (fermented
soybean and grain soy sauce)
Nuts roasted and seasoned with barley malt
Nuts roasted and seasoned with rice malt
Nuts used in cookies, crackers, and as an ingredient in other
baked flour products

SEED-BASED SNACKS
Seeds roasted and seasoned with sea salt
Seeds roasted and seasoned with tamari soy sauce (fermented
soybean and grain soy sauce)
Seeds roasted and seasoned with barley malt
Seeds roasted and seasoned with rice malt
Seeds used in cookies, crackers, and as an ingredient in other
baked flour products

SEAWEED-BASED SNACKS
Seaweed crackers
Baked seaweed
Fried seaweed
Seaweed also as an ingredient in crackers, cookies, and other
grain flour products

FRUIT-BASED SNACKS
Fresh fruits
Cooked fruits
Dried fruits
Fruit used as an ingredient in cookies, muffins, and other grain
flour products
Other traditionally used and commonly consumed fruit snacks

CONDIMENTS

The Standard Macrobiotic Diet uses a wide variety of condiments
for daily, regular, or occasional use. They are sprinkled on or

added in small amounts to food as an adjustment to taste, seasoning, and flavoring as well as an addition to the nutritional value of the food and a stimulant to appetite. Condiments are commonly used for grains, soups, vegetable dishes, bean dishes, and sometimes with desserts.

Kinds of Condiments

Gomashio (roasted sesame seeds and sea salt)
Seaweed powder
Seaweed powder with roasted sesame seeds
Tekka (condiment made from soybean miso, sesame oil,
   burdock, lotus root, carrots, and gingerroot)
Umeboshi plum (pickled plum)
Umeboshi plum and raw scallions or onions
Shio kombu (kombu cooked with tamari soy sauce and water)
Chopped shiso leaves (pickled beefsteak plant leaves)
Roasted shiso leaves (pickled beefsteak plant leaves)
Green nori
Yellow mustard (used mainly for fish and seafood)
Green mustard (used mainly for fish and seafood)
Cooked miso with scallions or onions
Cooked nori condiment
Roasted sesame seeds
Other traditionally used and commonly consumed condiments

SEASONINGS

The Standard Macrobiotic Diet uses both regularly and occasionally a variety of seasonings in cooking and before serving. The seasonings are all vegetable-quality and naturally processed. These seasonings have been used traditionally throughout the world. The use of seasonings should be moderate and adequate for personal needs. The following seasonings are commonly used within the Standard Macrobiotic Diet.

Kinds of Seasonings

Unrefined sea salt
Soy sauce
Tamari soy sauce (fermented soybean and grain soy sauce)
Miso (fermented soybean and grain paste)
  Rice miso
  Barley miso
  Soybean miso
  Sesame miso
  Other traditionally used and commonly consumed miso
  Note: Dark miso has been fermented for a longer period of
    time. Light miso has been fermented for a shorter
    period of time.
Rice vinegar
Brown rice vinegar
Umeboshi vinegar
Sauerkraut brine
Mirin (fermented sweet brown rice sweetener)
Amasake (fermented sweet brown rice beverage)
Barley malt
Rice malt
Grated gingerroot
Grated daikon
Grated radish
Horseradish
Umeboshi paste
Umeboshi plum
Lemon juice
Tangerine juice
Orange juice
Freshly ground black pepper
Red pepper
Green mustard paste
Yellow mustard paste
Sesame oil
Corn oil
Safflower oil
Mustard seed oil

Kinds of Seasonings (cont.)

Olive oil
Sake (fermented rice wine)
Sake lees (residue in making sake)
Other natural seasonings that have been traditionally used and
commonly consumed

GARNISHES

The Standard Macrobiotic Diet emphasizes balance of qualities,
tastes, nutritional factors, and energetic harmony. For that purpose, garnishes are frequently used in small volume to balance
some dishes, especially for the purpose of creating easier digestion.

Kinds of Garnishes

Grated daikon
  Used mainly as a garnish for the following:
    Fish and seafood
    Mochi (pounded sweet brown rice)
    Buckwheat noodles and pasta
    Natto
    Tempeh
Grated radish
  Used mainly as a garnish for the following:
    Same as above
Grated horseradish
  Used mainly as a garnish for the following:
    Same as above
Chopped scallions
  Used mainly as a garnish for the following:
    Noodle and pasta dishes
    Fish and seafood
    Natto
    Tempeh
Grated ginger, green mustard paste, freshly ground pepper,
    lemon pieces

Used mainly as a garnish for the following:
Noodle and pasta dishes
Soup
Fish and seafood
Red pepper, freshly ground pepper, green mustard paste
Used mainly as a garnish for the following:
Soup
Noodle and pasta dishes
Fish and seafood
Natto (fermented soybeans)
Tempeh (fermented soybeans)

DESSERTS

The Standard Macrobiotic Diet includes frequent use of a variety
of desserts usually served at the end of a major meal.

Kinds of Desserts

Azuki beans sweetened with barley malt or rice malt
Azuki beans cooked with chestnuts
Azuki beans cooked with squash
Kuzu sweetened with barley malt, rice malt, fresh fruit, or
    dried fruit
Agar-agar cooked with barley malt, rice malt, fresh fruit, or
    dried fruit
Cooked fruit
Dried fruit
Fruit pies, including apple, peach, strawberry, berry, and other
    temperate climate fruits
Fruit crunch, including apple, peach, strawberry, berry, and
    other temperate climate fruits
Grain desserts sweetened with dried fruits, barley malt, rice
    malt, amasake (fermented sweet rice beverage), or fresh
    fruit, such as couscous cake, Indian pudding, rice pudding,
    and other similar naturally sweetened desserts
Baked flour desserts such as cookies, cakes, pies, muffins,
    breads, and others prepared with natural sweetners,
    including fruits and grain sweeteners

BEVERAGES

The Standard Macrobiotic Diet recommends various beverages for daily, regular, or occasional consumption. The amount of beverage intake varies according to the individual's needs and the climate change. Beverage consumption should comfortably satisfy the person's desire for liquid in terms of kind, volume, and frequency of intake.

Kinds of Beverages

Bancha twig tea
Bancha stem tea
Roasted rice with bancha twig tea
Roasted barley with bancha twig tea
Kombu tea
Spring water
Well water
100 percent cereal grain coffee
Amasake
Dandelion tea
Lotus root tea
Burdock root tea
Mu tea
Other traditionally used and commonly consumed
    nonstimulating, nonaromatic natural herb teas (made from
    seeds, leaves, stems, bark, or roots)

Infrequent-Use Beverages

Fruit juice
    Apple juice
    Grape juice
    Apricot juice
    Other temperate-climate fruit juices
Cider
Soybean milk
Vegetable juice
    Carrot juice

Celery juice
Juice from leafy green vegetables
Beet juice
Barley green juice
Other juices made from fruits and vegetables that have been
traditionally grown in a temperate climate
Alcoholic beverages
Sake (fermented rice wine)—more naturally fermented
quality
Beer of various kinds—more naturally fermented quality
Wines of various kinds—more naturally fermented quality
Other grain- and fruit-based weak alcoholic beverages that
have been fermented naturally

REMARKS

In some instances and under certain conditions, the Diet can be
further modified to include temporarily some other foods such as
salmon, tuna, other red meat, blue skinned and fatty fish, organic
fertilized fowl eggs, caviar and other fish eggs, white meat poultry, skim cow's or goat's milk, traditionally naturally fermented
cheese and yogurt, unrefined honey, maple syrup, and beet
sugar. These modifications are to be made according to individual requirements and necessity, though within the Standard
Macrobiotic Diet, these foods would not be regularly and commonly required in daily practice to maintain health and well-
being.

WAYS OF EATING

To establish well-being, Standard Macrobiotic Dietary practice
recommends following the manner of eating and practice outlined
below:

1. Eat regularly. Two to three meals a day can be consumed.
In the case of vigorous physical labor, the frequency of meals can
be increased to four times per day.

2. Every meal is to include grain or grain products. Grain and

grain products should represent, more or less, 50 percent of the daily intake of food.

3. Variety in food selection and preparation, proper combinations of foods, and the correct way of cooking are essential.

4. Cooking is to be done with a peaceful mind, with love, and with care.

5. Snacks are to be taken only in moderate amounts. They should not replace a regular meal.

6. Beverages can be consumed comfortably as one desires.

7. Refrain from eating before bedtime, preferably three hours, except in unusual circumstances.

8. Chew very well. Chew each mouthful until it is liquid.

9. The volume of food varies depending upon the individual's needs.

10. Eat with the spirit of gratitude and appreciation for people, society, nature, and the universe.

7

Nutritional Studies
and the Heart

Over the years concern has been expressed in the United States
and Canada about the nutritional adequacy of vegetarian and
semivegetarian diets, including the macrobiotic diet, which includes foods such as sea vegetables and miso soup and some condiments such as sesame salt that may be unfamiliar to contemporary
Westerners. In recent years, as more North Americans and Euro-
peans have begun eating whole wheat bread, brown rice, stir-fry
vegetables, tofu, fresh garden salads, and other natural foods, initial apprehension has subsided, and nutritional research has shown
that a balanced grain and vegetable diet provides all the essential
nutrients, including protein, calcium, iron, and vitamins B_6, B_{12},
and C. Several studies on the nutritional aspects of the macrobiotic
diet have appeared in the *Journal of the American Dietetic Association.* [1] *Atherosclerosis,* a professional heart research journal,
recently published the results of a major European study showing
that the Standard Macrobiotic Diet not only had no nutritional
deficiencies but also that on the basis of cholesterol and other
blood value tests, those who consumed it appeared to have healthier hearts and circulatory systems than both those eating the regular modern diet and vegetarians who ate eggs and dairy foods.[2]
We shall look more closely at the macrobiotic heart studies in
Chapter 9.

During the last twenty years, the dietary guidelines of national
and international public health organizations have rapidly moved
closer to the macrobiotic recommendations. For example, in 1980

the American Heart Association published a large *Heartbook* that advised:

> Habitual excesses in eating habits—especially of fats, salt, and possibly sugar—are high on the list of controllable factors that have been linked to cardiovascular disease. . . . it is recommended that the proportion of fat to the total caloric intake be kept to somewhere between 30 and 35 percent, and that vegetable (polyunsaturated) fat be substituted for that from animal sources as an important means of lessening the risk of atherosclerosis and coronary disease. . . . Most people in the United States consume more protein than they need. To lessen the risk of cardiovascular disease, the balance should be shifted in favor of more complex carbohydrates, such as are found in fresh fruits and vegetables. On the other hand, overindulgence in the chemically simpler sugars, in the form of desserts, soft drinks, and snack foods, is to be avoided. . . .[3]

In this book, the American Heart Association recommends brown rice and tofu along with a wide variety of other whole grains, beans, vegetables, and vegetable oils.

Table 11 compares the nutritional content of the Standard American Diet, the diet recommended in *Dietary Goals for the United States* (similar to the guidelines of the American Heart Association, the National Academy of Sciences, and other scientific and medical organizations), the Standard Macrobiotic Diet, and the diet of the Tarahumara Indians of Mexico (which as we have seen are the largest remaining traditional society in North America completely free of heart disease and the other ills of modern life). As we can see from this table, the major difference between the macrobiotic and Tarahumara approaches on the one hand and the modern diet on the other is in the amount of fat, especially saturated fat from animal sources, and the amount of carbohydrate ingested, especially from complex carbohydrate sources such as whole grains, vegetables, and fruit and that from simple sugars such as refined cane sugar, corn syrup, and fructose.

The Standard American Diet currently consists of about 42 percent fat and oil, including 16 percent saturated fat. Table 12 lists the sources of total fat consumption, and it is interesting to observe that the largest category includes cooking oil, salad dressings, and other lighter forms of oil and fat. Consumer guidelines, such as those of *Dietary Goals for the United States* and the American Heart Association, calling for cutbacks in fat consumption to 25 to 35 percent of total food intake represent only a "prudent" first step toward a more balanced diet. Most medical associations now agree that further reductions in fat and sugar intake (which is converted to fat in the body) and corresponding increases in complex carbohydrate consumption are justified. For example, in *Diet, Nutrition, and Cancer*, the National Academy of Sciences linked a majority of cancers with excessive fat consumption and in its interim dietary guidelines called for a reduction in fat consumption to a maximum of 30 percent of total calories in the diet. Explaining this figure, the Report noted, "The scientific data do not provide a strong basis for establishing fat intake at precisely 30 percent of total calories. Indeed, the data could be used to justify an even greater reduction. However, in the judgment of the committee, the suggested reduction (i.e., one-quarter of the [current] fat intake) is a moderate and practical target, and is likely to be beneficial."[4]

In this chapter we shall look briefly at the different categories of foods in the Standard Macrobiotic Diet, with special reference to their value in preventing heart and circulatory diseases.

WHOLE GRAINS

Whole cereal grains contain a balance of protein, carbohydrate, fat, and vitamins and minerals ideally suited for human consumption.[5] Their high-fiber content has been increasingly recognized as beneficial to digestion and as a protection against colonic troubles, some forms of cancer, and other chronic diseases. Whole grains are also high in protein, niacin and other B vitamins, vitamin E, and vitamin A. A multitude of studies have indicated that whole grains strengthen the heart and circulatory system. Reviewing the medical evidence, epidemiologist Jeremiah Stamler, M.D., one of the world's leading authorities on heart disease, concluded, "People subsisting on cereal-root diets have low levels of serum cholesterol and little atherosclerotic coronary disease (clinical or morphological). This correlation has been consistently observed in every economically less-developed country to date."[6] In a 1979 editorial, "Sensible Eating," the *British Medical Journal* stated, "Few nutri-

Table 11. A NUTRITIONAL COMPARISON BETWEEN THE CURRENT AMERICAN DIET, THE U.S. DIETARY GOALS, THE STANDARD MACROBIOTIC DIET, AND THE TARAHUMARA DIET

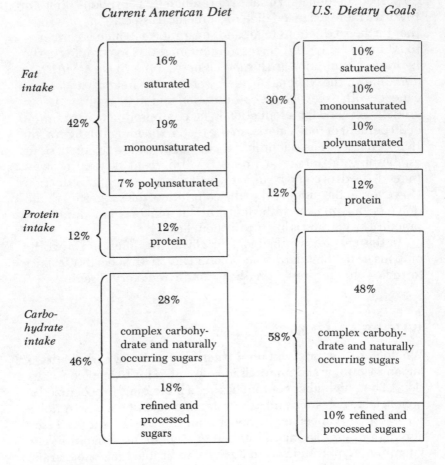

tionists now dispute that Western man [and woman] eats too much meat, too much animal fat and dairy products, too much refined carbohydrate, and too little dietary fibre. Epidemiology studies of heart disease suggest that some at least of the deaths in the middle ages from myocardial infarction could be cut by a move towards a more prudent diet—which means more cereals and vegetables and less meat and fat."[7]

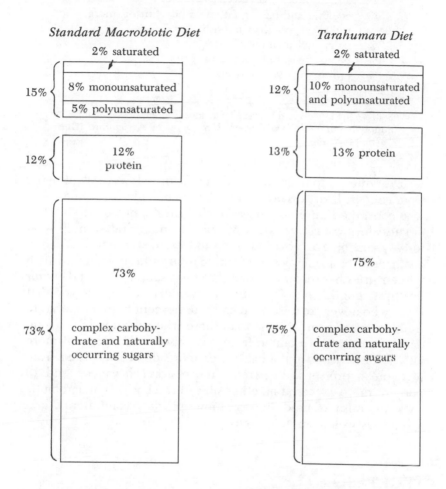

Standard Macrobiotic Diet

2% saturated

15% { 8% monounsaturated
5% polyunsaturated

12% { 12% protein

73% { 73%
complex carbohy-
drate and naturally
occurring sugars

Tarahumara Diet

2% saturated

12% { 10% monounsaturated
and polyunsaturated

13% { 13% protein

75% { 75%
complex carbohy-
drate and naturally
occurring sugars

MISO SOUP

Miso is made from fermented soybeans, grains, and sea salt and contains living enzymes that aid digestion, strengthen the blood, and provide a nutritious balance of complex carbohydrate, essential oils, protein, vitamins, and minerals. In 1982, the National Cancer Center Research Institute in Japan reported that people

Table 12. SOURCES OF FAT CONSUMPTION IN THE AMERICAN DIET

43%	cooking and baking fat, salad oils, butter, margarine
34%	red meat, poultry, and fish
12%	dairy, not including butter
4%	beans, peas, nuts, soy flour, grits
4%	grains, vegetables, fruits
3%	eggs

Source: R. Marstow and L. Page, "Nutrient Content of National Food Supply," *National Food Review*, U.S. Dept. of Agriculture (Dec. 1978), pp. 28–33.

who ate miso soup every day had significantly lower risk of dying from cancer, heart disease, and other major illnesses than those who consumed miso only occasionally, rarely, or not at all.[8] The large-scale prospective study of 265,000 men and women over forty years of age covered a period from 1966 to 1978 and confirmed the principles of traditional Oriental medicine, which for centuries has recommended that miso soup be taken daily for health, strength, and longevity. The modern survey showed that those who never ate miso soup had a 43 percent higher death rate from coronary heart disease than those who consumed miso soup daily. Those who abstained from miso also had 29 percent more fatal strokes, three-and-a-half times more deaths resulting from high blood pressure, 33 percent more stomach cancer, and 19 percent more cancer at all other sites in the body. In macrobiotic cooking, miso is used in seasoning, pickles, condiments, and spreads as well as in daily soup.

VEGETABLES

Fresh vegetables are high in complex carbohydrate, fiber, vitamins, and minerals. The National Academy of Science's cancer and diet report especially recommended consumption of yellow and orange vegetables such as carrots, and green leafy vegetables such as cabbage, broccoli, cauliflower, and brussels sprouts.[9] In macrobiotic cooking, these vegetables as well as a wide variety of other root, round, and leafy green vegetables are prepared daily. Since citrus fruits are generally limited except in semitropical and tropical locations where they grow naturally, macrobiotic persons receive vitamin C in lightly cooked greens that provide an ample source of this nutrient.

One of the few studies that correlated overall vegetable protein, vegetable fat, and vegetable fiber to cardiovascular health involved the Tarahumara society of Mexico. The Tarahumara eat primarily whole corn, beans, squash, other local vegetables and fruit, and almost no animal foods except occasionally for eggs. In 1978 a medical study of this traditional culture, published in the *American Journal of Clinical Nutrition,* reported that the Tarahumaras displayed no evidence of high blood pressure, obesity, coronary heart disease, stroke, or other circulatory disorders. Their high intake of vegetable protein, unsaturated fat, and fiber were associated with substantially lower concentrations of cholesterol in their blood. "The customary diet of the Tarahumara is adequate in all nutrients, is hypolipidemic [low in fat and oils], and is presumably antiatherogenic [protective against hardening of the arteries]," the investigators concluded.[10]

One vegetable-quality food that has been specifically studied and found to protect against both heart disease and cancer is shiitake mushroom, the large edible mushroom native to the Far East and now grown in the United States, Canada, and Europe. In laboratory experiments, researchers discovered that shiitake mushrooms lower cholesterol levels in the blood and markedly inhibit the growth of sarcoma, a soft-tissue tumor, resulting "in almost complete regression of tumors . . . with no sign of toxicity."[11] In Japan, shiitake mushrooms are traditionally cooked with kombu sea vegetable and tamari soy sauce to prepare a soup stock called dashi. In addition to broth, shiitake mushrooms are occasionally added to stews, casseroles, or salads in macrobiotic cooking and consumed medicinally as a small side dish to help eliminate from the body excess fat and protein that have accumulated over the years from overconsumption of animal food.

BEANS

Beans are high in fat, calcium, and phosphorus and contain about twice as much protein as a comparable volume of meat, poultry, or dairy food. Combined with whole grains, they provide all the needed amino acids. Among beans, soybeans are highest in protein and have been the bean most studied by medical researchers. Heart studies in the 1940s first noted that animals fed a diet high in soy protein remained free of atherosclerotic lesions while those on a diet high in dairy protein contracted hardening of the arteries.[12] More recent studies on humans have shown similar benefits. In 1980, Swiss researchers reported that a soy protein diet significantly reduced the risk of heart disease in patients with dangerously high cholesterol levels.[13] In 1982, scientists at the University of Western Ontario gave human volunteers both cow's milk and soy milk and found that "both cholesterol and triglyceride [fatty acid] values dropped substantially during the soy period."[14] In macrobiotic cooking, a wide variety of beans and bean products is consumed daily, including soybeans in whole form or naturally processed into miso, tofu, tempeh, natto, or tamari soy sauce.

SEA VEGETABLES

Edible seaweeds, or sea vegetables, are high in carbohydrate, protein, vitamins, and especially minerals (up to 30 percent by volume). Compared with dairy foods, sea vegetables provide up to ten times more calcium and iron by weight and contain other important trace minerals. For thousands of years, Far Eastern civilizations have recognized the importance of sea vegetables in the diet, and they have traditionally been eaten to strengthen the blood, heart, and circulatory system. Recent scientific studies have begun to confirm this practice and find sea vegetables to have antibacterial, antifungal, antiviral, and anticancer effects.[15]

In laboratory experiments in Japan, kombu, wakame, nori, hiziki, and other common sea vegetables reduced cholesterol levels in the blood, inhibited the development of high blood pressure and arteriosclerosis, and improved fat metabolism.[16] Several varieties of sea vegetables also have been discovered to have blood anticoagulants similar to heparin, the body's natural blood thinner, which is often given intravenously to heart patients to prevent clotting.[17]

In Japan, the highest incidence of longevity is found in the village of Oki Island whose inhabitants eat large amounts of sea vegetables on which their local economy partly depends.[18] Compared with other regions of Japan, these villagers also have unusually low rates of stroke. In Okinawa, sea vegetables are also eaten in plenty, and in this southwestern group of islands women live longer than in any other prefecture of Japan.[19]

Sea vegetables also offer protection against nuclear radioactivity. At McGill University in Canada, medical researchers reported in the 1960s and 1970s that sea vegetables contained a substance that helped eliminate radioactive strontium from the body. The substance, sodium alginate, was prepared from kombu, kelp, and other brown sea vegetables off the Atlantic and Pacific coasts. "The evaluation of biological activity of different marine algae is important because of their practical significance in preventing absorption of radioactive products of atomic fission as well as in their use as possible natural decontaminators," the researchers concluded in an article in the *Canadian Medical Association Journal.*[20]

For external use, the algae Eisenia and Eckloniane are added by some Japanese to hot bath water to help relieve hypertension.[21] In macrobiotic home care remedies, sea vegetables are used externally in hip baths to help loosen accumulations of fat and mucus in the lower abdominal and reproductive regions.

SEA SALT

In cultures free of heart disease, cancer, and other chronic disorders, salt is usually evaporated from seawater or obtained by burning sea vegetables or swamp plants and retaining the crystallized sediment in the ashes.[22] Natural sea salt contains six major salts of sodium, magnesium, and calcium, compounds of eight elements, and minute traces of sixty other elements found in the ocean. The commercial table salt consumed in modern society is either mined land salt or refined sea salt from which most of the minerals other than sodium chloride have been eliminated.[23] Both types are commonly iodized with potassium iodide and stabilized with dextrose, a form of refined sugar. Anticaking substances are also often added.

Modern medicine is unclear about the role of salt in raising blood pressure and contributing to heart and circulatory diseases. Some clinical tests have shown that a low-sodium diet reduces blood pressure, while other studies have shown no important association. The American Heart Association and other medical bodies recommend prudently reducing salt intake until further data are available, and heart researchers point out that in traditional societies at low risk for heart disease, salt intake tends to be about half that of modern society. For example, the Tarahumaras ingest about 4 to 5 grams of salt a day versus 10 to 20 grams in the United States. Sodium, the most contractive element in salt, is naturally found in abundance in the organs and tissues of animals, and sodium from this food source is possibly more directly associated with high blood pressure than salt added in cooking or at the table. Many fast foods contain excess salt as well.

While natural sea salt has not yet been especially singled out in nutritional studies as part of a balanced whole foods diet, it does not appear to raise blood pressure or otherwise adversely affect the heart and circulatory system. In macrobiotic cooking, unrefined natural sea salt is used in moderation in seasoning, as is miso, tamari soy sauce, and umeboshi plums, all of which contain unrefined sea salt.

UNREFINED VEGETABLE OIL

Polyunsaturated vegetable oils (see Table 13) provide essential fatty acids that strengthen cells and capillary membranes, lower

Table 13. TYPES OF OILS AND FATS

Saturated	Monounsaturated	Polyunsaturated
Beef	Olive oil	Whole grains
Pork	Peanut oil	Beans
Lamb		Corn oil
Chicken		Sesame oil
Lard		Soybean oil
Butter		Sunflower oil
Milk		Mustard seed oil
Dairy food		Safflower oil
Coconut oil		Many white-meat fish
Palm oil		and some seafood

blood cholesterol, control clotting, and lubricate the hair and skin. They are also major sources of vitamins A and E and aid in the metabolism of the B vitamins. Nutritionally, the body has no need for saturated or monounsaturated oils, which are heavier, greasier tasting, and less digestible than polyunsaturated oils.

All the major cardiac associations now recommend substantial reductions in consumption of saturated fats and increased consumption of polyunsaturated fats and oils, but they still fail to distinguish between unrefined vegetable oils and refined vegetable oils. Unrefined oils (often labeled "cold-pressed" to indicate processing at low temperatures) are extracted from raw seeds by nonchemical methods that retain the plants' rich color, flavorful aroma, cloudy consistency, and original nutrients. Refined vegetable oils are chemically extracted, bleached, and deodorized, losing most of their vitamin E, lecithin, and other nutrients in the process. Some refined oils are also hydrogenated to keep them solid at room temperature. This process saturates the fatty acids and is used in manufacturing margarines, nut butters, chips, and other fried foods. Macrobiotic cooking makes use of unrefined vegetable oils, such as dark sesame oil, corn oil, mustard seed oil, and occasionally other polyunsaturated or monounsaturated oil in a moderate amount. Saturated oils such as palm and coconut oil, refined vegetable oils, and hydrogenated products such as soy margarine are minimized or avoided.

FISH AND SEAFOOD

The Inuit (Eskimos) and other societies that traditionally consumed high volumes of fish and seafood showed no signs of cardiovascular disease until contact with modern society introduced into their diet sugar, white flour, and other processed foods. Recently, scientists have identified EPA (eicosapentaenoic acid), a marine fatty acid found in fish, some marine oils, and possibly sea vegetables as protective against thrombosis, a blood clotting in the blood vessels of the leg or other extremity that can lead to fatal complications. In 1981, the *Journal of the American Medical Association* reported that a ten-day diet in which salmon was ingested in substantial volume lowered serum cholesterol up to 17 percent in relatively healthy subjects and 20 percent or more in patients with high levels of fat in their blood.[24] The British medical journal, *The Lancet*, reported that in a Japanese clinical trial, when fish was substituted for meat in the diet, bleeding time in heart patients increased 42 percent and platelet aggregability decreased significantly. "We suggest that a seafood diet reduces blood viscosity, that the effect of the diet may be attributable mainly to EPA, and that ingestion of EPA-rich seafood may be of use for the prevention and treatment of thrombotic disorders."[25]

For those in good health who desire animal food, the macrobiotic dietary approach recommends white-meat fish or low-fat seafood a few times a week on average. Depending on the case, some individuals suffering from circulatory disorders may also eat fish and seafood.

FRUIT

Fruit contains moderate amounts of fiber, carbohydrate, and vitamins, especially vitamin C. The Standard Macrobiotic Diet includes seasonal fruit (fresh or dried and preferably cooked) several times a week. In general, the volume of fruit consumed in modern society is excessive, and the forms in which it is taken are often imbalanced. This imbalance includes most tropical and semitropical fruits that are not part of our native ecosystem, canned and frozen fruits that retain little of their original natural energy and nutritional content, and fruit juice, which is an extremely concentrated product. Although there have been few medical studies on the effects of fruit, excessive consumption of fruit and fruit juice contributes to a wide variety of sicknesses ranging from colds and flu to arthritis, rheumatism, diabetes, and heart disease. Fructose, the simple sugar in fruits, taken in excess, has adverse physiological effects and generally weakens the blood and vital organs. The National Academy of Sciences' cancer and diet report noted that one epidemiological study found an association between high fruit consumption and cancer in female reproductive organs.[26] Further studies in this area are needed. In moderation, fresh fruit that grows in the local environment and that is eaten in the season in which it is grown is an enjoyable part of a healthy diet and should not be the cause for any concern.

SEEDS AND NUTS

Seeds are high in vitamins E, B, and A; protein; fat; carbohydrate; and fiber. Nuts include proportionately higher amounts of protein and fat. The fat in nuts is generally neutral in saturated quality, except for walnuts, which contain a polyunsaturated oil. Cancer studies have recently identified an ingredient in seeds called a *protease inhibitor* that protects against tumor development.[27] This factor is also found in some beans, especially soybeans. In macrobiotic cooking, lightly roasted seeds and nuts are occasionally used as snacks, garnishes, or in cooking.

NATURAL SWEETENERS

In traditional societies free of heart disease and cancer, white sugar (sucrose), and other refined sweeteners are virtually unknown. The epidemic of sugar consumption in modern society has been increasingly recognized by the medical profession as a cause or contributing factor to dental cavities, hypoglycemia, hyperactivity, diabetes, several forms of cancer, mental illness, and aggressive antisocial behavior.[28] Sugar currently accounts for about 50 percent of carbohydrate intake in the Standard American Diet.

Studies in the 1950s first associated sugar with heart disease. "There is a better relationship with intake of sugar than with any other nutrient we have examined in the relationship between diet and the incidence of death from coronary disease," John Yudkin, M.D., a British nutritionist, reported in *The Lancet*.[29] Subsequent studies have confirmed that sugar increases cholesterol levels in the blood and triglycerides (fatty acids in the blood that may also contribute to some forms of heart disease), but the strong association with coronary atherosclerosis that Yudkin found has not been generally repeated. While the exact role of sugar remains unclear, the American Heart Association, *Dietary Goals for the United States*, and most other national and international health organizations have called for substantial reductions in sucrose intake and the intake of other refined sweeteners.

The comparatively mild grain-based natural sweeteners used in macrobiotic cooking—rice syrup and barley malt—offer practical alternatives to white sugar, brown sugar, molasses, fructose, corn syrup, saccharin, and other refined sweeteners, as well as honey, which is a natural product of animal origin and generally too concentrated for usual consumption.

A CHANGE IN DIRECTION

Taken separately, all the categories in the Standard Macrobiotic Diet contain foods that are wholesome and nutritious and have been increasingly shown by modern scientific and medical studies to protect against heart disease, cancer, and other chronic illnesses. The popularity of whole natural foods and their demonstrated value to the health of the cardiovascular system have prompted the major medical organizations to encourage their consumption, at the same time decreasing the consumption of items high in fat, refined carbohydrates, and animal protein.

The evidence presented in this chapter is persuasive. However, the real proof lies not in the parts but in the macrobiotic dietary approach taken as a whole. *Dietary Goals for the United States* brought to national consciousness the finding that of all risk factors in heart disease "the strongest and most consistent risk factor was elevated serum cholesterol."[30] Beginning in the next chapter with a discussion of cholesterol, we shall look at how medical researchers became interested in studying the Standard Macrobiotic Diet as a whole and how their discoveries of its benefits are revolutionizing modern society's understanding of nutrition, health, and the human heart.

8

Cholesterol and the Heart

Although comparatively rare before the twentieth century, heart disease did affect a tiny minority of the population in ancient and medieval times, especially those in the more well-to-do strata of society who could afford to eat rich, highly refined or imported food. Thus, hardening of the arteries has been found in a few of the mummies from ancient Egypt. Traditional physicians appear to have recognized the underlying nutritional origin of this disorder and suggested dietary modifications for their patients. For example, in the Ebers Papyrus, dating to 1552 B.C., there is a diagnosis suggestive of angina pectoris:

> When you examine a man for illness in his cardia, he has pains in his arm, in his breast, on the side of his cardia; it is said thereof: this is the wzd-illness. Then you shall say thereof: it is something which entered his mouth; it is death which approaches him. Then you shall prepare for him stimulating herbal remedies, fruits of pea, bryony [and other vegetable remedies]; let them be boiled [in beer] and be drunk by the man.[1]

In India in the ninth century B.C., the Vedic medical sage Sushruta identified excessive intake of hot spices, half-cooked food, prohibited articles of diet, overeating, and consumption of decomposed substances with abnormal functioning of the heart.[2]

During the Renaissance, Leonardo da Vinci depicted hardened arteries in his anatomical drawings and described the diffi-

culty of examining hearts "surrounded by waxy fat." In his note-
books, he observed that "the artery and the vein in the aged which
extends between the spleen and the liver acquires so thick a covering that it contracts the passage of the blood which comes from the
mesanteric-portal vessels."[3] These observations may have contributed to the development of Leonardo's vegetarian philosophy
and celebrated maxim, "You are only as old as your arteries."
Leonardo's own artistic and scientific imagination, as well as the
physical strength and reservoirs of energy for which he was re-
nowned, appear to have been nourished primarily by whole grain
millet and brown rice, which entered southern Europe from
China in the late Middle Ages and flourished in the region around
Florence and Milan at this time.[4] Leonardo summed up his own
way of life in verse:

> To keep in health this rule is wise:
> Eat only when you want and sup light.
> Chew well, and let what you take be well cooked and
>   simple.
> He who takes medicine is ill advised.
> Beware of anger and avoid grievous moods.
> Keep standing when you rise from table.
> Do not sleep at midday.
> Let your wine be mixed [with water], take little at a time,
>   not between meals and not on an empty stomach.
> Go regularly to stool.
> If you take exercise, let it be light.
> Do not be with the belly upwards, or the head lowered;
> Be covered well at night.
> Rest your head and keep your mind cheerful.
> Shun wantonness, and pay attention to diet.[5]

By the late nineteenth century, the modern scientific world that
Leonardo helped conceive had reached its early adolescence, and
measurement of the constituents of the blood, organs, and tissues
had developed into an exact science. The earliest nutritional theories linked heart disease with excess protein consumption, especially from foods high in nitrogen as well as from the
overconsumption of fat and sugar. In 1880, Henry Kennedy, an
Irish physician, noted in *Observations on Fatty Heart*:

To subject the human frame to a particular kind of food—more especially animal food—is sure to lead to serious results. . . . all highly nitrogenized foods, such as eggs, cheese, etc., are to be forbidden. Of milk I have already spoken. As far as possible the oily foods are to be avoided. . . . All writers are agreed that, as far as may be, fatty food is to be avoided. It need scarcely be observed that sugar, in its varied forms, is to be used with great reluctance, or even given up entirely.[6]

In 1898, Sir William Broadbent, physician to the Prince of Wales, tried to explain the mechanism underlying this process in his book, *Heart Disease,* and also focused on protein metabolism:

Excess should be avoided, but, subject to this condition, the diet may be liberal and varied. It is important, however, that there should be a due proportion of farinaceous [cereal grain] and vegetable articles of diet; when the food is highly nitrogenized, as when it consists largely of meat, imperfectly oxidized waste accumulates in the blood, and there is a great cause of resistance in the capillary circulation, which constitutes a serious addition to the work imposed upon the heart, and puts a continued strain upon the compensation by which it adjusts itself to the imperfect state of the valves.[7]

THE CHOLESTEROL CONNECTION

Over the next decade, heart research shifted from considerations of protein to the effects of fat and fatlike substances, including cholesterol. Cholesterol had been discovered in the mid-nineteenth century, but it was not until the turn of the new century that it was recognized as the major constituent of clogged arteries. In St. Petersburg, then the capital of Russia, A. I. Ignatovskii discovered in 1908 that rabbits fed on a high-protein diet of meat, milk, and eggs developed lesions resembling those of human atherosclerosis.[8] In 1913, another Russian scientist, Nicolai Anitschkov, linked the effects of the experimental diet fed the animals to elevated cholesterol in the blood.

Cholesterol is a member of a family of fats, oils, and fatlike substances called *lipids* or *lipoids*. Lipids are essential to digestion but can be harmful to the body if consumed or manufactured in the body in excess. One of the chief lipids is cholesterol, a naturally occurring substance in the body that contributes to the maintenance of cell walls, serves as a precursor to bile acids and vitamin D, and also serves as a precursor to some hormones.

Cholesterol is classified into two types: dietary cholesterol and serum (or blood) cholesterol. Dietary cholesterol is scarcely found in plant foods but is contained in all animal foods, especially eggs, meat, poultry, and dairy products. Since cholesterol is insoluble in the blood, it attaches itself to a protein that is soluble in order to be transported through the body. This combination is called a *lipoprotein*. Excess cholesterol in the bloodstream tends to be deposited along artery walls and, as hardened plaque, eventually causes constriction of the arteries and reduces the flow of blood. This buildup of cholesterol is the atherosclerotic process and the underlying cause of most heart attacks, strokes, and peripheral artery disease. As we shall see in further chapters, the lipoproteins bearing cholesterol are further divided into several forms, so that some are more beneficial to the body and others are more harmful. Until recently, the controversy surrounding cholesterol has been whether dietary cholesterol (consumed in the form of animal fats and oils) influences the level of blood cholesterol or whether blood cholesterol is independent of dietary cholesterol intake and manufacturered entirely or controlled by the liver. The early Russian experiments showed a definite causal relationship between dietary cholesterol and blood cholesterol, at least in animals, and set the stage for a half-century of research.

During World War I, researchers noted a sharp decrease in the incidence of and mortality from heart disease, cancer, and other degenerative diseases and hypothesized that this may have resulted from wartime restrictions on milk, meat, cheese, eggs, sugar, and other luxury items in Europe. In 1924, Ludwig Aschoff, M.D., a German pathologist and professor of anatomy, delivered a series of medical lectures in the United States in which he singled out dietary cholesterol and other lipids as the primary factors in the human atherosclerotic process. For this condition to develop, he declared, there needs to be "a sufficient concentration of lipoids, especially of cholesterin esters in the plasma. From plasma of low cholesterin content no deposition of lipoids will occur. . . ."[9] Aschoff said that he knew of no population studies measuring blood cholesterol levels, although the reduction of animal food intake in the later years of the war and in the postwar period in Germany appeared to account for the substantial decrease in heart disease. "The character of the diet remains the most important factor," he concluded. "There is no doubt in my mind that the lipoid concentration of the plasma is essentially influenced by the nature of the diet determined both by the richness and character of its lipoid content."[10]

Despite these early clinical findings, animal experiments, and epidemiological reports, modern medicine largely ignored the importance of nutritional factors in the formation of heart disease until after the Second World War when similar dietary restrictions in Europe resulted in another sharp drop in deaths and new cases of heart disease. Meanwhile, during the first half of the twentieth century, genetics, virology, and immunology commanded most research attention and grants, and advances in electrocardiology, pharmacology, and surgery shifted the emphasis from the prevention of heart ailments to their cure. During these decades, moreover, most heart disease was associated with the effects of rheumatic fever and to a lesser extent syphillis, which were substantially reduced or controlled by the early 1950s.

Most modern doctors believed that coronary heart disease was a natural part of the aging process and that the rise in atherosclerotic disease could be attributed primarily to the fact that modern people were living longer as a result of the conquest of infectious diseases. The Standard American Diet was considered sound, and its high proportion of fat and cholesterol was believed to prevent potentially fatal infectious illnesses and to contribute to the elimination of the nutritional deficiency diseases such as pellegra, rickets, and beriberi. A few dietary pioneers, such as Ancel Keys, an epidemiologist at the University of Minnesota; Weston Price, a dentist who investigated primitive cultures and wrote *Nutrition and Physical Degeneration;* and George Ohsawa, the macrobiotic educator, linked the modern diet with the emerging epidemic of coronary disease, but their warnings were not taken to heart.

THE FRAMINGHAM HEART STUDY

Following the Second World War, neglect of nutritional factors started to ease as coronary disease and other atherosclerotic forms of heart disease displaced that caused by rheumatic fever and as the relation of wartime dietary restrictions to unexpectedly improved health was recognized. In 1949, the National Institutes of Health established a long-term study of all the possible factors associated with the development of cardiovascular disease and selected Framingham, Massachusetts, a small community 18 miles west of Boston, to be the site of this experiment.

From the town's 28,000 inhabitants, the Framingham Heart Study enrolled 5,127 generally healthy adults between the ages of 30 and 59. At the start of the study, doctors ascertained that the participants were free from any clinical signs of cardiovascular disease other than high blood pressure, a factor in the development of heart disease that was not fully understood at the time. The participants were examined every two years for twenty years and the incidence of and mortality from heart attack, angina, stroke, and other conditions carefully recorded. The original study was later extended to a total of twenty-four years and has subsequently enrolled several thousand offspring of the original participants. Of the original study group, 2,950 were still alive at the beginning of 1983. More than 50 percent of the others had died of cardiovascular illness.[11]

Now in its thirty-sixth year, the Framingham Heart Study has become the longest and the most influential heart study in the world. Largely as a result of its investigation of the health and life-styles of nearly 10,000 people, atherosclerotic disease is no longer viewed as the inevitable result of the aging process. The Framingham Heart Study identified three primary risk factors in the development of heart and circulatory disease: (1) high blood cholesterol, (2) high blood pressure, and (3) smoking. (Other major risk factors included diabetes and obesity.)

In each of the three age groups observed—30 to 39, 40 to 49, and 50 to 59—total incidence of coronary heart disease among males significantly increased with elevated blood cholesterol levels. In the youngest group, men with cholesterol levels 260 or above had over four times the risk of heart attack than those with cholesterol levels below 200. In women, a relative increase in risk similar to men was observed in the middle decade. Cholesterol was also associated with greater incidence of stroke and peripheral arterial disease, but the rate of increase was not uniform.

Meanwhile, other studies around the world investigated the types of fats that contributed to the rise of high serum cholesterol levels and their relationship to the incidence of coronary heart disease. Hard saturated fats, such as those found in beef, pork, eggs, and other animal foods, were found to raise serum cholesterol levels independent of the dietary cholesterol content of these and other foods. For example, the Seven Countries Study, the most influential of these international epidemiological surveys, involved 12,000 men between the ages of 40 and 59 in eighteen communities around the world. The Seven Countries Study found that communities with low consumption of animal food and other saturated fats and oils had both lower cholesterol levels and lower incidence of coronary heart disease (see Tables 14, 15, and 16).[12] The studies found that men from eastern Finland and the United States had the highest cholesterol levels and the

Table 14. SATURATED FATS AND CORONARY HEART DISEASE

Areas	Percent Calories Saturated Fatty Acids	Coronary Deaths. Infarcts per 100
Corfu	5.4	1.3
Crete	8.6	0.1
Velika Krsna	8.8	0.2
Montegiorgio	8.9	1.7
Dalmatia	9.5	1.1
Crevalcore	9.7	1.8
Zrenjanin	10.0	0.5
Belgrade	10.0	0.9
Slavonia	13.0	2.0
United States	17.0	3.2
Western Finland	18.8	2.2
Zutphen	19.5	3.4
Eastern Finland	22.2	4.4

Source: *Seven Countries Study*, Harvard University Press, 1980.

Table 15. SERUM CHOLESTEROL AND CORONARY HEART DISEASE

Areas	Average Serum Cholesterol (mg per 100 ml)	Coronary Deaths, Infarcts per 100
Velika Krsna	156	0.2
Dalmatia	186	1.1
Montegiorgio	196	1.7
Corfu	198	1.3
Slavonia	198	2.0
Crevalcore	200	1.8
Crete	203	0.1
Zrenjanin	208	0.5
Belgrade	216	0.9
Zutphen	230	3.4
United States	237	3.25
Western Finland	253	2.25
Eastern Finland	264	2.4

Source: *Seven Countries Study*, Harvard University Press, 1980.

Table 16. SERUM CHOLESTEROL AND FIRST CORONARY EVENT

Serum Cholesterol level mg/100cc	10-Year Rate per 1,000 Men 30–59
under 175	45
175–199	52
200–224	53
225–249	67
250–274	112
275–299	115
300 and over	162

Source: The Pooling Project Research Group, American Heart Association, 1978.

highest rates of coronary heart disease. They also consumed the highest proportion of saturated fats in their diet, 22 and 19 percent respectively. In contrast, the Greeks consumed only 8 percent saturated fat and the Japanese, 3 percent.

As a result of studies such as this in the 1950s and 1960s, the American Heart Association and other medical societies began to modify their dietary guidelines. Over the last twenty years, these scientific bodies have progressively called for further reductions in consumption of food high in dietary cholesterol and in saturated fats and oils. In their place, they have recommended an increased consumption of whole grains, vegetables, fruits, and polyunsaturated fats and oils.

The typical American man consumes about 500 mg of dietary cholesterol a day and the typical woman about 350 mg (one egg, for instance, equals about 274 mg). These amounts are about 60 percent higher than the American Heart Association's current recommendations and about 90 percent higher than the dietary cholesterol intake of traditional cultures and the macrobiotic community.

CLINICAL TRIALS

Until the late 1970s and early 1980s, when the impact of dietary guidelines began to filter into cardiology clinics and hospital kitchens, most heart patients or patients at high risk for coronary disease were routinely served or advised to eat bacon, eggs, whole milk, beef, custard, and other high-cholesterol and high-fat items. The concept of a Prudent Diet for heart patients began as early as 1957 in the Anti-Coronary Club Trial sponsored by the Nutrition Department of the New York City Department of Health. After a fifteen-year period, those in the study group eating a diet high in polyunsaturated fat and low in total fat, saturated fat, and dietary cholesterol had a coronary disease rate only two-thirds that of a control group on the Standard American Diet.[13] The results of other studies involving slight dietary modifications have also been encouraging. A five-year study of 1,232 men with elevated serum cholesterol levels in Oslo found that dietary control of cholesterol intake and cessation of smoking resulted in 47 percent fewer deaths from heart attack and stroke than experienced by a control group.[14] Several other Scandinavian studies, involving actual heart patients, have also shown significant declines in mortality among the low dietary cholesterol groups.[15]

In *The Framingham Study: The Epidemiology of Atherosclerotic Disease*, Thomas Royle Dawber, M.D., the project's original director and now a professor of medicine at Boston University School of Medicine, reviewed the cholesterol controversy:

> The Framingham data provide overwhelming evidence that the level of cholesterol in the blood is a powerful factor in development of the major manifestations of coronary heart disease, myocardial infarction, and angina pectoris. This evidence is so convincing that it is difficult to understand how any reasonable person could question the relationship.[16]

In 1984, the cholesterol controversy was finally resolved to the satisfaction of most scientists and doctors with the results of a comprehensive study of the National Heart, Lung, and Blood Institute. The ten-year survey followed 3,806 men between the ages of 35 and 59 who had serum cholesterol levels above 265 mg, putting them in the moderately high risk category for heart attack and stroke. Half the participants were put on a daily dose of cholestyramine, a drug that lowered cholesterol in the blood, and half received a placebo. At the end of the study, the cholestyramine group had serum cholesterol levels 8.5 percent lower than the placebo group and experienced 19 percent fewer heart attacks. Total death rate from heart disease was 24 percent lower than that of the control group. The researchers used a drug to lower cholesterol rather than diet because diet would have been very difficult to control in such a large study. However, the results were designed to apply to diet, and the researchers emphasized that dietary modifications, rather than drugs, were the method of choice to lower cholesterol. Basil Rifkind, M.D., the project director, said, "It is the turning point in cholesterol-heart disease research."[17]

Shortly afterwards, in the most comprehensive public health recommendations on cholesterol and heart disease to date, the National Institutes of Health called for an all-out campaign to reduce cholesterol levels and implement its dietary recommendations. For the first time the national government's top health organization cited elevated serum cholesterol as a direct cause of heart disease rather than as an associated risk factor. It called upon the food industry and the restaurant trade to serve healthier foods and to label the fat and cholesterol contents of their products. Programs to educate the public and physicians were also recommended. The N.I.H. noted that it was especially important for children and people in their early twenties to reduce their cholesterol levels, since heart disease starts early in life, though symptoms rarely show up before middle age.[18]

Finally, in a study designed to explain why coronary heart disease in America has fallen about 20 percent since 1968, the *Annals of Internal Medicine* reviewed the findings of 130 coronary studies and reports and concluded that dietary changes resulting in reduced serum cholesterol levels have been the single biggest factor in the improved cardiac health of the American public.[19]

In addition to high cholesterol, the Framingham Heart Study discovered that high blood pressure was a major factor predisposing individuals to the development of heart and circulatory disease. In a remarkable series of experiments begun in the early 1970s to evaluate the Standard Macrobiotic Diet, researchers at Harvard Medical School and the Framingham Heart Study found that high blood pressure, as well as high serum cholesterol levels, appeared to have a nutritional foundation.

9

The Macrobiotic
Studies at Harvard

The first study of the Standard Macrobiotic Diet, conducted by
Edward H. Kass, M.D.; Bernard Rosner, M.D.; and Frank M. Sacks,
a graduate student and later medical doctor at the Harvard Medical School, examined the relationship between blood pressure and
consumption of food from animal and plant sources. High blood
pressure had been identified by the Framingham Heart Study as
one of the three primary risk factors in the development of cardiovascular disease.[1] For example, the risk of coronary heart disease
is seven times greater among men with high blood pressure than
among men with normal blood pressure. Both men and women
with high blood pressure have a three times higher risk of developing stroke.

Blood pressure is expressed by two numbers separated by a
slash. The first number indicates the relative pressure when the
heart is pumping and is called the *systolic pressure*. The second
number measures the heart's pressure during the resting phase
and is referred to as the *diastolic pressure*. In testing, blood pressure is computed by observing the rise of millimeters (mm) in a
column of mercury (Hg) much like the fluctuation of temperature
in a thermometer. For diagnostic purposes, high blood pressure
(hypertension) is defined medically as a measurement of 160/95
mm Hg or higher. Normal blood pressure (normotension) is
defined as 140/90 or below. Borderline is above 140/90 but below
160/95. These figures are not absolute and do not necessarily
indicate the presence or absence of heart and circulatory disor-

ders. Some people in the high blood pressure range will not develop symptoms of heart disease over their lifetimes, while some of those in the normal blood pressure range may develop serious heart trouble and die. However, in general, as with serum cholesterol levels, the higher the blood pressure, the higher the risk of cardiovascular illness, and elevated values warrant concern and remedial attention. Medical researchers have advanced several theories to explain how high blood pressure contributes to diseases of the heart and circulatory system, but there is no scientific consensus on the mechanism involved.

Several dietary factors had been hypothesized to contribute to high blood pressure, but except for salt (which the Framingham Heart Study found unrelated to blood pressure), there had been little direct investigation of specific food items. Epidemiological studies of primitive societies suggested an association between their generally low blood pressure levels and their low-fat, high-fiber diets. However, so many other variables and life-style factors in these nonindustrialized societies could account for these low blood pressure values that controlled experiments of the traditional dietary approach in an industrialized setting seemed necessary. Furthermore, most heart studies on vegetarian or semivegetarian diets had been carried out on communities that had lived together for many years and shared religious, familial, ethnic, or other special ties. The macrobiotic group in Boston consisted mostly of ordinary middle class Americans who had grown up on the Standard American Diet and only recently changed their way of eating. Some of them were interested in Eastern philosophy, holistic health, preservation of the environment, and meditation, but there was no religious creed, political belief, social orientation, or other formal membership requirement for belonging to the macrobiotic community other than eating macrobiotic food. The researchers felt that significant changes in the blood pressure of these ordinary American men and women could have practical effects on setting guidelines for public health and dietary policy.

THE FIRST MACROBIOTIC STUDY

The initial study involved 210 individuals living or eating at seventeen large households in the Boston area.[2] These households were known as macrobiotic study houses, where persons from around the country and abroad could come and study macrobiotic cooking, attend my lectures at the East West Foundation on the contemporary meeting of the Occident and the Orient, and generally pursue their own physical, psychological, intellectual, and spiritual development. Experienced cooks at each house provided balanced daily meals based on the Standard Macrobiotic Diet.

In the test group, 127 subjects were male and 83 female. Age ranged from 16 to 68, with the majority under 30. The racial structure of the participants was 93 percent white, 6 percent Oriental, and 1 percent black. Ethnic background was 78 percent northern European, 6 percent Mediterranean, 6 percent Asian, 2 percent Latin American, and 8 percent mixed extraction. Seventy percent grew up in the northern United States, 13 percent in the South or West, 7 percent in Europe, 2 percent in Latin America, and about 8 percent elsewhere or mixed. Forty-three percent had immediate family in the Boston or New York City corridor. Marital status was 56 percent single, 23 percent married, 11 percent living together, and 10 percent divorced, separated, or widowed. The mean length of time the participants had followed the macrobiotic dietary approach was two years. Twenty-four percent meditated daily. The men engaged in a variety of occupations requiring a wide range of physical activity. Some of them were employed in manufacturing or distributing natural foods at the Erewhon Trading Company warehouse or retail stores in Boston and Cambridge. The women either worked outside the home or were involved in child and home care.

From November 1972 through February 1973, the participants were subjected to a wide range of medical tests by the Harvard medical researchers. Overall, the researchers found that the men had mean systolic blood pressures of 109.7 mm Hg and diastolic pressures of 60.9. The women had slightly lower readings, 100.9 and 58.2 respectively. Both of these measurements fell well within the normal blood pressure category and approached the systolic level of 100 under which, the Framingham Heart Study director theorized, there would develop virtually no coronary heart disease.[3] In fact, the blood pressure values in macrobiotic individuals turned out to be the lowest ever recorded for any group in modern industrial society.

In assessing blood pressure fluctuation, the researchers looked at several variables, including the amount of animal food consumed. In the Standard Macrobiotic Diet, animal food is optional and, for those who consume it, consists primarily of low-fat fish or seafood two or three times a week. On the basis of dietary histories, the investigators divided the macrobiotic group into two categories: those who ate 5 percent or more animal food per day and those who consumed 5 percent or less. Adjusting for other variables, the scientists discovered that those who ate 5 percent or more animal food had significantly higher blood pressure. The systolic rates were generally 2 to 10 mm Hg higher, depending on age and weight. The researchers further found that the addition of salt at the table was not associated with changes in blood pressure in those examined, and those individuals who abstained from coffee or cigarette smoking had lower systolic but not diastolic pressures. Married persons also had lower systolic pressures, as did those who meditated. The Framingham Heart Study had found systolic pressure to be the more reliable indicator of potential coronary heart disease, while diastolic pressure did not emerge as a significant determinant in most cases.[4]

The unexpectedly low blood pressure of the macrobiotic group was considered all the more remarkable because of the relatively short time the participants in the study had been on the new diet. "The generally short duration (less than 2 years) of adherence in half suggests that dietary effects on BP [blood pressure] become established relatively earlier," the researchers noted in their final report, published in the *American Journal of Epidemiology* in 1974.[5] "Perhaps of greater interest," the researchers concluded, "is that the declared intake of food from animal sources is significantly associated with higher pressures in individuals and there is significant clustering of systolic BP among the members of communal households, a phenomenon hitherto observed only in relation to first-degree relatives of an individual and with varying degrees of association for spouses. . . ."[6] The implications of these findings for a pluralistic society composed of many different racial and ethnic backgrounds were far-reaching.

THE SECOND MACROBIOTIC STUDY

The results of this first study led to a second experiment comparing the blood values of macrobiotic individuals with those of a control group of the same age and sex eating the Standard American Diet.[7] Seventy-three men and 43 women eating macrobiotically in the Boston area were matched with a randomly chosen group of offspring of the original Framingham Heart Study. William P. Castelli, M.D., medical director of the Framingham project, and Allen Donner, Ph.D., of Harvard Medical School, joined Dr. Kass and Frank Sacks in conducting the second study.

The macrobiotic group was similar to the first test group in racial, socioeconomic, and ethnic background, and their mean time following the diet was three years. The results of the second experiment were consistent with those of the first. The levels of blood pressure and serum cholesterol in the macrobiotic group were found to be strikingly low in all age groups, and the rise of lipid values with age was slight. The macrobiotic group had mean cholesterol levels of 126 mg dl versus 184 for the Framingham control group, a difference of 58 mg dl, or 32 percent less. Blood pressure in the macrobiotic group averaged 108/63 mm Hg compared with 119/77 in the control group, about 10 percent less.

Overall consumption of animal products by the macrobiotic individuals was directly related to the levels of total cholesterol and to LDL cholesterol, a type of cholesterol strongly identified with coronary heart disease. In the late 1960s and early 1970s, scientists differentiated serum cholesterol into five types. The kind that contributes most to the atherosclerotic process is called LDL (Low Density Lipoprotein) cholesterol and is found chiefly in animal foods. The kind of cholesterol that is beneficial to the body and helps reduce LDL and other forms of cholesterol is called HDL (High Density Lipoprotein) cholesterol and is associated with eating nutrients available in whole grains, vegetables, and vegetable oils as well as fish. The three other types of cholesterol are called chylomicrons, IDL (Intermediate Density Lipoprotein) cholesterol, and VLDL (Very Low Density Lipoprotein) cholesterol, and in excess they are also believed to contribute to hardening of the arteries. Good health depends upon a proper balance among the five cholesterols. The higher the level of LDL or VLDL cholesterol, which comprise about 90 percent of the plaque-forming cholesterol in the blood, the higher the subsequent rate of coronary heart disease. Conversely, the higher the HDL cholesterol in the blood, the lower the total body cholesterol and the lower the risk of cardiovascular troubles.

The Framingham researchers found that one of the most accurate ways to measure an individual's risk of heart disease is to compare the total cholesterol in his or her blood to the amount of HDL cholesterol. Most men and women who suffer a heart attack have ratios from 4.6 to 5.7. As a practical first step, the Framingham Heart Study physicians recommend that Americans reduce their ratio to 4.5 or less.[8] "The macrobiotic vegetarians we studied, incidently, had a ratio of 2.5," Dr. Castelli later noted. "Boston marathon runners are at 3.4. These are ratios at which we rarely, if ever, see coronary heart disease."[9]

In evaluating the effects of animal food, the researchers found recent intake a more useful indicator than overall intake in predicting elevated cholesterol levels—another indication of the day-to-day impact of diet on health and the possibility of reversing imbalanced conditions. For example, those macrobiotic individuals who ate no eggs or dairy products during the week prior to testing had lower levels of serum cholesterol than those who said they generally consumed 5 percent or less animal food. The researchers found that among those who ate animal products, fish, which was consumed as much as dairy products and eggs combined, had significantly less effect on raising cholesterol levels than either dairy products or eggs measured separately. Those who drank coffee also exhibited higher cholesterol levels than non–coffee drinkers.

The results of the second study were published in the *New England Journal of Medicine* in 1975. The researchers concluded that the low levels of blood pressure and serum cholesterol found in the macrobiotic group were unique in modern society. In contrast to semivegetarian groups such as the Seventh Day Adventists, which have relatively low rates of heart disease compared with the nation as a whole, "the present study encompasses persons who came from middle-class backgrounds and who were taking the [macrobiotic] diet for an average of 3 years, with many who were taking the diet for but a few months."[10] Comparing the macrobiotic diet with the restricted and generally unappetizing therapeutic diets of the past, the researchers concluded that it "offers a wide range of flavors and textures" and "may help to determine the nature of the food restrictions that may be of value in selected persons."[11]

Four other medical studies in the United States and Europe substantiated the Harvard and Framingham findings (see Tables 17 and 18). In Belgium and the Netherlands, a survey of 168 men and boys found that macrobiotic males had lower lipid levels than those on the ordinary modern diet, semivegetarians who ate meat or fish products less than once a week, and vegetarians who regularly consumed eggs and dairy products. The ratio of total cholesterol to HDL cholesterol further showed the macrobiotic men and boys to have healthier hearts and circulatory systems, based upon this measurement, than all the other categories. The results of the Flemish study were published in 1982 in the professional cardiac journal *Atherosclerosis*.[12]

THE THIRD MACROBIOTIC STUDY

In Boston, the Harvard and Framingham researchers conducted a third experiment to evaluate the effects of meat consumption on the unusually low cholesterol and blood pressure values of people eating macrobiotically.[13] Also participating in the study, along with the original researchers, were James Gronemeyer, D.O. of Harvard Medical School; Peter Pletka, M.D., University of Massachusetts Medical School (Worcester); Harry S. Margolius, M.D.,

Table 17. BLOOD PRESSURES IN MACROBIOTIC PEOPLE

Reference	Number of people	Systolic blood pressure (mm Hg)	Diastolic blood pressure (mm Hg)
Sacks et al. (1974)			
men	127	109.7±11.5*	60.9±10.8
women	83	100.9±9.3	58.2±12.0
Sacks et al. (1975)			
macrobiotic	115	108.0±12.0	63.0±10.0
nonvegetarian	115	119.0±11.0	77.0±8.0
Sacks et al. (1981)	21	104.0	60.3

*Values are mean ± standard deviation.

Table 18. CHOLESTEROL LEVELS OF
MACROBIOTIC PEOPLE

Reference	Number of people	Total cholesterol (mg/dl)	HDL cholesterol (mg/dl)	Total/ HDL
Sacks et al. (1975)				
macrobiotic	115	126±30*	43±11	2.9
nonvegetarian	115	184±37	49±12	3.8
Bergan & Brown (1980)				
men	44	148±32		
women	32	154±30		
East West Journal (1980)	11	121 (range: 102–147)		
Sacks et al. (1981)	21	140	31**	4.5**
Knuiman & West (1982)				
men				
macrobiotic	33	146±35	46±12	3.2
non-vegetarian	52	212±39	46±12	4.3
boys				
macrobiotic	6	131±20	46±12	2.86
non-vegetarian	54	162±20	54±12	2.94

*Values are mean ± standard deviation.
**Since the HDL cholesterol in this study was measured in blood specimens which had been frozen for three-and-a-half years, there was probably some deterioration of the HDL cholesterol. These figures are therefore unreliable.

Medical University of South Carolina; and Lewis Landsberg, M.D., Beth Israel Hospital in Boston. In the medical literature considerable data were accumulating on the relationship between total fat, saturated fat, dietary cholesterol, polyunsaturated fat, and blood cholesterol but no information, surprisingly enough, was available on meat in its intact form or on the relation of meat to blood pressure.

In a supervised setting in which one of the investigators was present at every meal, twenty-one macrobiotic persons were monitored over an eight-week period. The first two weeks they followed their usual diet, which contained little if any animal food but no meat. During the middle four weeks, 250 grams of beef were substituted for part of the grain portion of the meal. During the final two weeks, the beef was discontinued and the ordinary diet resumed.

The twenty-one individuals included fourteen men and seven women ranging in age from 20 to 55. The participants had been eating macrobiotically for an average of three years, with one as little as one month and others five months and nine months. The meat used in the experiment came from range-fed animals and was purchased in the fresh-frozen state from a local farm. Each portion was weighed before cooking by the head chef. The beef added 170 mg of dietary cholesterol to the usual 30 mg consumed every day on average by the participants.

At the end of the study, the researchers found that blood cholesterol rose an average of 19 percent during the period when beef was added to the diet. Within ten days after the meat was discontinued, cholesterol returned to previous levels. Systolic blood pressure and pulse rate also went up significantly (about 3 mm Hg) during the meat stage and returned to previous levels when meat was discontinued. Diastolic pressure did not substantially change during the study.

The researchers also evaluated the emotional state of the participants during the meat-eating stage. Each person was asked to fill out weekly a standard psychological questionnaire prepared by the Educational and Industrial Testing Service, profiling their mood. During the meat-eating stage, the perception of anxiety, depression, anger, and fatigue were higher than during the non-meat stages, and vigor and activity were felt to be lower. The intensity of these moods was five times higher during the final weeks of the meat stage than during the earlier weeks. Mood swings were not found to be correlated with changes in blood pressure or serum cholesterol.

This landmark experiment strongly suggested that both serum cholesterol and blood pressure, two of the three major high-risk factors in coronary heart disease and stroke, were directly related to dietary changes. By contemporary standards, the volume of meat consumed by the macrobiotic individuals for purposes of the test was relatively moderate, about ½ pound daily. Yet, as the researchers concluded in their report, published in the *Journal of the American Medical Association* in August 1981, the addition of this modest amount of meat changed blood values "characteristic of persons of low risk to those of high risk for myocardial infarctions [heart attacks]."[14]

OTHER STUDIES

The three macrobiotic studies have contributed significantly to modern medicine's understanding of the origin and development of heart and circulatory diseases. Other projects have been completed by the Harvard researchers, including a study of the effect of protein on blood values, which we shall look at in the next chapter.

Other medical centers have also been studying the relationship between the macrobiotic diet and heart disease. In a preliminary clinical study in New York City in 1984, physicians at Columbia Presbyterian Hospital reported that heart patients with symptoms of angina showed significantly improved blood pressure values and lowered coronary risk factors after ten weeks on a macrobiotic diet and treatment with biofeedback. The chief researcher, Dr. Kenneth Greenspan of the hospital's Laboratory and Center for Stress Related Disorders, reported that cholesterol levels dropped from an average 300 to 220, levels of blood pressure also dropped, patients could walk about 20 percent farther in stress tests, and three patients with severe angina showed no symptoms at the end of the study. The participants, mostly businessmen, and their wives learned how to cook and ate together at the Natural Gourmet Cookery School under the direction of long-time macrobiotic and natural foods cook Annemarie Colbin. Dr. Greenspan noted that there was "tremendous enthusiasm and adherence" to the new diet.[15] The study was funded and closely monitored by the New York Cardiac Center, the first research group in the country to distinguish among the various cholesterols. Its director, George Barasch, noted that New York Cardiac Center has been studying the relationship among such factors as diet, exercise, and stress for many decades, and he said he hoped that Dr. Greenspan's pioneer clinical work with the macrobiotic diet would be followed up by other doctors.[16]

Meanwhile, in Belgium, researchers at the Academic Hospital of Ghent University studied the influence of the macrobiotic diet on the blood composition of adult males. Twenty men working at Lima Natural Foods Factory in Ghent who had an average age of thirty-six and had been macrobiotic for about eight years were studied. According to the blood tests, all the men were very healthy. Their blood pressure values and body weight were low, their hormone level was favorable, they had normal values for most important nutrients, including vitamins, minerals, and proteins, their cholesterol levels were low, and their HDL cholesterols were higher than ordinary people. One of the researchers, J.P. Deslypere, M.D., concluded, "In the field of cardiovascular and cancer risk factors this kind of blood is very favorable. It's ideal, we couldn't do better, that's what we're dreaming of. It's really fantastic, like children, whose blood vessels are still completely open and whole. This is a very important matter, deserving our full attention."[17]

In an Oregon study, six borderline diabetics were put on a macrobiotic diet for thirty days. Excluding the one obese subject, the researchers reported a significant drop in cholesterol levels from a mean of 140 to 110. The subjects were primarily lacto-ovo vegetarians, accounting for their low cholesterol levels to begin with. A control group of ten macrobiotic subjects showed average cholesterol levels consistent with the Harvard Medical School findings.[18]

Meanwhile, researchers at the University of Rhode Island have published several studies on the nutritional aspects of the macrobiotic diet and are conducting chemical analyses of the Standard Macrobiotic Diet from a sampling of macrobiotic study house meals to determine the exact composition of protein, fat, carbohydrate, vitamins, minerals, and other nutrients.[19]

FUTURE STUDIES

In the future, the Kushi Foundation and Macrobiotics International hope to cooperate with medical researchers in a full clinical study of the possible value of the macrobiotic diet in reversing coronary heart disease in actual heart patients. Individually, many people have reported relief of serious cardiovascular conditions when changing to a macrobiotic diet. However, for medical purposes, this way of eating needs to be carefully monitored and the results compared with those of a control group of patients on the usual modern diet. After several years, survival rates and blood values could be compared and the possible therapeutic value of the macrobiotic approach determined.

Macrobiotic educational organizations also plan to cooperate with scientists in evaluating the effects of other natural foods, including unrefined vegetable oils, unrefined sea salt, sea vegetables, soy foods, and natural sweeteners such as barley malt. The discovery that these foods cause significant reductions in blood pressure and serum cholesterol would provide a scientific basis for substituting them for margarine and other refined polyunsaturated oils, refined salt, low-fat dairy foods, and honey, fruit sugar, and dairy sugar in national and international dietary guidelines.

The Harvard and Framingham studies suggest that a practical solution to heart disease and blood vessel disorders is within easy reach of every American. The macrobiotic experiments have demonstrated that people of different racial and ethnic backgrounds, religious faiths, and social, economic, political, and sexual orientations can unite around the dinner table to strengthen their hearts and improve their common health and well-being.

10

Diet and the Development of Heart Disease

The macrobiotic approach to heart disease is not limited to the relief and prevention of symptoms. It is equally concerned with educating people toward an understanding and practice of a way of life in harmony with the order of the universe. Health and happiness result from living in harmony with nature, while sickness results from acting, thinking, and living in a manner that is imbalanced or extreme. The most fundamental way of approaching sickness is to restore ourselves to a condition of harmony with our environment, including our family, our community, world civilization, and the universe as a whole, as well as our deepest aspirations and dreams.

Proper eating is the most basic way of establishing harmony with our environment. If our daily food is in accord with our surroundings, our blood, cells, and tissues—and therefore our emotions, thoughts, and consciousness—will also be in accord. Harmony is created through the union of opposites: for example, hard and soft, light and shadow, man and woman, and countless other complemental phenomena in the universe. The union of man and woman is referred to as love and sex, while the union of human beings with the vegetable kingdom is known as eating. Proper eating is the essence of natural healing, and without it sickness cannot be fundamentally cured. Sickness is also an indication that our way of life has become too sedentary and we need to be more active. In the next chapter, we shall look more closely at the important roles that emotions and exercise play in maintaining health.

Sickness is the mechanism by which our bodies seek to restore balance if we continue living disharmoniously. The repeated over-consumption of incorrect food causes a variety of adjustment mechanisms in the organism that lead progressively toward high blood pressure, heart attack, stroke, and other circulatory disorders. Since the body at all times seeks balance with the surrounding environment, the normal process is for this excess intake to be eliminated in chronic discharges, especially through the skin, or to be restored in and around the inner organs when it exceeds the body's capacity for normal or abnormal elimination. As the body's network for transporting oxygen and nutrients to all the cells and tissues, the circulatory system may be subjected to further functional changes as it labors under additional pressure, increased cardiac output and rate of heartbeat, and localized blockages in the arteries to meet the increased needs of other impaired organs.

YIN AND YANG FORMS OF HEART DISEASE

Cardiovascular disease encompasses about one hundred clinically recognized illnesses. These are divided into several major categories according to criteria established by the International Classification of Diseases. This is a registry designed to standardize incidence, mortality, and survival rates so that uniform medical data and statistics are available around the world. The main categories include rheumatic heart disease, hypertensive disease (high blood pressure and its complications), ischemic heart disease (degenerative heart disease, including myocardial infarction, angina pectoris, and hardening of the coronary arteries), pulmonary heart disease, valve disorders, cardiac arrhythmias (abnormal heartbeats and murmurs), heart failure, cerebrovascular disease (stroke), diseases of the arteries, diseases of the veins, and congenital heart defects. In Part II we shall look at some of the specific forms that heart disease may take within these categories, examining their underlying dietary origin and development and offering recommendations for their relief and prevention.

Although there are thousands of seemingly unrelated diseases of the digestive, circulatory, and nervous systems, all sicknesses share a common origin and can be classified according to their symptoms and causes into three major categories: (1) those caused by excessive yin—centrifugal and expansive tendencies, (2) those caused by excessive yang—centripetal and contractive tendencies, and (3) those caused by both excessive yin and excessive yang factors together.

Expansive yin qualities include dilation, swelling, inflammation, enlargement, loosening, softening, and increased speed, flow, and vibratory rate. Contractive yang qualities include constriction, narrowing, tightening, blocking, hardening, and decreased speed, flow, and rate of vibration. On this basis, we can easily see that diseases that involve enlargement and swelling of the heart or blood vessels are primarily yin in origin and development, while those that involve constriction of the heart and blood vessels are primarily yang. In respect to blood flow itself, thinning and bleeding are more yin, while thickening and clotting are more yang. A fast pulse is generally yin and a slow pulse, yang. However, in excess a quality can turn into its opposite, so that occasionally a fast pulse is yang and a slow pulse, yin. High blood pressure is an example of a condition caused by excessive consumption of both factors: The blood vessels are generally constricted and narrowed while the heart itself is swollen and enlarged.

Using this compass of complemental opposite forces, we can readily identify the predominant type of excess energy in any form of illness. Modern nomenclature makes them seem very complex, but in truth they are really very simple to understand. For example, an aortic aneurysm is a ballooning out of the wall of the large artery leading away from the heart. This happens when the wall of the aorta expands and creates a small sac that fills with blood. Ballooning is an outward, expansive symptom characteristic of yin. Other seemingly abstruse entries in the heart disease lexicon can be similarly treated. Left ventricular hypertrophy is a big word for enlargement of the lower left side of the heart—this is more yin in origin and development. Myocarditis refers to the inflammation of the heart muscle—a swollen, yin condition. Coronary occlusion signifies an obstruction of a coronary artery impeding the flow of blood to the heart itself—a narrowing or yang condition. Pulmonary embolism indicates the lodging of a blood clot in the artery of a lung—a condensed yang disorder. Atrial fibrillation refers to uncoordinated contraction of the upper heart muscles—a yin loss of contractive power.

In this way, the predominant quality of any specific heart ailment can be easily identified (see Table 19). Still, there are exceptions. For example, mitral stenosis signifies the narrowing of the

Table 19. A YIN/YANG CLASSIFICATION OF CARDIOVASCULAR DISEASE

More Yin Cause	Yin and Yang Combined	More Yang Cause
Cushing's Syndrome	Diastolic hypertension Renal hypertension	Systolic hypertension Eclampsia hypertension
Some low blood pressure		Some low blood pressure
		Coronary heart disease
	Prinzmetal angina	Angina pectoris
		Myocardial infarction
Some cerebral thrombosis	Some cerebral thrombosis	
Cerebral hemorrhage		
Some heart failure	Some heart failure	Some heart failure
	Cardiomyopathy	
Valve disorders	Irregular heartbeats	
Pulmonary heart disease	Rheumatic heart disease	
	Infectious heart disease	
	Arteriosclerosis Obliterans	
	Acute thrombosis or embolism	
Raynaud's Phenomenon	Aneurysm	Buerger's Disease
	Varicose veins Phlebitis	
Congenital heart defects		

heart valve in the left side of the heart. This is a constrictive yang symptom; however, it is often the result of rheumatic fever, a disorder involving extreme yin as well as yang factors, and thus is an example of a malfunction caused by an opposite tendency as hardened scar tissue covers over loose, diseased valves.

An expanded heart—an overly yin condition—arises from drinking too many liquids, particularly soda pop, fruit juice, milk, alcohol, coffee, and other stimulants, and eating too much fruit and sugar and too many refined and tropical foods. This type of eating results in a swollen heart and may lead to a heartbeat that is weak, irregular, or fluttery. This form of heart disease is usually characterized by high blood pressure, or occasionally low blood pressure, and may lead to stroke or contribute to a heart attack.

A contracted heart—an overly yang condition—is the result of consuming foods high in saturated fat and cholesterol. This causes narrowing and hardening of the arteries and accumulations of stagnated fat deposits in and around the heart. As a result, the heart and arteries lose their elasticity and vitality, and the heart labors excessively to do its job of pumping blood throughout the body. The fat and cholesterol that collects in the arteries reduces blood and oxygen to the heart and brain. Eventually, enough of these fatty deposits build up and cause a heart attack or stroke.

When one factor clearly predominates in the development of heart disease, we should keep in mind that the other factor is always involved, and they must be approached as a dynamic unity. Excessive consumption of imbalanced yin and yang foods and beverages usually go together, and the modern diet, which is high in meat and sugar, may produce disorders that result from a combination of both extremes. Atherosclerosis, the underlying condition for most heart attacks and strokes, is a good example. On the one hand, atherosclerosis is a contractive yang disorder involving the hardening, thickening, and narrowing of the arteries. This is caused primarily by the consumption of meat, eggs, poultry, dairy food, and other excessively yang substances. On the other hand, the buildup of plaque inside the arteries—its physical growth—is an expansive yin process and one that is enhanced by excessive yin foods and fluid, leading to enlargement of the heart muscle as it works harder to pump blood through the obstructed blood vessels.

THE HEART AND OTHER ORGANS

The relationship of the heart to the other organs of the body must also be kept in mind. According to traditional Far Eastern medicine, the heart and the small intestine are complementary and antagonistic organs. In addition to their corresponding anatomical locations in the central upper torso and the central lower torso, the small intestine is thought to be where absorbed nutrients become initially transformed into blood, while the heart serves as the center of the blood distribution network. The small intestine is more yin in structure—hollow and expanded—while the heart is more yang—solid and compact. The intestines govern the deep, internal, largely invisible transmutation of electromagnetic energy that flows between the celestial bodies and Earth along the meridians, or pathways of energy radiating through the body, while the heart coordinates more external, visible sources of nourishment and vitality.

When the heart is weak or overactive, the small intestine is usually impaired. When the small intestine is functioning smoothly, the heart and blood vessels usually function likewise. The villi in the small intestine consist of a forest of minute hairlike projections in which billions of bacteria and viruses digest, absorb, and transmute absorbed food particles into blood. The consumption of excessive food and drink, including meat, dairy products, sugar, and alcohol, kill these microorganisms and lead to indigestion, reduced blood production, and possibly an imbalance in the proportion of red and white blood cells. As in the heart and arteries, the lining of the small intestine can become coated and clogged with hardened fat and mucus. Depending upon the combinations of food consumed regularly, the intestinal walls can become either hardened and lose their natural ability to expand or swollen and lose their natural capacity to contract. When peristalsis—the smooth, rhythmic alternative contraction and expansion of the digestive tract—is interrupted, metabolism is further impaired. Consumption of overly yin substances, including excessive liquids and especially icy cold beverages on top of sweet, sticky, fatty foods, produces intestinal stagnation, leading to a swollen lower abdominal region and overweight. Consumption of overly yang food can lead to appendicitis, duodenal ulcers, putrefaction of excess protein in the intestines, gas formation, constipation, and a wide variety of colonic disorders. The end result of this degenerative process is often cancer of the colon or rectum.

Interestingly, cancer affects every part of the human body except usually the heart and the small intestine. This is because these two organs are the centers of the circulatory and digestive systems respectively. To prolong life and limit degeneration, the storage and accumulation of excess fat, protein, carbohydrates, and minerals will be directed (by the liver) elsewhere, first to peripheral areas such as the skin, then around reproductive organs, and finally in vital organs such as the kidneys and in the deep tissues such as the innermost regions of the brain and the central nervous system. So long as the small intestine can still absorb and transport foodstuffs to the bloodstream and the heart can still pump, even under severe strain and injury, there is a possibility of reversing the degenerative process through dietary means and restoring the whole body to health. To extend the metaphor from the Yellow Emperor's Classic of Internal Medicine, the liver, the body's general, will even sacrifice a large part of itself if necessary on behalf of its commander-in-chief, the heart, and the minister of basic life energy, the small intestine.

The kidneys and heart are also related, though in a different way. According to traditional Oriental medicine, there is a cycle of complementary energy and a cycle of antagonistic energy flowing among the five pairs of major organs. The heart and small intestine are said to be nourished by the liver and gallbladder and controlled by the kidney and bladder. In turn, the heart and small intestine strengthen the stomach and spleen and weaken the lungs and large intestine. Modern medicine has long recognized the heart–kidney relationship. When the kidneys are overtaxed by a diet high in saturated fat and high in salt, they can no longer cleanse the blood efficiently. When the kidneys become overcontracted, the blood gets backed up in the arteries, resulting in high blood pressure. This increases the demands on the heart. The toxins that are normally filtered by the kidneys remain in the bloodstream longer, where they are often absorbed by cells and tissues, contributing to imbalance in other areas of the body. These complications put an additional burden on the heart. Meanwhile, heart and small intestine problems interfere with the smooth functioning of the lungs and large intestine. Pulmonary troubles often result from heart disease, which increases the demand for oxygen, and additional stress is put on the blood vessels in the lungs.

Thus, we can begin to see the fundamental unity and interrelationship among the various organs. Circulatory ailments may be localized in one region of the heart or a remote artery, but the sickness affects the body as a whole.

Heart disease generally develops over a period of years, passing through a series of recognizable stages. Later in the process, as external symptoms appear, these stages are not necessarily sequential but more like limbs of a tree branching off a common trunk. Let us look at this general process.

NORMAL BLOOD CIRCULATION

Our slightly salty bloodstream is a replica of the ancient sea in which life developed during most of its biological history, and each cell is surrounded by fluid similar in composition to seawater.[1] The blood consists of liquid in the form of plasma and of formed elements consisting of red blood cells, white blood cells, and platelets. Several dozen other nutrients and compounds also circulate in the bloodstream, including fat, cholesterol, glucose, sodium, potassium, and urea. The transport of oxygen and nutrients in the blood is essential for life, and the efficiency with which it is accomplished directly influences our health and well-being.

Normal blood is slightly alkaline, with a pH between 7.3 and 7.45, thus giving rise to its mildly salty taste. A pH of less than 7 is acid, while one more than 7 is alkaline. If the pH of the blood dips below its normally weak alkaline level and becomes acidic, acidosis arises. Acidity is classified as an expanded or yin condition. Sickle-cell anemia, leukemia, and in my experience AIDS are examples of blood disorders in which the acidity is so great as to be life-threatening. When the pH factor of the blood moves into the high pH range, the more yang condition of alkalosis occurs. An example of a potentially lethal blood disorder involving high alkalinity is scurvy—a disease associated historically with British sailors living on a diet high in salt pork, dried fish, and other contractive yang foods with almost no counterbalancing yin factors such as the vitamin C in pine-needle tea, leafy green vegetables, or citrus fruits.

Daily diet is the principal determinant of the blood's relative acidity or alkalinity. Whole grains, vegetables, beans, and sea vegetables are the most centrally balanced foods and produce strong, healthy blood that is neither too acid nor too alkaline. Through the network of capillaries, this strong blood—neither too thick nor too thin—is distributed to the cells and tissues of the body, including the brain cells, creating harmonious day-to-day, month-to-month, and year-to-year health, a bright outlook, and vitality.

More expansive yin foods and beverages such as sugar, white flour, fruits, juices, milk, soft drinks, coffee, black tea, alcohol, and artificially processed and chemicalized foods, though in some cases extremely alkaline, thin the blood and make it more acidic. Contractive, overly yang foods, including meat, eggs, poultry, hard cheese, fish, and refined salt, are extremely alkaline and may thicken the blood, making it more alkaline, or may change into their opposite quality (acid) and in most cases serve to weaken it. The body compensates for momentary imbalances in the blood by several mechanisms. For example, when we exhale, excess acids are discharged in the form of carbon dioxide. The liver and kidneys filter toxins and excess acids from food and drink and discharge them through urination, respiration, and perspiration. The blood also contains a variety of buffers, such as sodium bicarbonate, which serves to neutralize acids. The autonomic nervous system also releases hormones that further regulate the balance of minerals and electrolytes in the blood and offset any momentary imbalances. In this way, the blood can maintain a weak alkaline condition despite occasional consumption of extreme foodstuffs.

ABNORMAL BLOOD CIRCULATION

So long as the amount of excess is light to moderate, normal discharge mechanisms such as urination, bowel movement, respiration, and perspiration can handle toxins or excess waste that enter the circulatory system. However, if the quantity of excess is large and continuous, the body is not capable of discharging it smoothly, and various abnormal processes begin. Today, for example, we all tend to overeat. We consume foods from geographic and climatic environments vastly different from our own. We eat local produce in seasons during which it does not naturally grow in our own area. We enjoy party food every day rather than just on special occasions.

These imbalanced practices can trigger a variety of abnormal discharge mechanisms in the body. For example, when we accumulate too much mucus and phlegm in our system to be eliminated through the urine or other normal channels, the body "catches" a cold, and it comes out through the nose and mouth. Mucus is produced by eating sugar; sweets; fatty, oily, and greasy food; and hard baked or softly cooked flour products. These foods are more yin in quality, and a cold is a more yin condition, characterized by swelling and upward, outward, expanding energy.

Fever, in contrast, is generally an example of a more yang symptom. Fever arises primarily from excess consumption of animal foods and is manifested as a more inward, downward, contractive energy. The main sign of fever is elevated body temperature. Compared with a cold, fever is a "warm." Sometimes, after the consumption of both excess yin and excess yang substances, we get a cold and a warm together. Fever can sometimes also be caused by excessive yin factors and is then another example of like producing unlike when there is excess, rather than the usual like producing like.

If we let it alone, a moderate cold will naturally clear up without our needing to take medication or pills. Similarly, unless it is dangerously high, fever should not be suppressed but allowed to run its course and either "burn off" excess imbalanced energy that has accumulated in the body and localized in the forehead or other region or "absorb out" by a cold application on the surface of the body. Suppressing symptoms of cold or fever only drives the excess deeper into other parts of the body, where it will eventually surface in a different form and usually with greater intensity.

In this way, mild symptoms such as cold, fever, diarrhea, too frequent urination, sneezing, and coughing can be seen as natural reactions of the body to restore balance. "Everything in excess is opposed by Nature," Hippocrates stated twenty-five hundred years ago. Through the beginnings of the modern age, this principle of the beneficial nature of disease largely guided traditional physicians and healers. "Disease is nothing else but an attempt on the part of the body to rid itself of morbific matter," Thomas Sydenham, a famous English medical doctor, noted in the seventeenth century.

HIGH BLOOD PRESSURE

The force that circulating blood exerts against artery walls is measured as blood pressure. Consumption of imbalanced foods and beverages, especially excessive yin substances but also overly yang items, can cause elevated blood pressure and lead possibly to stroke, coronary heart disease, congestive heart failure, kidney failure, peripheral artery disease, or other serious circulatory condition (see Table 20).

Systolic pressure—the pressure of the heart when pumping— is determined by the volume of the blood pumped by each stroke, the heartbeat, and the elasticity of the aorta and other large arteries near the heart that receive the full force of the ejected blood. Diastolic pressure—the pressure of the heart at rest—is governed by the resistance to the flow of blood from the arteries to the capillaries, where the nutrients and gases essential to cells and tissues are transported. The mechanism by which high blood pressure develops, especially the relationship between blood pressure and diet, is not completely understood by modern science. Traditional Oriental medicine, however, provides some insight into this

Table 20. DIASTOLIC BLOOD PRESSURE AND FIRST CORONARY EVENT

Blood Pressure in mm Hg	10-Year Rate per 1,000 Men 30–59
under 75	48
75–84	52
85–94	87
95–104	99
105 and over	188

Source: The Pooling Project Research Group, American Heart Association, 1978.

process, indicating how excessive dietary factors can affect one or more of these functional blood pressure determinants (cardiac output, heartbeat, elasticity of arteries, and resistance of arterial walls), raising or lowering either systolic pressure or diastolic pressure, or both.

The consumption of excessive yin foods and beverages such as sugar, sweets, refined flour, milk, light cheese, tropical fruits, spices, stimulants, and certain tropical vegetables can produce a significant elevation in blood pressure. In the digestive system, simple sugars from many of these foodstuffs are broken down into glucose and stored in the liver as glycogen. When the amount of glycogen exceeds the liver's storage capacity, it is released into the bloodstream in the form of fatty acids, or triglycerides. This fatty acid is stored first in the inactive places of the body such as the buttocks, the thighs, and the midsection and is a primary cause of overweight and obesity. Then, as these more peripheral areas become saturated, excess fatty acid becomes attracted to deeper, more central organs such as the heart and kidney, which gradually become encased in a layer of fat and mucus. This accumulation can also penetrate the inner tissues, weakening the normal functioning of organs, causing blood vessels to lose their elasticity, and diminishing diastolic blood pressure. In the bloodstream, fatty acids adhere to plasma and red blood cells and make them sticky. The red blood cells must normally bend and fold in order to pass through the tiny capillaries. If the red blood cells are encased in fat, they will stick together, clump, and clog the capillaries, depriving the cells of oxygen and raising both systolic and diastolic blood pressure.

The intake of excessive yin factors also influences the sympathetic nervous system, which extends from ganglia in the vertebrae region of the chest to the blood vessels of the stomach, liver, kidneys, and other vital organs. Stimulation of these nerves releases yin hormones that produce a rise in diastolic pressure. Other hormones and substances in the kidneys, adrenals, and endocrine system can also affect blood pressure levels.

Fluctuations in blood pressure can also be caused by the repeated consumption of meat, eggs, poultry, and other excessively yang substances. The saturated fat and cholesterol from these foods constricts arterioles, the small arteries connecting the arteries and the capillaries. This hardening is an example of arteriosclerosis and involves differing degrees of narrowing, thickening, or closing of the artery walls. As a result of diminished contractive power, resistance to blood flow in the capillaries will increase, forcing diastolic pressure to rise. As diastolic pressure rises, systolic pressure also rises to maintain equilibrium.

The intake of extreme yang factors can also harden the aorta and larger arteries, including the coronary arteries of the heart itself. As these larger vessels rigidify, they lose their normal flexibility and cannot distend when blood is ejected from the left ventricle. To compensate, the systolic pressure against the walls of the artery will increase. In this type of hypertension, arteries lose their ability to contract between heartbeats, and diastolic pressure consequently falls. This form of high blood pressure is more commonly observed in middle-aged or elderly persons, as hardening tends to start in more peripheral blood vessels and over the years moves inward toward more central vessels and the heart itself.

In the macrobiotic experiments by a research team at Harvard Medical School, we saw that those who regularly consumed a small volume of fish had significantly higher systolic and diastolic pressures than those who consumed little or no animal food at all. However, when a half-pound of beef was added to the diet for a month, systolic pressure rose significantly but diastolic pressure remained about unchanged.

At the American Heart Association's annual scientific sessions in Anaheim, California, in 1983, my son, Lawrence Kushi, presented results of an epidemiological study comparing diet and mortality from coronary heart disease among groups of men born and living in Ireland, men born in Ireland who had emigrated to Boston, and men born in the Boston area of Irish immigrants. He and his co-workers at the Department of Nutrition, Harvard School of Public Health; the Department of Preventive Cardiology and the Department of Community Medicine and Epidemiology, University College, Dublin; and the Department of Nutrition, Trinity College, Dublin, found many interesting relationships. In respect to blood pressure, they found that vegetable-quality foods may operate at least in part through reducing blood pressure and other factors to modify risk of coronary heart disease.[2] Though only suggestive, these results tended to parallel several other more conclusive studies showing that feeding a diet high in fiber, especially cereal grain fiber, decreases both systolic and diastolic blood pressure.[3] In a clinical trial, Dutch doctors recently reported a slight decrease in blood pressure among angina patients with hypertension put on a special vegetarian diet.[4]

The effects of high blood pressure on the cardiovascular system are usually injurious and potentially lethal. First, the load on the heart, especially the left ventricle, is increased as it labors to pump against increased pressure. For example, in the arterioles, a decrease in the diameter of a small vessel by 50 percent increases resistance by sixteen times. To offset this resistance, the heart must pump harder and the normally thicker wall of the left ventricle may enlarge several times. The heart muscle's own demand for oxygen is correspondingly increased.

High blood pressure also increases the strain on artery walls, and like an overinflated inner tube the arteries may burst or rupture. When this happens in the brain, it produces a type of stroke called a *cerebral hemorrhage*. Persons with high blood pressure are from about seven to twenty times at greater risk of developing stroke than persons with normal blood pressure. Earlier, we saw how high blood pressure could be caused by blood backing up from overworked kidneys. The path of injury can also move in the other direction, as reduced blood flow from high blood pressure sometimes leads to kidney failure.

High blood pressure also accelerates the development of atherosclerosis, a kind of arteriosclerosis in which the inner layer of the artery wall is thickened with deposits of hardened fat and cholesterol that impede blood flow and may close the artery. It is believed that the turbulence, or excessive force, of the blood under high pressure can lead to injury of the arterial walls and affect the rate of plaque buildup or thrombosis (clot formation). This is theorized to be especially localized around the openings and branches of the blood vessels and along major curves of arteries, where the flow is most disturbed. In experiments with monkeys, modest increases in blood pressure significantly increased atherosclerotic lesions.[5]

Finally, by itself high blood pressure can lead to a hypertensive crisis in which a sudden extreme elevation of pressure can produce headache, seizures, vision disorders, unconsciousness, and even death. Table 21 indicates some of the ways in which different

Table 21. A YIN/YANG GUIDE TO METABOLIC CHANGES

	YANG STIMULI		YIN STIMULI	
	External	*Internal*	*External*	*Internal*
	Temperature increase, pressure increase, exercise	*Salt, animal food, deep inward meditation*	*Temperature decrease, pressure decrease, rest*	*Sugar, alcohol, drugs, emotional stress*
Heartbeat	+	−	−	+
Arterial resistance	−	+	+	−
Breathing	+	−	−	+
Cardiac muscle	+	−	−	+
Systolic BP	−	+	+	−
Diastolic BP	+	−	−	+
Stroke volume	+	−	−	+
Cardiac output	+	−	−	+

+ = Increases, stimulates, or expands
− = Decreases, inhibits, or contracts
Note: At extremes, + changes to − and vice versa. That is, in the first column, the heart values and respiratory rate of a trained athlete are often the opposite quality. Also, in practice, systolic blood pressure rises when diastolic blood pressure rises. Thus, an external yang stimulus and an internal yin stimulus will raise both blood pressures. However, at their extremes, they will change into their opposite and result in low blood pressure.

stimuli influence fluctuations in blood pressure and other metabolic changes.

LOW BLOOD PRESSURE

If the person with high blood pressure continues to take extreme foods and beverages, especially sugar, soft drinks, coffee, and other excessively yin items, the heart may become so swollen and loose that it no longer has sufficient contractive power. As a result, blood pressure often becomes dangerously low, producing what is called *hypotension.* Strain and overwork on the part of the heart muscle can lead to irregular or fluttery heartbeats. Hypotension can also lead to the excessive accumulation of fluids in the body, congestive heart failure, or sudden death.

Low blood pressure can also be produced by an excessively yang way of eating, which causes the heart to become so contracted and tight that it slows down and pressure diminishes. In modern society, low blood pressure from this cause is not so common as that from excessive yin factors. However, it can arise, and when it does needs to be properly evaluated to make correct dietary adjustments slightly emphasizing the quality of food opposite to the underlying cause.

ATHEROSCLEROSIS

Atherosclerosis is the underlying cause of most heart attacks, strokes, and peripheral artery disease and is the most common cause of death in modern society. Atherosclerosis occurs when deposits of hardened fat and cholesterol build up in the inner linings of artery walls and obstruct the flow of blood transporting oxygen and nutrients to the brain, heart, kidneys, or lower limbs. As this plaque continues to accumulate, the diameter of the blood vessels narrows, impeding the flow of blood, increasing blood pressure, and causing partial or total obstruction of the artery (see Figure 10). If oxygen is cut off in a part of the brain, the result is a *stroke*. If one or more coronary arteries is deprived of oxygen, the result is the death of a portion of the heart muscle. This is called a *myocardial infarction*, or *heart attack*. If a blood clot forms around an atherosclerotic deposit, it is called a *thrombus*, and if a blood clot breaks off it is called an *embolus*. Floating through the bloodstream, an embolus may eventually become lodged in the smaller arteries of the brain, lungs, legs, or other region. Sometimes this is fatal, as often in the case of the head. Other times, as in the case of the feet, gangrene may set in, requiring amputation. A hemorrhage or abscess also may form (see Figure 11).

The atherosclerotic process illustrates the complementary and antagonistic relationship of yin and yang. Hardening of the arteries is considered a predominantly yang disorder because it constricts and narrows the blood vessels and is caused primarily by the

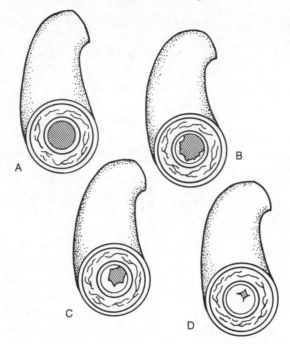

**Figure 10. Hardening and Narrowing of Arteries through
Buildup of Atherosclerotic Plaque**

overconsumption of meat, eggs, poultry, dairy food, and other
animal food. However, the growth of fatty deposits in the arteries
is an expansive yin phenomenon and one that is accelerated by the
consumption of excessive yin foods and beverages. Moreover, the
added strain put on the circulatory system by hardened arteries
tends to enlarge and swell the heart. As the heart labors under
demands for oxygen, the heartbeat and blood pressure tend to
rise, and a larger volume of blood is pumped to constricted blood
vessels and other organs.

The mechanism by which atheromata, or masses of fat and
cholesterol, develop in modern humans is the subject of intensive
medical research and hypothesis. Scientists have tentatively identified several stages in this process, which extends from infancy to
adulthood.[6]

1. Within several months of birth, abnormal physiological
changes begin to take place within the circulatory systems of most

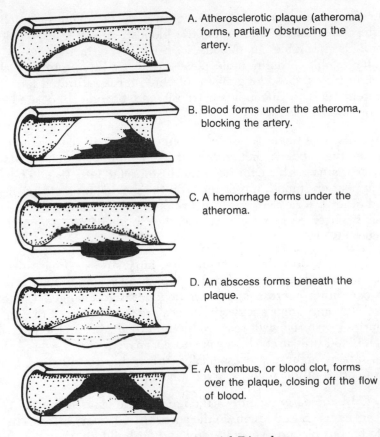

A. Atherosclerotic plaque (atheroma) forms, partially obstructing the artery.

B. Blood forms under the atheroma, blocking the artery.

C. A hemorrhage forms under the atheroma.

D. An abscess forms beneath the plaque.

E. A thrombus, or blood clot, forms over the plaque, closing off the flow of blood.

Figure 11. Arterial Disorders

modern infants. Tiny injuries to the endothelial linings of the medium and larger arteries develop, possibly as the result of turbulent blood flow occasioned by the quality of metabolized foodstuffs. As a result of these injuries, blood platelets begin to accumulate, along with isolated monocytes and macrophage foam cells, and begin to fill in with excess cholesterol and fats. Monocytes are a type of leukocyte, or white blood cell, and macrophages are cells that combat inflammation, degrade old red blood cells, and perform other functions to strengthen the body's immunity to disease. Normally the human liver produces sufficient serum cholesterol for smooth metabolism. However, when excessive dietary cholesterol or saturated fats are consumed, too much serum cholesterol is available and enters the bloodstream. Because cholesterol is insoluble in blood, it normally attaches itself to water-soluble protein molecules and forms lipoproteins. Like freight trains, these long chains of cholesterol, saturated fat, and protein tend to uncouple in transit and become deposited on artery walls.

2. By about age three and through age ten in many children eating the modern diet, the lipid-filled monocytes and macrophage foam cells have formed into clusters, and fatty streaks begin to appear on smooth muscle cells on the inside lining of the aorta and other arteries. At first, the streaks localize around the openings of arteries, especially where they branch into connecting blood vessels.

3. In the next decade of life, the fatty streaks progressively increase, and many teenagers develop raised lesions in their arteries exhibiting necrosis and other degenerative changes. Cholesterol, fat, and other sticky substances are also attracted to minor injuries in arterial walls that are thought to arise from the force of high blood pressure. The aorta and coronary arteries, where the pressure is highest, are especially susceptible to injury and accumulation of intra- and extracellular lipids.

4. By the early twenties—though in some cases sooner and in others later—raised lesions in the aorta and coronary arteries turn into fibrous plaque. As cholesterol and fat build up, they become encapsulated by scarlike fibrous tissue that binds them firmly to arterial walls. Plasma proteins such as fibrin and fibrinogen also accumulate in atheromata. Meanwhile, tiny blood vessels in the artery walls continue to supply more fat and cholesterol to fibrous tissues so that the deposits continue to grow. As we have seen, hardening tends to increase blood pressure and augments the vessels' susceptibility to further injury and more fatty buildup. In this way, like sediment in a riverbed, layers of fat, cholesterol, protein, and minerals coagulate and change from soft, spongy clusters to hardened, rocklike strata. It is estimated that atheromata spread or develop over the surface area of the major blood vessels, especially the coronary arteries, at the rate of about 2 percent a year in persons on the modern diet. As noted earlier,

a medical study of U.S. soldiers killed in Korea and in Vietnam showed evidence of atherosclerosis in the coronary arteries of 45 to 77 percent of presumably healthy young Americans. The soldiers' mean age was twenty-two. Autopsies of young Asians the same age who had eaten a diet consisting primarily of grains and vegetables revealed almost no plaque.

5. By the mid-thirties and early forties, the atherosclerotic deposits in many people have calcified, as chalky minerals fill in the fibrous scar tissue. Most young adults have plaque not only in the heart vessels but also along the entire length of the ascending aorta, leading toward the brain, and along the iliac and femoral arteries nourishing the organs in the pelvic region. These complicated lesions set the stage for stroke, heart attack, or peripheral vascular disease. Usually, the plaque obstructs only a part of the arterial opening, which is called the *lumen.* Oxygen supply is generally not imperiled until about 50 percent of the lumen is blocked, though in some cases heart attack can occur with only minimal narrowing of the coronary vessels. To compensate for the diminished supply of oxygen, the heartbeat, cardiac output, and blood pressure tend to rise. When about 70 percent of the coronary arteries are occluded, or obstructed, severe pain and discomfort may arise in the chest area and be felt radiating to the neck and down one or both arms. This chronic chest pain, which reaches a threshold at certain levels of activity, is called *angina pectoris.* Partial or total narrowing of the coronary arteries by the buildup of plaque or the formation of blood clots can cause a myocardial infarction in the heart or a cerebral infarction in the brain. By the onset of a heart attack or angina, two or three main vessels in the coronary circuit are usually obstructed by one or more deposits.

In addition to narrowing the arteries, atherosclerotic plaque may ulcerate and form thrombi made up chiefly of coagulated blood platelets. These blood clots may form when blood circulation is slowed, or they may develop around atheromata and further obstruct the arteries. Blood clots may also be swept away by a surge of elevated blood pressure or other motion and lodge in distant parts of the circulatory system. From the lining of the aorta, neck vessels, and coronary arteries, thrombi can develop and be propelled up to the brain or down to the legs and feet. An embolus, or detached thrombus, will continue to drift to smaller-diameter blood vessels where it may eventually become lodged like a boulder in a stream. When this happens, blood supply may be completely shut off, producing an infarction, or localized death, of a segment of the brain, the heart muscle, the legs, or the feet.

Other complications may also result from the buildup of atherosclerotic plaque. When tissue in the wall of an artery under an atheroma bleeds, hemorrhaging may result. An abcess, or localized infection, may also develop beneath the hardened deposit, leading to injury and disease.

FAT, CHOLESTEROL, AND PROTEIN METABOLISM

To understand the role of fat, cholesterol, and protein in the development of heart and circulatory disease, we need to consider the relative balance of yin and yang in the nutrients that are absorbed into our bodies. Minerals are classified as very yang because they are comparatively small, hard, and dense in structure (put a pinch of salt on your tongue and your tongue will contract). Complex carbohydrates are metabolized gradually in the digestive tract and fall in the center of the yin/yang spectrum. Complex carbohydrates are found primarily in whole grains, beans, vegetables, sea vegetables, and seasonal fruit, and their energy is generally balanced. Refined carbohydrates, including white sugar and white flour, are more yin in structure since the compact parts of the original plant, such as the germ, are removed in processing. Protein is also more yin in structure, and at the far end of the yin scale fall fat, oil, and other lipids, including cholesterol. Their molecules are relatively large, volatile, and soft and may be classified as extremely yin.

As we can see from this analysis, some food items contain both extreme yin and extreme yang nutrients. Red meat, for instance, is high in sodium and other yang minerals as well as large amounts of protein, saturated fat, and dietary cholesterol, which are highly yin. In the arteries, it is the excessively yin factors—the fats and cholesterol—that initially accumulate, impeding the flow of blood. The more yang nutrients in animal food—such as sodium and other minerals—then harden the fat and cholesterol as it builds up in the blood vessels. Thus, in the human body, food of animal origin breaks down into highly volatile yin and yang factors that can combine to create imbalance in the organs and tissues.

Within the lipid family, there are different subdivisions. Saturated fats are the most yang variety and make cells harder. Monounsaturated fats are less hard, and polyunsaturated fats are relatively soft. In addition to hardened fats from meat and dairy food, triglyceride (fatty acid) levels in the bloodstream, as we have seen, are elevated by the consumption of cane sugar (sucrose), fruit sugar (fructose), dairy sugar (lactose), white flour, alcohol, and other excessively yin substances. Glucose, the end result of metabolized sugar, changes to fatty acid in the liver when it exceeds the liver's regular storage capacity as glycogen, and in the bloodstream where it is neutralized by insulin glucose is easily converted to hardened fat. Elevated triglycerides in the blood are associated with about a 30 percent higher risk of death from cardiovascular disease.

Because of increased public awareness of the connection between cholesterol, saturated fat, and heart disease, many people have increased their consumption of polyunsaturated fats and oils, including vegetable cooking oils, mayonnaise, corn or soy margarines, salad dressings, and artificial creamers and spreads. These unsaturated fats, however, appear to redistribute cholesterol from the blood to the tissues and combine with oxygen to form free radicals. These are unstable and highly reactive substances that can interact with proteins and cause the loss of elasticity in artery walls and general weakening of cells and tissues. In cancer studies, researchers have found that unsaturated fats and oils actually enhance tumor development at a slightly higher rate than do saturated lipids.[7] In addition, some of these refined polyunsaturated products, especially margarine, nut butters, potato chips, and other fried foods, are hydrogenated in order to allow the oils they contain to remain solid at room temperature. Hydrogenation changes the molecular structure of the oils, saturating the fatty acids to varying degrees and making the oil harder.

Whole grains, beans, and seeds also contain polyunsaturated fats and oils, but they are naturally balanced by the right proportion of other nutrients, including vitamin E and selenium, which are lost in the refining process. Similarly, unrefined vegetable cooking oils, such as naturally processed dark sesame seed oil, retain the vitamin E and other nutrients that make them a balanced food product. If used in small to moderate volume, unrefined vegetable cooking oils will contribute to smooth metabolism, make arteries more flexible, provide lubrication, and generally harmonize the heart and circulatory functions.

As saturated fat and dietary cholesterol become deposited in the arteries, sodium from salt and other minerals in the bloodstream accumulate, making arteries even harder. This is a good example of the attraction of yin and yang. In the arteries, yin deposits of fat and cholesterol are covered and filled in by yang fibrous tissue and calcium. In turn, more fat and cholesterol gravitate to these mineral deposits, so that excessive yin and yang substances continually combine and interact to progressively harden and narrow the vessels.

Yin and yang can also help us understand the role of the various types of cholesterol. As we saw, the two basic types of lipoproteins are Low Density Lipoprotein (LDL), containing about two-thirds cholesterol and one-third fat and protein, and High Density Lipoprotein (HDL), containing proportionately more protein and lesser amounts of fat and cholesterol. LDL is strongly associated with atherosclerotic plaque formation, while HDL is associated with lowering total serum cholesterol levels in the body, especially LDL cholesterol.

From a yin/yang perspective, HDL is the more yang form of cholesterol because it is physically smaller and contains the most protein, which is less yin in quality than fat and cholesterol. About 90 percent of the cholesterol in atheromata is of the LDL type. Medical tests indicate that the higher the HDL in the blood, the lower the total serum cholesterol. While the precise mechanism is still unclear, HDL appears to pick up LDL in the arteries and initiate a process that brings it back to the liver for disposal through regular eliminatory channels.[8] We may say that HDL, the more yang lipoprotein, serves to neutralize or balance LDL, the more yin, and is another example of the body's natural capacity to adjust itself and eliminate excess.

Over the last decade or two, it has been discovered that a diet high in whole grains and vegetables raised HDL levels in the blood. These findings provoked a flurry of experiments to ascertain the possible reversibility of atherosclerosis, which until then had been generally considered irreversible. Studies have shown that in most animals with 90 percent of their blood vessels blocked by fatty deposits and scar tissue, 80 percent of the lesions will disappear in about four years if low-fat diets are substituted and serum cholesterol is reduced to 150 mg dl or lower.[9] Case-control studies on human heart patients with advanced atherosclerosis are beginning to show similar results, and the reversibility of coronary heart disease by dietary methods is now gradually being accepted by the medical community.[10]

THE PROTEIN CONTROVERSY

While most researchers and physicians agree on the the role of saturated fat and cholesterol in increasing the risk of coronary heart disease, the influence of protein in the atherosclerotic process is still debatable. As early as 1923, laboratory studies showed that rabbits fed beef containing 36 percent protein developed lesions in two to three months, while those fed beef with 27 percent protein did not get lesions for 11 months.[11] In the 1940s, investigators found that rabbits fed on a high-protein diet from dairy sources developed atherosclerotic plaque, while those fed on a high-protein diet from soybean sources did not form deposits.[12] Subsequent studies also showed that in many animal species animal-quality protein from beef, egg yolk, and milk elevated serum cholesterol levels, but vegetable proteins such as soy, wheat, and sunflower did not.

In human beings, however, the results of protein modification were less conclusive. Some studies suggested a similar effect as in animals, while others showed no such effect. In the early 1980s, Drs. Sacks and Kass and colleagues at Channing Laboratory, Brigham and Women's Hospital, Harvard Medical School, and Children's Hospital Medical Center in Boston decided to test the effects of different amounts and types of protein on members of the macrobiotic community. A test group ultimately consisting of thirteen macrobiotic students from the Kushi Institute and related organizations were given 27 grams of cascin (the main protein in dairy food) a day for a period of 20 days. The casein amounted to the equivalent of 1.1 liters of skim milk, about twice the daily average American intake. After the initial period, the test subjects were given 27 grams a day of soy protein isolate for an additional 20 days. No other animal protein was consumed during the study period, and the protein additives were cooked either in muffins or oatmeal.

In their report in the *Journal of Lipid Research* in 1983, the investigators noted that they observed no significant differences in the effects of the two proteins on the levels of cholesterol in the blood or in different types of lipoproteins, including LDL and HDL.[13] The conclusion seemed to suggest that the protein in non-fat dairy products was not an independent risk factor. However, as the final report noted, "There is no way of knowing whether the [macrobiotic] diet of the subjects somehow protected them from the possible effects of the protein supplements."[14]

In Canada, K. K. Carroll, an internationally noted heart disease and cancer researcher, has concluded from epidemiological studies that animal-quality protein is a major factor in the development of heart disease:

> Epidemiological data derived from human populations show that the positive correlation between animal protein in the diet and mortality from coronary heart disease is at least as strong as that between dietary fat and heart disease. . . . The trend toward increasing mortality from coronary heart disease in the United States during this century coincides with a doubling in the ratio of animal protein to vegetable protein in the diet. . . .[15]

Carroll speculates that vegetable protein reduces total cholesterol by reducing the absorption of cholesterol from the intestines into the bloodstream. One of the benefits of fiber in whole grains and vegetables is that it increases the body's ability to excrete bile acids, which are made from cholesterol. From a yin/yang point of view, vegetable protein is more centrally balanced than animal protein and contributes to more flexible maintenance and growth of body cells and tissues.

How do we account for the difference between the epidemiological data and the clinical evidence? From a holistic perspective, the often contradictory results of modern medical research can be explained by looking at the balance of energy as a whole rather than just one fragment of the equation. In *The Cancer-Prevention*

Diet we devoted a chapter to the limits of the scientific method, showing that by measuring only one isolated element or nutrient the exact opposite effect could often result as excess yin or yang energy turned into its opposite.[16]

Because modern experimental science is based on looking at matter as substance rather than as energy, it is forced to look at ever smaller substances to explain behavior rather than examine the overall balance of energy. For example, in the field of heart disease research, while most studies have shown that consumption of saturated fat and dietary cholesterol increases the risk of coronary disease, there are a few exceptions. The Masai of Africa and a few other tribes eat proportionately more animal food than most other traditional societies yet have low rates of heart problems. Contradictions such as this have led scientists to differentiate among HDL, LDL, and other types of cholesterol. However, once again a few studies do not fit the general pattern. For example, the Tarahumara Indians have much lower levels of HDL, the generally protective cholesterol, and much higher triglyceride levels than are expected for a group with a complete absence of heart disease.[17] The lipoproteins in turn have been broken down into further subcategories in the search for the specific component that may be responsible for elevating risk.

In the field of cancer research, the search has reached infinitesimally small levels as the focus has shifted from systems, functions, and organs to the nucleus of the affected cells, the DNA in the nucleus, the chromosomes that make up the DNA, the chemical elements that make up the chromosomes, and so forth, to ever more refined levels.

The whole, of course, is more than the sum of its parts, and it is the whole that is left out of such scientific pursuits. Moreover, the nutrients, vitamins, and minerals in our bodies are not the same as those synthesized in a test tube. In any experiment, we must look at the overall balance and quality of all the factors rather than a single determinant or a constant variable. Several research groups are beginning to do this. In the Ireland-Boston Diet-Heart Study, Lawrence Kushi, Professor Fredrick J. Stare, M.D., and other co-workers noted that "while risk of coronary heart disease has been reported to be related to intake of dietary lipids, an equally consistent finding has been the [inverse] relationship with starch and complex carbohydrates."[18] They noted that during the period from 1909 to 1976, the rise in heart disease among the American people appears to be more closely associated with a sharp decrease in the consumption of grains, vegetables, and other high carbohydrate foods (excluding sugar) than with a modest rise in dietary fat and cholesterol intake.

In another recent protein study, the *American Journal of Clinical Nutrition* reported in the summer of 1984 that the substitution of vegetable-quality protein for animal-quality protein in the diet for the first time significantly affected cholesterol metabolism in clinical tests on human beings.[19] The researchers noted that their study was something of a scientific landmark because it involved feeding subjects food prepared from whole soybeans rather than soy protein isolate, as has been commonly used in earlier experiments such as the Harvard test, which showed no significant effect.

Thus, in evaluating the effects of the foods we eat, we must weigh the energy and quality of all factors together. It is not enough to look just at fat or cholesterol consumption, components of cholesterol, triglyceride levels, blood pressure levels, amount and type of protein, salt intake, or other independent variables. We must look at the overall balance of yin and yang energy together and come to a determination that reflects the whole.

BALANCING ENERGY

In this chapter, we have seen that some nutrients, including animal salts, minerals, animal protein, cholesterol, saturated fat, refined polyunsaturated fat and oils, and simple sugars, when taken in excess, contribute to imbalance and the development of abnormal blood circulation, high blood pressure, and atherosclerosis. Over time, as imbalance progresses, soft turns to hard, porous turns to dense, and strong turns to weak. Predominantly yin factors such as leukocytes and macrophage foam cells, fat, cholesterol, and protein combine and interact with relatively yang factors such as blood platelets, sodium, calcium, and other minerals to weaken the circulatory system and eventually cause the heart to stop beating.

The eternal play of opposites, however, governs health as well as sickness. Heart disease is now known to be not only a disease of old age but also a condition that begins at birth and progressively develops during childhood, adolescence, and early adulthood into middle life and beyond. High blood pressure and atherosclerosis, once thought to be irreversible, are increasingly recognized to be both preventable and curable. By balancing centripetal and centrifugal energies in the daily selection and preparation of our food, as well as balancing our activity, thinking, feelings, and way of life, we can set ourselves free from disease, stress, and worry. By unifying yin and yang in our heart, we harmonize with the universal rhythms of nature and the cosmos.

11

Evaluating the Heart Naturally

Modern medicine has developed many methods to diagnose the heart. These range from simple lab tests for measuring blood pressure and cholesterol levels to more detailed electrocardiograms (EKGs) of the heart's activity to very intricate coronary arteriography. In some cases, heart tests are highly accurate and can locate precisely the obstruction, weakness, or other irregularity. In other cases, these diagnostic methods give misleading results. It is well known, for example, that the electrocardiogram may register normal for someone with known heart disease, while in some healthy persons it may indicate the presence of abnormalities. For angina pectoris, moreover, there may be no special electrocardiogram pattern of unusual activity. Exercise testing on the treadmill may also be subject to error. Cardiologists are increasingly concerned about the hazards of some of the more invasive methods and are seeking to limit their application.

The expense of some of these techniques has also been questioned. Coronary arteriography, including doctors' fees, lab tests, and an overnight stay in the hospital, costs about $2,000 and is thus not available to everyone. Finally, despite the introduction of these new methods, the art of detection appears to have steadily declined over the last fifty years rather than improved as might be expected. The *Journal of the American Medical Association* reported that in one long-term hospital survey medical examiners found that in 1938 65 percent of heart attacks had been correctly diagnosed as shown by subsequent autopsies on patients who died. By the early 1980s this figure had fallen to 53 percent.[1]

Studies such as this remind us that the advanced technology at our disposal depends upon the consciousness and health of those who use it. The results of X-rays, EKGs, and angiograms must still be interpreted by individual technicians and physicians. Unless their own condition, judgment, and experience are sound enough, errors may arise. Even relatively simple procedures, such as taking blood pressure, are susceptible to wide fluctuations depending upon who is administering the tests and in what setting. In a recent Italian study, forty-seven of forty-eight subjects showed a rise, often pronounced, in blood pressure stimulated by the arrival of the doctor. In some cases, the physician's presence even caused tachycardia, an abnormally rapid heartbeat.[2]

In comparison with some other forms of modern diagnosis, such as biopsies and CAT scans, heart tests are generally less invasive and less dangerous. However, the more complex heart procedures are potentially life-threatening and may result in the condition they are designed to prevent. X-rays, computers, and nuclear technology allow us to look into the inner workings of our hearts. However, they cannot measure the quality of our minds, which ultimately must interpret all the gathered data and come to a determination.

PHYSIOGNOMY

One of the universal features of modern life is our declining ability to evaluate our own health without recourse to complex, expensive, and often dangerous techniques. In past eras, health and well-being were evaluated on the basis of more qualitative considerations through direct observation or other simple methods. All aspects of life, including mental, emotional, and spiritual tendencies, were seen as interrelated. The traditional educator could identify potential problems and offer practical dietary and lifestyle suggestions to correct the imbalance long before visible symptoms of illness appeared.

The principal tool of macrobiotic evaluation is physiognomy, which the *Oxford English Dictionary* defines as "the art of judging character and disposition from the features of the face or the form and lineaments of the body generally." Physiognomy is based on understanding the dynamic relationship between complementary and antagonistic structures and functions within the body and psyche. During embryonic development, all major systems—the digestive, circulatory, and nervous—gather and form the entire facial structure. As the fetus grows, the upper and lower parts of the body undergo parallel development, as do the inner and outer parts, the harder and softer parts, and the more expanded and more contracted parts. After birth and in later life, each area of the face corresponds with an inner organ and its functions, as well as emotions and character traits associated with the underlying physiological condition. When an internal organ or system is imbalanced, symptoms of disorder will appear on the face as well.

Prior to the beginning of the Industrial Revolution, the art of physiognomy was well developed in both East and West. In the Bible, for example, we read:

> Yet you can tell a man by his looks
> and recognize good sense at first sight.
> A man's clothes and the way he laughs
> and his gait reveal his character.
> —Ecclesiasticus 19:29–30

Shakespeare makes extensive use of face reading in almost all his works to delineate character and show the underlying unity of mind and body. In *Measure for Measure*, the Duke says to the Provost:

There is written in your brow, provost, honesty and constancy:
if I read it not truly, my ancient skill beguiles me.

(4.2.154–55)

In the poem "The Rape of Lucrece," we read:

> In Ajax and Ulysses, O, what art
> Of physiognomy might one behold!
> The face of either cipher'd either's heart;
> Their face their manners most expressly told:
> In Ajax' eyes blunt rage and rigour roll'd;

But the mild glance that sly Ulysses lent
Show'd deep regard and smiling government.
(lines 1394–1400)

Today as members of modern society, we have largely lost the ability to recognize health and good sense at first sight. We place our trust in X-rays and angiograms rather than our own perception and judgment. We can no longer tell at a glance whether someone is generally well or seriously sick. As a result, we tend to perceive everyone as potentially ill, disturbed, or hostile, and our fear and mistrust of one another contributes to even more sickness and social disorder. Finally, we perceive the whole universe as chaotic, random, and meaningless and create an educational system, scientific method, and foreign policy to support our separation from the natural world.

FACIAL COLOR AND THE HEART

To evaluate the condition of the heart, we need look only at our own faces and hands, listen to our voice, observe our body movements, and reflect on our way of thinking and eating. The first thing we generally observe in visual evaluation is overall facial color. The color of the skin is different in every person. There are also commonly known differences in skin color among persons of different racial and ethnic backgrounds: white for Caucasians, darker for Latins, yellow for Orientals, coppery for Middle Easterners, brown for East Indians and Central and South Americans, dark or black for Africans, and blue-black for native Australians. However, these differences in skin color are not primarily racial, since skin color is the result of the influence of the external environment and internal conditions and nourishment. The principles of skin color can be summarized as follows: (1) a colder and cloudier climate produces lighter skin, and a warmer and sunnier climate produces darker skin; and (2) animal foods, salt, and hard baked goods, as well as stronger cooking, produce lighter skin, while fruits, sweets, and fluids, as well as lighter cooking or raw foods, produce darker skin.

For example, people living in Africa develop a dark or black skin color due to the warm climate and to the consumption of such foods as tapioca, yams, bananas, and other expansive tropical foods. Their color tends to change if they move to North America or Europe and consume more animal products, including dairy foods. Among Asians it is well known that their skin color tends to change toward white if they move to a more snowy region and consume saltier foods that are cooked for a longer time. A colder climate and large amounts of dairy food create the distinctive pale and creamy complexion of the Scandinavians.

Aside from these natural skin colors, many abnormal colors may appear because of disorders in the physical condition. An overly expanded heart is usually accompanied by a reddish color to the face. Except in cold weather or when blushing, when this color naturally arises, a red face shows that the heart and circulatory system are overworked and expanded, causing irregularities in the blood pressure and a tendency toward hypertension. The redness results from expansion of blood capillaries beneath the skin toward the surface. Often accompanied by a puffy, swollen appearance, redness of the face indicates that the heart muscle is expanded and loosened from excessive intake of excessively relaxing substances, including sugar, fruit, salads, spices, and white flour, along with the overconsumption of fluid, including coffee and alcohol.

After many years of dietary abuse, the red color of the face may change to purple. This color is an indication of a dangerous overexpansion of the heart muscle and of the low blood pressure that often follows. Persons with this color, especially on the tip of the nose, face the possibility of a sudden heart attack or stroke. If the face is pale, the heart has become very tight from overconsumption of excessive contractive foods including meat, dairy food, and refined salt.

Other abnormal colors may appear on the face, the hands, or other surface areas of the body. A yellow hue or patches often indicates bile, liver, or gallbladder disorders. Milky or grey white indicates lung, lymphatic, or spleen troubles. Blue may accompany liver problems, brown and dark shades signify kidney ailments, and green is a sign of developing cysts, tumors, or cancer. Because sickness may take many different forms, more than one color or a blend of colors will sometimes appear. Normal healthy skin should be clear and pinkish or with a light touch of natural color, and should be smooth, slightly shining, and slightly moist but not wet to the touch.

NOSE AND HEART

After checking overall facial color for sign of developing heart disease, we can determine in more detail the condition of the heart by examining the nose. Located in the center of the face, the nose develops parallel to the heart, which is located in the center of the chest region. At the beginning of the second month of fetal development, the nose consists of two shallow pits of specialized skin that overlie the front end of the brain. The nasal pits deepen during the second month to form the nasal cavities. They are originally located far out on either side of the face but through a gradual process of contraction grow closer together until they are enclosed in the ridge of tissue that becomes the nose. A similar contracting process takes place in the heart, which begins as two separate tubes that fuse into a single organ. By the end of the second month, the embryonic nose has a broad, flat shape, with the nostrils pointing forward. The heart also changes from a simple bent tube to the normal adult form with four internal chambers—two atria and two ventricles—separated by partitions known as septa.

Like the heart, the nose is a central meeting place of the respiratory, circulatory, and nervous systems. After birth, when the embryonic organs have reached maturity, swellings, hardness, discolorations, and other irregularities of the nose indicate corresponding irregularities of the heart. The shape and size of the nose are primarily determined in the fetal stage, reflecting the biological quality of the ancestors and parents, and especially the mother's way of eating during pregnancy. After birth, the condition of the nose is significantly affected by the individual's way of life and especially of eating. In traditional Oriental diagnosis, the specific shape of the nose indicates corresponding physical and mental conditions (see Figure 12).

A *normal, well-formed nose*, displaying average length and roundness, shows a balanced mental and physical condition, including the heart and circulatory system. As a result of climate,

Figure 12. Various Forms of the Nose

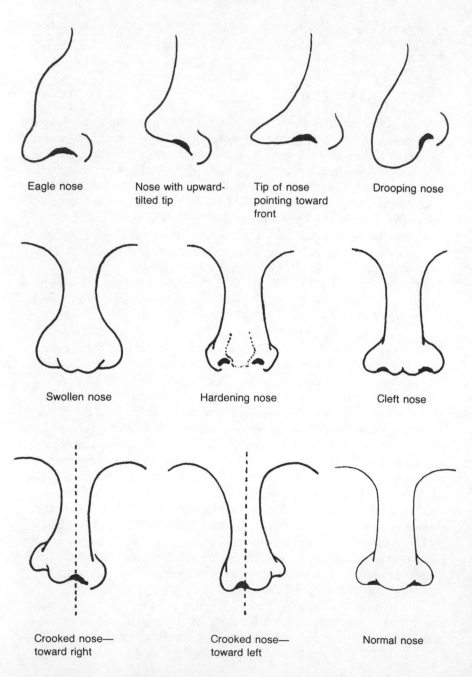

Eagle nose

Nose with upward-tilted tip

Tip of nose pointing toward front

Drooping nose

Swollen nose

Hardening nose

Cleft nose

Crooked nose—toward right

Crooked nose—toward left

Normal nose

diet, and other environmental factors, the shape of healthy noses will vary somewhat geographically tending toward a broader, flatter nose in the tropics, the Orient, and among other traditional societies and a narrower, raised nose in North America and Europe.

A *high, rounded nose*, sometimes called an eagle nose, is caused by the consumption of much poultry, including eggs, resulting in a tendency to be aggressive, self-centered, and restless. This shape indicates the development of atherosclerosis and the accumulation of layers of fat around the heart muscle.

A nose with an *upward-tilted tip* results from an excessive intake of animal food, especially fish and seafood, during the time of the mother's pregnancy, causing a tendency toward sharpness in thinking, as well as narrowness and shortsightedness. There is a tendency toward hardening of the arteries, especially if animal food is consumed regularly in childhood and in later life.

A *pointed nose* whose tip points toward the front like Pinocchio's is caused by the overconsumption of certain kinds of fruit, including melons and berries, resulting in weakness of the heart and an excitable nervous condition.

A *drooping nose* is caused by an excessive consumption of fruits and salad, as well as liquid and sweets, resulting in weakness of the heart as well as kidneys and bladder functions.

A *swollen nose*, caused by the excessive intake of sugar, fluid, fruits, and some vegetables of tropical origin, as well as excess animal fats and oils, indicates that both the circulatory and excretory systems are in disorder. A swollen nose indicates a swollen, overworked heart and circulatory system laboring to provide oxygen to cells and tissues. The swelling results from a combination of the overconsumption of meat, poultry, or eggs and of soft drinks, juice, sugar, coffee, and other fluids. Liquid is retained in the body because of excessive salt and mineral intake, primarily from animal sources. A swollen nose is often a sign of developing congestive heart failure.

A *nose with a hardened tip* is caused by the intake of excessive saturated fat and cholesterol from such foods as beef, pork, poultry, eggs, cheese, and other dairy products. This results in hardening of the arteries and muscles and the accumulation of fat around the heart and other major compacted organs, including the liver, kidneys, spleen, and prostate or ovaries. Together with the swollen condition described above, this hardening of the end of the nose is a sign that a heart attack or stroke may occur.

A *cleft nose* is caused by nutritional imbalance, especially a shortage of minerals and complex carbohydrates during the fetal stage and childhood development. This split or indentation at the tip of the nose can also be produced in childhood or later life by an excessive intake of simple sugars such as fruits, juices, sucrose, or honey, as well as soft drinks, all of which deprive the body of minerals and complex sugars. A cleft nose indicates that the heart is beating irregularly or murmuring. This type of nose is becoming more common among modern people.

A *crooked nose* indicates a general imbalance in the mental and physical constitution as a result of ancestral or parental disharmony. A nose bending toward the person's left shows that the left side of the body, including the left atrium and ventricle of the heart, the left lung, the left kidney, the descending colon, and the left ovary or testicle, are stronger and more tolerant of stress and abuse than the organs on the right side. Generally, this constitution shows that the father's hereditary factors or influence were stronger. A nose bending toward the right shows more activity in the right chambers of the heart and other organs on the right side of the body. In this case, the mother's hereditary factors or influence on the person's development were usually stronger.

Sometimes these conditions overlap. For example, a swollen nose can be either hard or soft. Within each category, there are many degrees of imbalance, from slight to very serious. In general, the right side of the nose corresponds with the right side of the heart and the left side with the left side of the heart. The bulb of the nose reflects the heart muscle as a whole. The upper bulbous region shows the atria and the lower region the ventricles. The tip generally corresponds with the coronary arteries that nourish the heart itself. The nostrils show the condition of the lungs and pulmonary vessels.

Pimples and patches on the nose also show circulatory disorders, and their location on the nose corresponds to their location in the heart. Yellow-white pimples or patches represent the discharge of excessive animal fat, especially dairy products. In this case, the digestive and excretory functions are also in disorder. Red or dark spots appearing on the nose show the discharge of excessive sugar, including refined sugar, honey, and fruit sugar.

In this case, the excretory and circulatory functions are also in disorder. These spots show that deposits of fat and cholesterol are accumulating in and around the heart and the coronary vessels.

Nasal irregularities may accompany serious heart conditions. For example, Barney Clark, the world's first artificial heart recipient, suffered moderate to severe nosebleeds following his operation. "Dr. Clark's nosebleeds are considered more serious than previously stated simply because they have not stopped," a Utah Medical Center spokesperson explained during one nosebleeding bout that lasted eight days.[3] The nosebleeding might have been enhanced by anticoagulants given to Clark to prevent general blood clotting in his body. However, removal of the natural heart probably had an underlying weakening effect on the nose.

In another first, the *Boston Globe* reported that a husband and wife had had identical triple coronary bypass operations at a local hospital there. From the photograph published with the article, it is interesting to observe the similarity between the couple's facial features. The noses are almost indistinguishable. After eating the same foods together, many husbands and wives, as well as other family members and even family pets, begin to look alike and to think and act alike. (An estimated 30 percent of all dogs in the U.S., and up to 75 percent of older dogs, have heart disease, according to veterinarians.) In this case, the pair with the twin triple bypass operation had been married for forty-two years.[4]

In another news clipping, a California doctor told an American Heart Association meeting that snoring had been identified as a high-risk factor in the development of high blood pressure and could lead to potentially life-threatening irregularities in the heartbeat.[5] Snoring or making snorting noises through the nose and mouth while sleeping can block temporarily the airways in the throat, shutting off breathing for up to three minutes. In response to this emergency, the autonomic nervous system increases blood pressure to circulate blood faster and provide oxygen to inhibited organs and tissues. For those with already elevated blood pressure or weakened hearts, the strain can result in heart rhythm disturbances and possibly sudden cardiac arrest. The doctor went on to recommend a new form of throat surgery for some snorers at high risk. According to traditional Oriental medicine and macrobiotic understanding, snoring is caused primarily by the overconsumption of liquids. Items such as milk, fruit juice, alcohol, and coffee expand and loosen the uvula in the back of the throat as well as the tissues of the mouth cavity, causing them to vibrate excessively. These fluids also contribute to the development of mucus in the nose and sinus cavities, which can obstruct breathing through the nasal passages. Snoring can be relieved very quickly by controlling liquid intake.

THE FACE AS A WHOLE

For a more magnified view of the heart and the regions affected, we can look at the face as a whole (see Figure 13). Areas A and B in the diagram correspond to the right and left sides of the face. The incoming flow of blood from the body to the right side of the heart is correlated with the canal from the outer right ear in toward the inner right ear (area x). The incoming flow of blood from the lungs to the left side of the heart is correlated with the

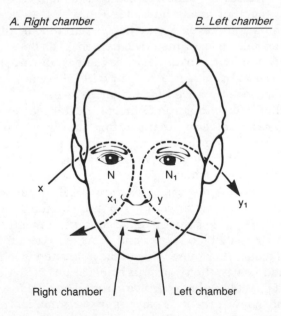

Figure 13. Diagnosis of the Heart in the Face

left nostril and nasal passage. The size of the ear's opening represents the size of the superior and inferior vena cavae carrying blood to the right side of the heart. If mucus or liquid is accumulating in that area of the ear, similar accumulations are taking place in the corresponding area of the heart. Similarly, if mucus occurs in the left nostril or nasal passage, accumulations arc also taking place in the region of the heart that corresponds to area y. The right nasal passage and the left ear canal, areas x_1 and y_1, correspond, respectively, to the flow of blood from the heart to the lungs via the pulmonary vein and from the heart to the body via the aorta.

The heart valves correspond to the eyes, as indicated by areas N and N_1 in Figure 13. For good strong heart functions, these valves should be tight and strong. If the eyes become weak and watery, with frequent blinking, then those valves are becoming loosened. If the eyes are swollen and red, some swelling or light inflammation is occurring in the corresponding valves. If the eyes are discharging mucus, mucus is also accumulating around the valves. If the eyes are narrowed or tend to be partly shut, the valves are becoming too tight and pressure is building in the corresponding heart chamber.

THE MOUTH AND SPEECH

The general condition of the right and left chambers of the heart can further be seen in the mouth. If the right side of the mouth is more swollen or loose, this reflects a similar condition in the right chamber. The same applies to the left. If the mouth as a whole is becoming swollen and loose, the entire heart is becoming loose and weak. To ascertain the condition of the heart rhythm and the balance between the two chambers, we can examine how well the two sides of the mouth coordinate when the person is speaking and the degree of balance or imbalance of the two sides while the mouth is at rest.

The activity of the heart can also be determined by listening to the person's voice or manner of expression. A very excitable or talkative individual often has an expanded, overactive heart. The sound of the voice tells us what kind of life the person is leading and the types of food being eaten. Salty foods, dry foods, and refined carbohydrates make the pitch of the voice higher and faster, while fatty and oily foods, dairy products, and excessive liquids make it lower and slower.

By listening to the resonance of the voice, we can tell where there is any blockage or inflexibility in the body, for even though sounds are produced in the throat, they vibrate different organs. This is why in ancient times chanting was used to harmonize the body and mind. Figure 14 illustrates some of the basic sounds and the areas they vibrate.

Sounds are more closed at the top of the body and become more open as we move down the body. (Notice how traditional chants and greetings such as Aum (Om), Amen, and Shalom harmonize all regions of the body and mind.) Once we understand how sound originates and develops, we can hear in which areas of the body the voice is vibrating or not vibrating. This tells us where there are deposits of fat and cholesterol. For example, people who either exaggerate or drop their *o*'s and *u*'s—the more rounded whole vowels corresponding to the heart region—have a tendency to develop cardiovascular disorders.

Speech difficulties, such as stuttering, stammering, and lisping, are also indications of underlying cardiac problems. Stuttering often shows a heart murmur, hyperactive heartbeat, or other irregular rhythm. Slow stammering speech shows a tired, overworked heart and disturbances in the electrical impulses that acti-

Figure 14. Sounds Resonating in the Body

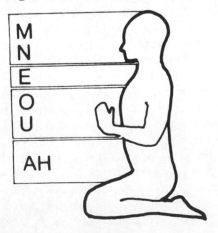

vate the heartbeat. False starts and stops in speech also may show skipped or missed beats. Speaking rapidly or falling over words shows a hyperactive heart and a tendency to develop high blood pressure. People in regions where spices, sugar, and oily food are frequently consumed often talk faster than people in regions where these foods are consumed less frequently. Slow speech is more a kidney problem than a heart problem, signifying loose and overactive kidneys. This condition, however, often combines with heart problems to produce a watery voice or streaming manner of expression, indicating excess liquid retention, overworked kidneys, and an enlarged heart.

By developing our listening ability, we can generally determine the condition of a person's heart and other internal organs. Even if we are not physically in their presence, we can often gauge fairly accurately their condition by listening to their voice on the telephone. Thus the proverbial expression of "the heart leaping into the mouth" has an underlying biological foundation.

HUMOR AND THE HEART

Excessive laughter, giggling, and humor often indicate a swollen, overactive heart. This tendency results from overconsumption of items such as sugar, sweets, fruit, juices, salad, tropical foods, coffee, stimulants, or alcohol, usually in combination with meat, poultry, dairy food, and eggs. In general, as the saying goes, laughter is good medicine. A healthy sense of humor is essential to living an active and happy life and for enduring times of adversity and sickness. However, in traditional Oriental medical diagnosis, excessive laughter, especially to the point of hysteria, is considered a telltale sign of a weakened heart.

Interestingly, the word *humor* comes from the four humors, or nutritive fluids, of traditional Western philosophy and medicine. A person was said to be "in good humor" when the four humors in the body were balanced. A person was "in bad humor" when there was an excess or deficiency of one of the humors. In Chapter 29, we shall look at the doctrine of humors more closely, though here it may be noted that environmental factors, especially daily food, were traditionally believed to give rise to the four fluids and influence the course of their development.

The word *humor*, which comes from the same root as *humidity*, signifying retention of a large amount of water or water vapor, has survived to modern times as a synonym for the comic or amusing. The ability to provoke laughter with a good joke is based primarily on the art of exaggeration. Listen closely to a good comedian and you will see that his or her technique involves hyperbole and overstatement. Our idioms for humorous anecdotes reflect this tendency: a tall tale, a big fish story, or a whopper. The cardiovascular counterpart to "wagging the tongue" and "pulling the leg" is "expanding the heart." In some cases, however, understatement is employed to produce a laugh. This pithy, dry sense of humor appeals to inhabitants of more northern climates, such as Scandinavia and parts of Great Britain, where there is a sparser natural environment and a higher intake of salted food, dry baked goods, and animal food.

THE HANDS AND THE HEART

The condition of the heart can further be diagnosed by examining the hands, which is a good way to confirm initial observations of the nose, the face as a whole, and the voice. In the embryo stage, the heart begins to pulsate on about the twenty-fourth day. One day later, tiny arm buds appear, radiating directly from the chest region. These little buds spiral out to become shoulders, arms, hands, and fingers. At maturity the heart is about the same size and shape as the fist, with which it has grown in parallel development. The two open hands approximate the size and shape of each lung.

The left chamber of the heart corresponds to the left hand, while the right chamber corresponds to the right hand (see A and B in Figure 15). A reddish color often appears around the periphery of the hand along the thumb and fifth finger. The flow of blood through both chambers corresponds to this region. In the right hand, the flow of blood from body to heart corresponds to the top of the thumb (area y). Its circulation is traced along the periphery of the hand and out along the little finger (area y_1). In the left hand, the flow of blood from lungs to heart corresponds to the top of the little finger (area x), while the flow from heart to body corresponds to the top of the thumb (area x_1). (The arrows in the diagram show

Figure 15. Diagnosis of the Heart in the Hands

A. Left chamber   B. Right chamber

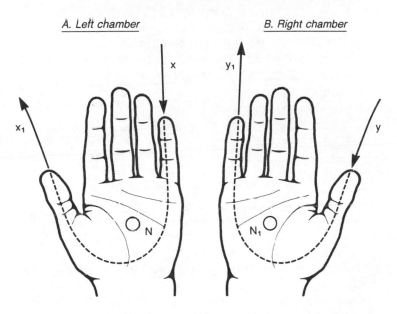

the direction of blood flow.) Any symptom appearing along this path is correlated with the corresponding region of blood flow in the heart. For example, a chipped or discolored nail on the thumb or on the fifth finger, or a dark discoloration in the fleshy part of the thumb, indicates stagnations within the flow of blood in the heart.

The condition of the two central valves between the atria and ventricles, marked N and N_1, appears directly in the center of each palm. If that area is swollen, expanded, or discolored or if the person experiences pain when that area is pressed, the corresponding tricuspid or mitral valve suffers from such problems as looseness, leaking, or weakness from excessive fluids or hardness and adhesive buildup from accumulations of fat and cholesterol.

The strength of the grip of each hand generally shows the strength of each chamber of the heart. A weak grip indicates general weakness or deficiency in the heart muscle, while an overpowering grip indicates high blood pressure and an overactive heart. High blood pressure and atherosclerosis may accompany either of these conditions. Shaking hands is an ideal opportunity to evaluate someone's heart and circulatory system.

A comparison of the two hands will further reveal how well the two chambers of the heart are coordinated and therefore how efficient the heart's activity is. In structural terms, if the size, shape, major lines on the palms, and other general features of the hands are very different, then the two chambers are very different. If the two hands work well together, the two chambers of the heart are in general harmony. If the two hands do not work together in a smoothly coordinated way, some irregularity of heartbeat may be present, and there will be a tendency for the emotions and the overall character to fluctuate between extremes rather than to be consistent, steady, and dependable. Such imbalance will also be reflected in all the various paired organs and functions, such as the two kidneys, the two lungs, the liver and spleen, the two halves of the brain, and the two sides of the face.

The complexion and temperature of the hands offers further indication of the condition of the heart. A reddish-pink shade or hot hands show an overactive heart, with a tendency toward high blood pressure. This condition results from an overconsumption of such items as sweets, sugar, fruit, juices, spices, or alcohol, usually in combination with some animal food. Pale hands indicate congested, underactive lungs. Cold, wet hands show an overly expanded heart weakened by long-term consumption of imbalanced foods and drinks, especially icy beverages and dairy foods. Cold, dry hands show contracted capillaries beneath the skin and in the heart as a result of too much salty animal food, refined flour, and hard baked goods.

Habitually keeping the hands in the back pockets often indicates deposits of fat and cholesterol in and around the heart muscle and small intestine. Keeping the hands in the front pockets may indicate stagnation and fatty buildup in the lungs and large intestine. Hands on the hips often show kidney and bladder disorders. Large hand gestures often indicate an overactive heart burdened from intake of too many spices, salt, tropical foods, liquid, or alcohol. Areas of the world where these foods are eaten frequently are especially known for this type of hand movement. Excessive gestures with the right hand often indicate liver problems, while those with the left hand indicate troubled spleen and pancreatic functions.

Unstable and uncoordinated body movements also show heart malfunctions. Jerky behavior; the inability to sit still or find a comfortable position; and frequent changes of residence, employment, or spouse or partner usually reflect irregular heart rhythms and developing heart disease.

A person with a rhythmic, relaxed heartbeat has calm, steady motions and even-handed gestures, a clear manner of expression, a well-modulated voice, and a simple, harmonious way of life.

THE PULSES, MERIDIANS, AND PRESSURE POINTS

The pulse may also be checked to evaluate the condition of the heart. In traditional Oriental medicine, there are three pairs of pulses on each wrist corresponding to the six pairs of internal organs and physiological functions. To feel the heart pulse, take the left wrist of a man or the right wrist of a woman. Placing your index, middle, and ring fingers lightly on the outside of the inner wrist just below the thumb, feel for the heart pulse with the finger nearest the base of the thumb (see Figure 16).

Feel for the deeper pulse in this location by slightly pressing the spot. This is the heart pulse. The superficial pulse in this spot is the small intestine pulse. Pulses felt with the other two fingers correspond with other organs and can be used to evaluate their condition. If the pulse is very strong, heavy, and rapid, the heart is laboring under elevated pressure and the arteries may be narrowed as a result of too much meat, poultry, dairy food, and refined salt. If the pulse is weak or fluttery, the heart is overly expanded or underactive from excessive consumption of sugar, oil, fruit, and liquids. Abnormally high or low blood pressure may also be present. A healthy pulse is calm, steady, and full, neither too rapid nor too slow. Evaluating the quality of the pulses takes some experience but can be learned fairly quickly.

The heart meridian, or channel of electromagnetic energy flow to and from the cardiac region, may also be checked for tension, tightness, and hardening or loosening of the heart. The heart meridian runs along the inside of each arm to the inside of the little finger. The meridians develop spirally in the embryonic stage and serve as channels for the flow of electromagnetic energy from the cosmos as well as rising energy from the spin of the Earth on its axis and its rotation around the sun. During a

Figure 16. Pulse Diagnosis

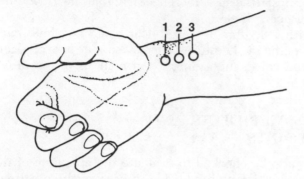

The heart pulse is felt in #1 position on the right wrist of a woman or the left wrist of a man.

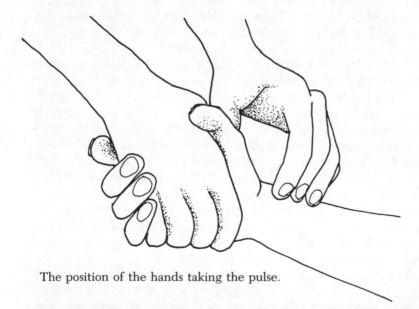

The position of the hands taking the pulse.

heart attack, pain is often felt running along this channel down the arms. Interestingly, in Coronary Pulmonary Resuscitation (CPR), practitioners are often taught to bite the nail of the little finger to stimulate the heart in case of heart attack, stroke, or sudden cardiac arrest. This location is the end of the heart meridian. While Western medicine has lost sight of the existence of internal energy flow through the body, it makes empirical use of pressure points along the meridians in many types of treatment, as this example shows.

To check the heart meridian, have the person raise his or her arm over the head and feel along the outside of the arm. A soft, flabby feeling along the heart meridian indicates a swollen congested heart, while a hard, stiff feeling indicates a contracted circulatory system and possible hardening of the arteries. A well-balanced meridian is firm but supple to the touch. The overall muscle tone is flexible and, when pressed, the muscle returns rapidly to its original shape.

The major pressure point for evaluating heart problems is located at the center of the breast bone about 1½ inches above the area where the sternum and rib cage meet. In traditional Oriental medicine, this point is called the Dan-shu. If you feel pain when you press firmly here, the heart is enlarged.

OTHER EVALUATIVE FACTORS

The condition of the feet can be used to evaluate the condition of the heart. For example, small square toenails are often a sign of developing heart troubles. The outermost ridge of the ears also reflects the condition of the circulatory system; redness here indicates a swollen and overactive heart. Sometimes fever or excessive sweating are signs of a hyperactive heart, while coldness or the inability to sweat show hypoactive circulatory functions. Cravings for burnt food, charcoal-broiled food, bread crusts, coffee and other stimulants, or alcohol all indicate the possibility of heart problems.

The time of day and season during which symptoms appear may also indicate cardiovascular disorders. According to traditional Oriental medicine, each pair of complementary and antagonistic organs is activated during a four-hour period of the day. In the case of the heart, the period of greatest stimulation occurs at midday, between about 10 A.M. and 2 P.M. Chest pains, cramps, lethargy, a feeling of unsettledness, hyperactivity, or other symptoms that arise during this time and subside at other times usually indicate heart and small intestine problems.

Similarly, heart problems are more common during the summer months than other times of the year. At this time, the sun's rays are directly overhead, and the kidney function, which is somewhat antagonistic to the heart, slows down. Water pressure builds up and the heart is forced to increase its output. Medical studies have shown that the peak period of heart attacks is about 1:30 P.M. and the month with the greatest number of attacks is July.[6] Fluctuating coronary activity is also related to the phases of the moon. During the full moon, the fluids in the body, like the tides, are increased, putting more stress on the heart. The incidence of physical and mental illness, as well as accidents and crime, all increase at this time, as most hospital emergency wards can attest.

Within the infinite order of the universe, we are infinitesimal. However, within each of us lives an infinite dream capable of infinite realization. The marvelous order that runs through creation includes patterns of unity and diversity, health and sickness, and the rise and fall of all phenomena from subatomic particles to far-distant galaxies, from individual lives and families to civilizations and epochs. Without any special equipment or training, we can understand this universal order with our own minds and hearts. This natural way of understanding is our birthright as free human beings and as citizens of the infinite universe.

12

Sex, Race, Genetics, and Smoking

While diet is the underlying cause of heart and circulatory disease, a variety of other factors are associated with its development. Coronary heart disease, for example, is much more prevalent among men than women, and high blood pressure is more common among blacks than whites. Heredity is often cited as a cause, and smoking is strongly linked with many forms of heart disease. Modern medicine has measured statistically the influence of these factors, but there is no consensus on the extent to which risk is increased, the physiological mechanisms involved, or the possible reciprocal relationship between these factors and diet. Traditional Oriental medicine may help clarify these relationships and enable us to look at multiple variables as part of a greater whole. In this chapter, we shall look at sexual, racial, and genetic influences on coronary heart disease, as well as the effect of cigarette smoking. In the following chapters, we shall look at the role of the emotions, stress, and physical activity.

SEX

Heart disease is strikingly higher among men than women. There are ten times as many heart attacks among men under forty-five than among women.[1] Between the ages of forty-five and sixty, the coronary heart disease rate among women rises dramatically, and the gap between the sexes is narrowed to 2 to 1.[2] After age sixty, the rate among men and women is about equal.

To understand why men are more susceptible to heart ailments than women, we need to look at the physiology of the two sexes. Traditionally, it is said that man represents Heaven and woman represents Earth. Consequently, the male body structure tends to be oriented by yang centripetal force, which comes from the distant galaxies and solar systems to the outer periphery of the atmosphere and spirals in toward the center of the Earth. In men, this force passes through the channel of electromagnetic energy, which runs from the central hair spiral on top of the head toward the penis. In the female body structure, centrifugal force expanding from the center of the Earth passes upward from the uterus and ovaries to the hair spiral on the head. Of course, both sexes receive both centripetal and centrifugal force, but in different degrees. In men, the predominance of Heaven's force produces a tall extended body, small breasts, sexual organs that are external and downward, and facial hair. In women, the expanding Earth's force passing through the body meets the incoming strong contractive force of Heaven, producing a short body, expanded breasts, sexual organs that are inward and upward, and abundant hair on the top of the head.

The relative influence of these two forces can be readily demonstrated by holding a pendulum over the hair spiral on the back of the head. Above men, the pendulum will generally begin rotating in a counterclockwise direction, showing the predominant influence of incoming celestial energy, while in women it will usually rotate in a clockwise direction, showing the predominant influence of upward terrestrial energy.

Traditionally, men and women ate the same or similar foods, although there were slight variations suitable for each sex. In addition to whole grains and vegetables, men ate an occasional side dish of fish or other animal food, more strongly cooked vegetables, and slightly more salt. These foods contributed to energy and strength and the more outward-directed physical, mental, and social activities produced by a yang constitution. Women naturally ate less animal food than men and more lightly cooked vegetables, more fruits, and desserts. These contributed to more developed emotional sensitivity, artistic expression, and a nurturing spirit.

In modern society, these natural tendencies have been taken

to unhealthful extremes. Among many men it is considered ideal to eat steak, ham and eggs, or other excessively yang foodstuffs at every meal. Conversely, many women subsist on cottage cheese, salads, fruit juice, milk chocolates, other sweets, and other excessively yin fare. In fact, there is so much chaos in the modern way of eating that either sex may go to either extreme. Boys and men may eat large amounts of dairy food, nut butters, raw vegetables, fruit, juices, and ice cream, while girls and women may consume large amounts of meat, poultry, eggs, cheese, and salt. Naturally, this tendency produces physical and psychological imbalance, and can lead to the breakdown of the family, which depends upon a harmonious interrelation among the sexes. Consumption of both extremes, such as meat and sugar, can also lead to wide swings in mood and perception, loss of center and direction, and the potential development of hostility, aggression, or withdrawal into a personal fantasy world.

Despite the overall imbalance in our modern way of eating, women are still comparatively healthier than men, living several years longer and suffering somewhat less from degenerative disease. This is because (1) women generally eat less total food in proportion to their size and weight, leading to more effective utilization of nutrients by the body; (2) women consume less animal food, including less saturated fat and cholesterol, which are the principal causes of heart disease and some forms of cancer; (3) women menstruate much of their lives, which provides an additional means of discharging excess accumulations in their body; (4) women are capable of giving birth and breastfeeding, which provide outlets for exchange of energy with the environment; (5) women are more in touch with their feelings than men, express their feelings better, and are more likely to adapt to their surroundings rather than trying to change them according to some philosophy or ideal; and (6) in most cases, women tend to assume responsibility for preparing daily food and bringing up children, putting them in closer touch with nature and the continuing spiral of life.

As a result of these tendencies, women are generally physically, emotionally, and mentally less chaotic than men. Their original, more yin constitutions and more loving nature predispose them to less illness, conflict, and stress. However, as women's consumption of animal food has risen in recent decades, accompanied by their entry into Type A high-pressure jobs, increased smoking, and reliance on more precooked meals and convenience foods, their rates of degenerative disease, especially cancer, have increased sharply. As the protective effects of menstruation and breastfeeding end in middle age, women's susceptibility to heart disease also dramatically increases. Younger women who have had hysterectomies or who take oral birth control pills, which interfere with the natural flow of energy in their body, have significantly higher rates of heart disease.[3] High blood pressure, generally a more yin form of cardiovascular disease, is experienced about equally by both women and men in all age groups.[4]

RACE

Black Americans, both male and female, have about a 10 percent higher incidence of high blood pressure than whites.[5] The reason for this is not racial but primarily dietary. "Soul food," the basis for eating still followed by many blacks in North America today, includes large quantities of inexpensive or scrap pork, such as necks, stomachs (hog maws), and intestines (chitterlings); sweet potatoes; and cornbread and greens cooked or laced with pork fat, lard, milk, eggs, butter, salt, sugar, or spices. This fatty, oily, greasy food is conducive to a variety of yin circulatory and blood disorders, including sickle-cell anemia, high blood pressure, and esophageal cancer.

Interestingly, soul food is not native to Africa but was developed in this country during slavery. As Dick Gregory explained in an interview with *East West Journal,* "For years we cooked for white folks, knew what they was eating. We would imitate pumpkin pie with sweet potatoes. We'd use salt to overcook everything to take the taint away, and then put the taste back in with more spices. Soul food is the worst food on the market. We [need to] return to a more natural way of eating."[6]

Today, as blacks have become more affluent, their consumption of beef and fattier forms of animal foods has increased, producing sharp rises in colon cancer, uterine and prostate cancer, atherosclerosis, and other contractive yang disorders. The traditional staples of Africa are sorghum and millet, and African cultures that still rely on these staples are free of heart disease and cancer. Blackeyed peas, butter beans, collards, mustard greens, turnip greens, and cornbread—derived from the American Indians—are still eaten by many blacks. As a complement to whole grains, these foods are very healthful, and everyone can benefit by incorporating them into their daily diet.[7]

GENETICS

Heart disease and cancer are often thought to be genetically caused. It is said that some people are genetically protected from or predisposed to disease. Population studies have largely disproved this theory. Researchers have found that people who migrate from societies low in degenerative disease to modern societies will attain the same rates of heart disease and cancer after one or two generations as they adopt the modern diet.[8] In the mid-1950s, pioneer heart disease researcher Ancel Keys wrote, "Granted that age and heredity may be final limiting factors, at least in some cases, there are compelling reasons to believe that for most of mankind the mode of life must, somehow, determine whether extensive and irreparable changes in the coronary arteries come early or late."[9]

However, some rare diseases still seem to be concentrated among members of the same family. For example, there is a form of chronically high serum cholesterol called *familial hypercholesterolemia* that appears to affect clusters of parents and children. To understand how this develops we need to consider both constitutional and conditional factors. Basically, the human physical and mental constitution at birth is derived from the biological quality of our parents, grandparents, and ancestors. Mental and physical influences from the mother, and especially her diet during pregnancy, are the single most important factor in our development. Constitutional traits include bone structure; muscle and skin condition; height; size of head, hands, and feet; and relative strength of the internal organs, including the heart. After birth, day-to-day, month-to-month, and year-to-year fluctuations in our health and vitality are referred to as conditional changes. These include changing skin quality, hair quality, voice and speech patterns, and the functioning of the internal organs, including the functioning of the heart.

After birth it is more difficult to alter one's inherited constitution than to alter one's condition. Yet within biological limits, there is considerable room for change, adaptation, and development. Many of the serious conditions described as genetic are correctable, at least to some degree. Whole foods can improve most of these conditions, and over time a natural way of life with the proper diet can modify even some constitutional traits. Thus, the degenerative process that has weakened the last several generations can gradually be reversed. In the future, children brought up on whole grains and vegetables will be far stronger than their parents, who may have stronger and better constitutions at their birth but abused them with poor-quality daily food and a more chaotic way of life.

Because families tend to eat together, it sometimes appears that they are suffering from the same hereditary illness. Even when the children grow up and leave home, they tend to eat in the same way and pass along the same imbalances to their children. Thus, diseases like hypercholesterolemia are not really genetically determined. What *is* passed along is the way of cooking. In the chapter on congenital heart defects in Part II, we will look at the embryological development of the heart and offer some dietary suggestions for constitutional weaknesses arising prior to birth.

SMOKING

Cigarette smoking, along with cholesterol and high blood pressure, is considered one of the three major risk factors in the development of heart disease. The Framingham Heart Study found that young and middle-aged men who smoked had from two to four times higher rates of coronary heart disease, sudden cardiac death, and peripheral vascular disease than nonsmokers. The effect on stroke and angina pectoris was slight. In women, they found no measurable relationship between smoking and heart disorders.[10] Combined with other factors, smoking sharply increases the risk of cardiovascular illnesses (see Table 22).

The subject of tobacco and its role in enhancing degenerative disease is also best understood in relation to daily diet. For centuries, North American native peoples have smoked tobacco without

Table 22. MULTIPLE FACTORS AND RISK OF HEART ATTACK AND STROKE

Factor	Risk of Heart Attack	Risk of Stroke
None	77	66
Cigarettes	120	100
Cigarettes and cholesterol	236	200
Cigarettes, cholesterol, and high blood pressure	348	700

Average risk = 100
Rates based on a 45-year-old man
Source: Framingham Heart Study

developing heart disease and have utilized the plant for medicinal purposes. One of the main differences between the Indians' use of tobacco and our own is that they observed a more natural way of life, including a balanced diet high in whole corn and corn products, wild rice and cereal grasses, flour made from acorns, locally grown or foraged vegetables, sea vegetables along coastal regions, fresh seasonable fruits, seeds and nuts, and a small to moderate amount of fresh fish, seafood, or wild game. Current medical studies show that in societies in Africa, Asia, and elsewhere where a traditional way of eating centered around whole grains and vegetables is still observed, there is no correlation between smoking and heart disease.[11] Nor is there a clear association between tobacco and lung cancer in these cultures.[12]

These findings suggest that cigarette smoking is not a substantial and primary risk factor in itself, but in conjunction with the modern diet will combine synergistically with saturated fat, cholesterol, and triglycerides to weaken the heart and circulatory system. Yin and yang can help us understand this mechanism. In Far Eastern medicine, tobacco is classified as very yang in quality due to its contracting and drying effects. Smokers are generally thinner (that is, more contracted and hence more yang) than nonsmokers, and most smokers put on weight (that is, they expand and become more yin) when they stop smoking. Thus, smoking contracts the body and has an alkalizing effect on the blood. As the Indians found, used in moderation pure tobacco can have a soothing effect and can increase immunity to colds, infections, and chronic ailments brought about by overly acidic (yin) conditions.

The quality of modern tobacco is quite different from that used by the Indians and is a contributing factor to the negative effects of smoking today. The original Indian tobacco was grown naturally without chemical fertilizers or artificial pesticides and was air-dried. Modern flue-cured tobacco is subjected to heavy amounts of chemicals during cultivation, and the drying process is speeded up from about three months to six days. Furthermore, commercial cigarettes usually contain from 5 to 20 percent sugar by weight, as well as humectants to retain moisture and other synthetic additives to enhance flavor and taste.

The effects of poor-quality tobacco on a circulatory system subjected to a regular intake of meat, sugar, and other volatile nutrients will be very different from the effects of Indian tobacco on a healthy heart accustomed to whole grains and vegetables. For one thing, the sugar and chemicals in refined cigarettes will produce a strong yin effect. Thus, in most people today even one or two cigarettes will increase the heartbeat (up to fifteen to twenty-five beats a minute). Blood pressure will also usually rise, as much as 15 percent.[13] Meanwhile, the tars and other heavier particles in tobacco will become coated with fat and mucus in the bloodstream. This can injure arterial walls and contribute to atherosclerotic plaque buildup. In lungs filled with fat and mucus, tar can become trapped in the alveoli, or tiny air sacs, setting the stage for emphysema or lung cancer. In addition to congesting the lungs and reducing oxygen flow, smoking also increases the level of carbon monoxide in the blood. Carbon monoxide combines with hemoglobin to displace the amount of oxygen in the blood. Reduced oxygen supply further strains a heart already overburdened by fat deposits and hardened arteries, enhancing susceptibility to irregular heart rhythms. Arrhythmia is the major symptom of sudden cardiac death and can be triggered by excessive smoking. Nicotine can also affect the rate of clotting, contributing to the development of thrombi and emboii. Platelets, the smallest and most concentrated of the formed elements in the blood, are classified as extremely yang in comparison with red blood cells (more yang) and white blood cells (more yin). Nicotine, which is also extremely yang, causes platelets to clump even more, forming clots.

The degree of synergism between tobacco and excess fat and cholesterol helps explain the varying heart disease rates in different societies. For example, in Japan about 75 percent of the men smoke compared with less than 50 percent in the United States. Yet the Japanese rate of coronary heart disease is only 15 percent of the American rate. The Japanese diet is proportionately lower in saturated fat and cholesterol, accounting for the reduced incidence of coronary heart disease despite more widespread smoking. Reviewing findings such as this, some medical researchers have come to the conclusion that coronary heart disease in cigarette smokers eating an affluent diet is possibly "potentiated by" serum cholesterol levels, whereas "cigarette smoking may not be as important in countries with relatively low levels of serum cholesterol."[14]

The absence of any measurable relationship between tobacco and heart disease among American women is also easy to understand when we look at the subject holistically. As we have seen, women generally have stronger hearts than men. Constitutional tendencies, along with menstruation and breastfeeding, help protect women from heart disease in the childbearing years. After middle age, however, American women begin suffering from dramatically higher levels of coronary heart disease and cancer. As we saw in the chapter on diet and the development of disease, excess fat and cholesterol in the body tend to accumulate first in more peripheral areas, such as the skin and the breasts, and then move inward to the reproductive organs, the digestive organs, and the lungs. From the perspective of the organism as a whole, these regions are less critical to survival than the continued functioning of the heart, on which everything else depends. By late middle age, the body's systems are often weakened and menstruation and lactation have stopped, and consequently women begin to experience similar rates of heart attacks and strokes as men.

Among the elderly it has been found that smoking does not increase the risk of heart disease after a certain age.[15] One reason for this is that the elderly naturally tend to consume less food, including proportionately less fat and cholesterol as the caloric requirements of their body decreases. The synergistic effects of tobacco seem to reach a plateau in later middle age and then taper off, although the same level of smoking may continue.

For everyone eating the modern diet—men and women,

boys and girls, young and old—cigarette smoking and, to a lesser extent, pipe and cigar smoking are definitely unhealthy. Anyone with a cardiovascular condition, cancer, or other serious illness should stop smoking or reduce it as much as possible. For those in good health, eating a balanced whole foods diet, the decision whether or not to smoke is a personal one. Biologically, there is no need to smoke, and most traditional societies existed happily without doing so. For those who wish to smoke for enjoyment or contemplation, like the native peoples of this continent, good-quality tobacco may be taken from time to time. Of course, air-dried tobacco free of chemicals and sugar is preferable, and the sensitivity of other people to the effects of smoking should be respected. Smoking extremely imbalanced substances such as marijuana should be strictly avoided.

For those who wish to stop smoking, physical activity or exercise will help compensate for the effects of withdrawing from nicotine. Miso soup is especially beneficial during this time to strengthen the blood, and a slightly greater quantity than usual may be consumed. In general, when quitting smoking, consumption of liquids should be reduced especially coffee, other beverages with stimulant effects, and alcohol, as well as desserts, fruits, and other more yin substances that can create an attraction for the strong counterbalancing energy of tobacco. In some cases, acupuncture on the ear has helped people to quit smoking.

In his classic treatise describing the circulation of the blood, William Harvey noted, "Every affection of the mind that is attended with either pain or pleasure, hope or fear, is the cause of an agitation whose influence extends to the heart." In the next chapter we will examine the role of the emotions in maintaining a healthy circulatory system.

13

Diet, Emotions, and the Heart

While improper diet is the underlying cause of heart disease, emotions play an important role in enhancing its development. Sudden cardiac death, in which the heart abruptly stops beating, can be provoked by emotional shock, trauma, or undue stress. This can occur without hardening of the arteries or a heart attack (the result of infarcted tissue). There is a great deal of current interest in the relation between the mind and the body, and psychologists have profiled several personality types most susceptible to degenerative disease.

To understand the role of the emotions in contributing to cardiovascular troubles, we need to examine the general relation between mind and body. In the modern world, mental and psychological problems are approached as though they were independent of physical problems. However, as traditional medicine instructs us, disorders of the mind and psyche are not separate from bodily ailments and afflictions. Physical ailments are the immediate cause of mental and emotional disturbances, and such disturbances immediately affect the physical condition. Mental and physical problems are two different manifestations arising from the same root: A disorderly way of life, including the habitual practice of improper diet and a lack of balance in mental, emotional, and physical activities. Over a thousand years ago, the Arabic philosopher Ibn Sina (Avicenna) noted, "Among the causes of heart disease are those connected with emotional disturbances."[1] As physician to caliphs and sultans, he witnessed considerable external stress brought about by the Crusades and the turbulent politics of the Middle East. He also observed considerable internal stress on the royal digestive and circulatory systems arising from consumption of sugar, spices, and other tropical foods arriving with the trade caravans. Dietary adjustments formed the core of Ibn Sina's approach, and his treatise on healing, *The Canon of Medicine*, served as the chief medical text in both Europe and Arabia until the advent of modern times.

In Oriental medicine, it has been traditionally known that each major organ in the body is connected with mental, emotional, and spiritual manifestations. These manifestations have been understood as progressive developments, taking place according to the five transformative stages of interaction between centrifugal (yin) and centripetal (yang) tendencies:

1. Healthy conditions of the liver and gallbladder are connected with patience and endurance, while unhealthy conditions produce short temper and anger.

2. Healthy conditions of the heart and small intestine are connected with gentleness, tranquility, intuitive comprehension, spiritual oneness, and a merry, humorous expression, while unhealthy conditions produce separateness, excitement, and excessive laughter.

3. Healthy conditions of the spleen, pancreas, and stomach are connected with sympathy, wisdom, consideration, and understanding, while unhealthy conditions produce irritability, skepticism, criticism, and worry.

4. Healthy conditions of the lungs and large intestine are connected with a feeling of happiness, security, and wholeness, while unhealthy conditions produce sadness, depression, and melancholy.

5. Healthy conditions of the kidneys and bladder are connected with confidence, courage, and inspiration, while their unhealthy conditions produce fear, lack of self-esteem, and hopelessness.

THE JOYFUL HEART

The heart is the central organ unifying mind and body. It is the seat where all thoughts and emotions meet and harmonize. The heart is where Heaven and Earth's forces are most balanced, and the heartbeat is not only an indication of our physical state but an expression of our mental, emotional, and spiritual condition. In all cultures, the heart is associated with joy. Joy is not a separate emotion but the result of all the other emotions being in harmony.

In the Yellow Emperor's Classic of Internal Medicine, the heart is described as the monarch of the body, commanding and receiving communications from the other organs.[2] The liver is compared to the general, the lungs to the prime minister, the gallbladder to the chief justice, the spleen and stomach to the ministers of agriculture and food storage, the large intestine to the official in charge of the imperial highways and roads, the small intestine to the port authority, the kidneys to the health department heads, and the bladder to the officer in charge of outlying districts. These officials are continuously in contact with the capital —the heart—reporting on conditions throughout the empire—the mind and body. When the liver brings good news, when the spleen is happy, and when everything else is functioning smoothly, there is joy in the heart. "The pericardium [the heart's sheath] is the sea of energy; thus, it acts as the messenger of the heart to spread the emotion of joy."[3]

Prior to modern times, the West recognized a similar relationship between the individual and society, between the microcosm and the macrocosm. In *The Anatomy of Melancholy*, written in 1621, Richard Burton voiced a similar metaphor:

Of the *noble* [organs] there be three principal parts, to which all the rest belong, and whom they serve, *brain, heart, liver;* according to whose site, three regions, on a threefold division, is made of the whole body. As first of the *head,* in which the animal organs are contained, and brain itself, which by its nerves give sense and motion to the rest, and is (as it were) a Privy Counsellor, and Chancellor, to the *Heart.* The second region is the chest, or middle *belly,* in which the liver resides as a hidden governor with the rest of those natural organs. . . .[4]

When there is harmony between the organs, there is peace and prosperity in the body and realm. Conversely, when there are bad tidings from the cabinet ministries and outlying provinces, sorrow and discontent spread throughout the land. Like their Eastern counterparts, Western philosophers and sages intuitively recognized the relationship between health, diet, and the emotions. For example, in the opening scene of *Richard III*, Shakespeare expresses in dialogue the mirror relationship between inner and outer order:

RICHARD: *What news abroad?*
HASTINGS: *No news so bad abroad as this at home:*
The king is sickly, weak, and melancholy.
And his physicians fear him mightily.
RICHARD: *Now, by Saint Joan, that news is bad indeed!*
O he hath kept an evil diet long
And overmuch consumed his royal person.[5]

To balance our physical, mental, and emotional activities, we need to select and prepare our daily food in an orderly way. When we include a large amount of meat, eggs, or other animal food, our mind contracts and narrows. As a result of this overly yang food, we become rigid and stubborn and behave more egocentrically and aggressively toward the outer world. On the other hand, if we eat a large volume of dairy food, sugar, fruit, and desserts or consume too much liquid, our mind overexpands and we begin to lose our strength, resolve, and direction. Our coordination diminishes, our reflexes are not so sharp, and we grow irritable and hyperactive. Over time, our thinking dulls, our memory fades, and we become sentimental or melancholy. As a result of too much yin intake, we tend to withdraw and take a defensive attitude to any strong stimulus coming from our surroundings. Of course, comparable changes are taking place physically in our organs, cells, and tissues as they become too tight from overcontraction due to yang intake or too loose from overexpansion due to yin intake.

EMOTIONS AND CONSCIOUSNESS

A holistic way of thinking that unifies mind and body has been in eclipse in the West for about four centuries. After this period of neglect, modern science is rediscovering the emotions. For a long time, mental, emotional, and spiritual phenomena were dismissed as too subjective to measure. Then physics discovered that the most solid substances turned out to be composed of waves of vibrating energy. Scientists also discovered that the objective structure of the natural world depended upon the relative standpoint of the observer. This meant that the experimenter is always part of the experiment.

To take a recent example, several years ago researchers at Ohio State University were studying the incidence of heart disease in different batches of rabbits. They fed the rabbits a diet high in fat and cholesterol in order to produce atheroscleroticlike lesions and then measured the precise amount of plaque buildup. They noticed that one batch of rabbits consistently showed about 60 percent fewer lesions than the other groups. The researchers were very puzzled because the rabbits had the same diet and blood pressure. As it turned out, the person who fed the healthier group of rabbits regularly took them out of their cages and petted, stroked, and talked to them. In this way, the scientists discovered an unforeseen variable: the handler and rabbits' mutual affection.[6] Modern medicine's approach to diet and nutrition is largely based on laboratory tests such as this on frightened and caged animals. The implications are worth contemplating.

Other laboratory studies have shown that while stress can enhance the development of serious illness, it cannot in itself bring about degeneration. In a survey of the role of the emotions on health, the *New York Times'* Science Section reported on research studies showing that "if no underlying disease is present, stress will have no effect on infections or cancers."[7]

THE AUTONOMIC NERVOUS SYSTEM

The mechanism by which emotions contribute to heart disease has been the subject of much investigation and speculation. In *Love's*

Labour's Lost, Shakespeare gives a whimsical description of the dulling effects of too much book learning on the human cardiovascular system:

> *Why, universal plodding poisons up*
> *The nimble spirits in the arteries,*
> *As motion and long-during action tires*
> *The sinewy vigor of the traveller.*[8]

To understand the physiological processes involved among the heart and the emotions, we need to look at the structure of the nervous system. The human nervous system has two anatomical divisions: the more yang central nervous system, which includes the brain and spinal cord, and the more yin peripheral nervous system, which includes all the nervous structures outside of the skull and vertebral canal. The central nervous system acts as a "switchboard" for incoming impulses from receptors and outgoing impulses to effectors; it regulates all body activities except for chemically controlled ones and of course is the seat for the processes of higher consciousness. The peripheral nervous system connects peripheral organs and tissues with the central nervous system.

The autonomic nervous system is not considered to be an anatomical division but rather a functional unit that handles the involuntary, nonconscious body activities, such as the beating of the heart, breathing, digestive peristalsis, and so on. The autonomic nervous system in turn is composed of two antagonistic branches, the parasympathetic (yang) and the orthosympathetic (yin). The parasympathetic nerves originate in a more central position in the body, beginning in the brain stem and sacral region of the spinal cord and passing outward through four pairs of cranial nerves and three pairs of sacral nerves. The orthosympathetic nerves have a more peripheral position, beginning in the central section of the spine and passing outward through the corresponding spinal nerves. In almost all organs, tissues, and smooth muscles there are pairs of autonomic nerves, one ortho- and one parasympathetic, which act in opposite ways. Thus, the whole body is held by an antagonistic and complementary system of nervous control. The parasympathetic is especially affected by the intake of strong yin such as drugs, medications, and sugar. Generally, these items reduce the polarity between the two branches, making all body reflexes and functions less sharp. The immediate effect can sometimes be observed in the eyes, where the pupils contract, and in the vascular system, where the blood vessels dilate. After continued abuse, the parasympathetic nerves become worn out, expanding more and more. The opposite then results: the pupils dilate and the vessels contract.

The action of the autonomic nervous system can be summed up as follows. When the parasympathetic nerves act on expanded organs, there is naturally a resultant contraction; their action on compact organs brings about expansion or dilation. The orthosympathetic nerves have a complementary, opposite effect, inhibiting the hollow organs and stimulating the compact organs. This is another example of how yin and yang are always interacting to maintain balance within the body and between the body and the surrounding environment.

In general, the parasympathetic nervous system governs homeostasis, the body's natural attempt to adjust itself to the environment through digestion, respiration, and fluctuations in response to temperature, pressure, and other external stimuli. The orthosympathetic nervous system responds to sudden disequilibrium caused by accidents, injuries, and emotional stress, including the "flight or fight" reaction.

To meet the emergency and restore balance, the orthosympathetic nervous system increases the heartbeat, contracts the muscles, steps up cardiac output, and raises the rate of breathing. In times of crisis, these processes are regulated by hormones. Hormones, which are secreted by an organ or gland, control specific chemical processes in an area remote from their origin. They may be classified, like all body structures and functions, as relatively yin or yang. Estrogen, the hormone that regulates the menstrual cycle in women, is yin. Testosterone, which regulates masculine development, is yang.

The quality of the nervous system, including the brain cells, spinal nerves, and hormones, are a reflection of our entire way of life, including our way of eating. Our susceptibility to stress and emotional illness is a reflection of our underlying health and vitality. If we are in generally good health, we can tolerate a lot of pressure. If we are weak and low in vitality, our nervous system will be poorly equipped to cope with even the mildest upset.

THE PRESSURES OF MODERN LIFE

There are many aspects of modern life that are stressful and may contribute to weakening an already overburdened heart. They include living in overcrowded cities, working in unventilated buildings, wearing synthetic clothing, living in structures made of concrete and plastic, and being constantly surrounded by machinery, excessive noise, and an electronic environment. In Great Britain, one medical researcher humorously compared the rising incidence of heart disease since 1930 with the ownership of radios and television sets and found an almost perfect correlation (see Figure 17).

Chronic stress can also be produced by economic factors. Such factors include living on credit, taking out a mortgage, paying high taxes, holding an unfulfilling job, being treated as a commodity, facing unemployment, and being surrounded by advertising. One sociological study found that beginning in the late 1940s for each 1 percent increase in the national unemployment rate, there have been on average 1.9 percent more deaths in the United States

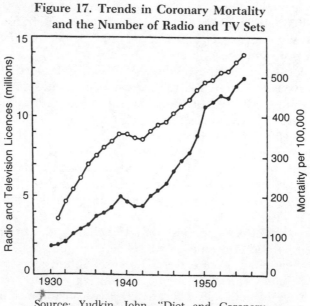

Figure 17. Trends in Coronary Mortality and the Number of Radio and TV Sets

Source: Yudkin, John, "Diet and Coronary Thrombosis: Hypothesis and Fact," *Lancet*, July 27, 1957, p. 161.

from heart disease.[9] New forms of anxiety exact an even greater toll on the modern psyche. The fear of nuclear war and the end of humanity is paramount. Others include the destruction of the natural environment, the extinction of numerous animals and plants, and displacement by computers and robots. Just reading the daily newspaper or listening to the nightly telecast amounts to a perpetual electrocardiogram of humanity's steady degeneration.

On the way to the hospital, in surgery, or while recuperating in a coronary care unit, heart patients often die of panic and feelings of helplessness, although their physical condition has stabilized. One study found that five times more hospitalized coronary patients died following visits by the chief physician than at other times.[10] Norman Cousins has written eloquently about the emotional causes and consequences of heart disease in his book, *The Healing Heart.*[11]

Modern medicine has developed many worthwhile emergency techniques and doctors are generally devoted to their calling. However, over the last four centuries, science has progressively eliminated the importance of the individual from the scope of its inquiry. Personal experience is commonly dismissed as "anecdotal evidence." Only double-blind case-control studies are considered valid. These are studies comparing two basically homogeneous groups of animals or people who are alike except for one or more variables. The loss of individual identity and personal meaning is a fundamental source of alienation and heartbreak in modern society. The notion that personal experience does not matter and that individuals are as interchangeable as parts of a machine is the cause of deep division within the psyche and loss of our human quality. This is expressed politically as totalitarianism, economically as planned obsolescence, and medically as the sovereignty of the double-blind experiment.

In contrast, traditional society respected the individuality of each of its members. Each person was seen not only as a unique being with thoughts and feelings to be respected but also as a microcosm of the world in its entirety. Everyone embodied the universal currents of Heaven and Earth and contributed to the health and well-being of the infinite universe. Traditional healers paid less attention to symptoms of disease than to the person's way of life: his or her thoughts, emotions, dreams, fears, way of speaking, way of relating to others, and of course daily way of eating.

Modern science has dismissed many of these factors because they cannot be measured in the laboratory. However, they can be measured by the enlightened mind.

As the importance of the emotions and consciousness in general has become more widely recognized, a variety of methods have been introduced to reduce tension and achieve balance. Some of these methods are useful and, in combination with a balanced diet, can help integrate mind and body. For example, a meditation program at New York Telephone helped reduce by half the number of employees with high blood pressure, from about 18 percent to 9 percent.[12] However, other methods of stress reduction are often artificially structured and based on false consciousness, excessive displays of feeling, or accompanied by ideological belief systems that can produce even more disharmony.

CORONARY SPASM

The process by which shock, fright, or stress can affect the heart is known as *coronary spasm,* or *vasospasm.* During a spasm, the smooth muscle cells of the artery linings suddenly and involuntarily contract, cutting down and potentially squeezing off the flow of blood. The artery abruptly closes like a bent soda straw (see Figure 18). This process may appear independently of the atherosclerotic process. However, the more plaque in the arteries, the

Figure 18. Coronary Spasm

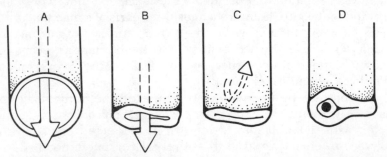

A. Normal blood flow
B. Spasm partially blocking artery
C. Spasm completely blocking artery
D. Combination of spasm, atherosclerotic plaque, and blood clot blocking artery

less intense the shock needed to induce spasm and close off the blood vessel. Spasms are also believed to lead to tears and ruptures of the arterial walls, acceleration of the atherosclerotic process, and clotting and the formation of thrombi. A single coronary artery thus may be blocked by a combination of plaque, clotting, and a spasm. Researchers estimate that spasms are implicated in 25 to 30 percent of coronary patients, though most have some degree of atherosclerosis.[13] Spasms are also believed to be a primary cause of Prinzmetal angina, a rare form of angina pectoris in which chest pains are felt at rest as well as during exertion.

Spasms are activated by two major hormones secreted through the function of the orthosympathetic nervous system. The first is norepinephrine, which is secreted from nerve endings or from the adrenal glands. The second hormone is epinephrine (commonly known as adrenalin), also secreted by the adrenals. These two hormones can also raise levels of free fatty acids in the blood, which increase the oxygen consumed by the heart. Norepinephrine and epinephrine are part of a group of powerful substances in the body called *catacholamines*. During times of fear, shock, or other strong emotion, the orthosympathetic nervous system automatically releases catacholamines to restore equilibrium. However, a nervous system that has already been desensitized by regular dietary abuse will flood the system with catacholamines. In such cases, the resulting spasm can be total, prolonged, and lead to fibrillation, the wildly rapid and erratic heartbeat that is the major manifestation of sudden cardiac death and the leading lethal consequence of a heart attack.

SELF-REFLECTION

Positive emotions can help strengthen the digestive, circulatory, and nervous systems. Beginning in the kitchen, where daily food —the staff of life—is prepared, feelings of gratitude and respect should radiate from our home in ever-widening spirals. Food that is prepared in a spirit of joy and thanksgiving passes along the calm and loving energy of the cook, while food that is prepared in a hurried or disorderly way will produce a chaotic vibration.

Our life should be well balanced between physical and mental activity. After an active day it is advisable to spend a few quiet hours developing our aesthetic, philosophical, and spiritual under-standing. We should continually refine our personality and deepen our understanding of art, literature, music, science, history, my-thology, and other aspects of life. As our health and judgment improve from proper eating, we are able to understand with ease any subject that we desire to learn without any special education or training. In addition to reading widely and contemplating na-ture, we should meet regularly with friends and associates to study together, and we should also seek out and talk with people from all walks of life and all levels of understanding, experience, and judgment.

Self-reflection is integral to our self-development. It involves using our higher consciousness to observe, review, examine, and evaluate our thoughts, feelings, and behavior and to contemplate the larger order of the universe, or what we might call the law of God. The more we reflect upon ourselves and the eternal order of change, the more refined and universal our awareness becomes. We begin to remember our infinite origin, foresee our common destiny, and understand what we came to accomplish upon this Earth.

Self-reflection may take many forms, including spending a short period in quiet meditation or prayer each evening before resting. Questions we might ask and areas we might seek guidance in include:

1. Did I eat today in harmony with my environment?

2. Did I think of my parents, relatives, teachers, and elders with love and respect?

3. Did I happily greet everyone today and express an interest in their life?

4. Did I contemplate the sky, the trees, and the flowers and marvel at the wonders of nature?

5. Did I thank everyone and appreciate everything I ex-perienced today?

6. Did I perform my tasks faithfully and thereby contribute to a more peaceful world?

Silence, solitude, and contemplating nature are conducive to quieting the heart. Walking in the woods or along the seashore puts us in touch with the larger rhythms of life. Everything we need to know may be found within our own hearts. We need only to listen.

LISTENING TO AND MAKING MUSIC

Music can produce emotional and mental states. Everyone knows how a tune, a melody, or a symphony can activate certain thoughts and feelings, subdue others, and influence our mood and perception. In general, singing, chanting, dancing, playing an instrument, or listening to music are excellent for stimulating the heart and circulatory system.

Basically, music can be divided into two categories: (1) music of the infinite, combining in a universal harmony all the sounds of the universe; and (2) music of the changing, relative world that expresses a cultural tradition or the mind and the emotions of an individual composer.[14]

The first category is all around us and can be experienced as our health improves and our consciousness naturally develops. Traditionally, this music was referred to as the music of the spheres and is often heard in deep solitude or reflected in natural sounds such as the wind in the trees, the waves on the seashore, or the melody of birds. The second category, the music of humanity, represents different combinations of high and low tones, loud and soft notes, fast and slow beats, repetitive rhythms and improvisations, and other pairs of centrifugal and centripetal tendencies within the world of creative sound.

The most developed human music seeks to express the eternal, invincible order of the universe and the celestial harmony out of which the complementary and antagonistic forces arise. The single note of a temple gong, for example, is far more powerful than an orchestra of one hundred instruments. The clear sound that it produces reverberates deep within our mind and body, conveying a sense of infinite peace and bringing us close to the melodious silence of infinity. Japanese koto and shakuhachi music, Gregorian chants and medieval madrigals, and some other traditional forms also approach this experience. Perfect harmony has very rarely been expressed by individual composers. Johann Sebastian Bach comes closest. Beethoven's Ninth Symphony, transcending the paired opposites, is another example.

Ethnic and folk music, arising out of the traditional experience of different cultures, represents the next highest level of development. This type of music expresses the awareness of humanity as a whole through the creative imagination of a specific society. Music, like language, differs from culture to culture and region to region because of variations in both climatic and geographical factors and diet. The quality of the celestial electromagnetic energy striking the Earth varies in different locations, contributing to the richness and diversity of natural growth, which includes human society and achievements. A few modern musical forms, such as classical blues, fall into the category of the music of humanity.

Most classical music and some popular music may be differentiated between the more active romantic or aesthetic music (yang) and the more reflective, abstract, intellectual music (yin). Mozart, Wagner, Tchaikovsky, and Chopin, as well as many modern composers and vocalists, fall into the first group, whose compositions or vocal sound expresses highly developed personal feelings and emotions. Most of Beethoven's works, jazz, and the Beatles fall into the latter category, expressing creative flights and explorations of the mind.

Less developed music expresses extreme emotions or utilizes sound in a discordant or artificial way. This includes much rock and popular music, some avant-garde and experimental music, synthesized music, and advertising jingles. At the lowest level is the music of discharge, or mechanical music. This kind of music constitutes a therapeutic release from the body of old toxins resulting from a long history of disorderly eating. Punk rock and other music that developed within the drug culture are examples. Muzak and other music lacking human quality appeals to a nervous system that has been desensitized by a history of improper eating or by anesthesia, as in the doctor's office.

To strengthen the heart, music from the higher levels is beneficial. Music from the intermediary levels can stimulate counterbalancing emotions and ideas and can also contribute to healing. When we are upset or overly active, quiet soothing music helps calm us down. It may even lower our blood pressure a little. When we are blue or low in energy, brisk, upbeat melodies will lift our spirits. Generally, cheerful, joyous music will help to charge the cardiovascular system of those with heart troubles. I recommend that everyone, sick or well, sing a happy song each day.

POETRY AND PROSE

Poetry, which derives from music, is also conducive to unifying the body and mind. Reciting verse—or strong, clear, rhythmic prose—out loud for a few minutes each day will strengthen the heart, expand the lungs, and stimulate the charge of electromagnetic energy to the internal organs. Like music, art, and other forms of human activity, literature may be classified into different levels of expression and judgment. The highest levels express the infinite order of the universe and include many of the world's scriptures, epics, and myths. The intermediate levels, expressing the truths of humanity, include folk and fairy tales, nursery rhymes, classical essays, plays, and novels, and traditional poetry. At the lower levels are most modern fiction, sentimental verse, experimental writing, the theatre of the absurd, and other expressions of the separation between mind and body, between self and cosmos.

Shakespeare is universally recognized as the supreme poet of the human heart. Like Bach in the world of tone, Shakespeare in the world of speech expresses the eternal order of the universe in a near-perfect unity of form and content. Even though Elizabethan English is difficult for us to understand today, we intuitively respond to Shakespeare's comedies, tragedies, histories, and romances, especially when performed on stage. We respond in this way for two reasons. The first relates to form, which is a more expansive yin tendency, and the second relates to content, a more yang contractive tendency.

The form of Shakespeare's verse speaks directly to our hearts. The plays are written primarily in iambic pentameter. Each line contains five pairs of syllables. The first syllable is unaccented, the second accented, and so on. This pattern of alternating stresses imitates the human heartbeat, the rhythmic expansion of diastole and contraction of systole. Furthermore, when recited out loud, iambic pentameter closely parallels the actual rate of the beating heart. The normal heart beats about 65 to 75 times a minute. Give or take a few lines, we can read about fourteen lines of iambic pentameter out loud a minute. Fourteen lines times five feet per line (a foot consists of one unstressed and one stressed syllable) gives seventy rhythmic expansions and contractions of metrical verse—the same as the heart. For example, when his mother accuses him of madness, Hamlet replies in a way that perfectly unifies form and content:

> *My pulse as yours doth temperately keep time*
> *And makes as healthful music. . . .*[15]

THE DECLINE AND FALL OF STRESS

Stress has become a byword referring to all the pressures, tugs, pushes, and pulls to which the modern human heart is subjected. The word *stress* comes from a family of Latin, Old French, and Old English words beginning with the sound *str*.[16] These include *strain, strong, strength, string,* and *strand. Str* means to draw tight, to press, to contract. The sound *str* itself is produced by contracting the lips. In both form and content, *str* is contractive or yang in quality. *Strain,* the common ancestor of the *str* family of words, refers physiologically to stretching, tensing, or otherwise contracting the muscles and organs of the body. *Strain* came to further signify the collective descendents of a common ancestor, such as a strain of wheat. Applied to sound, *strain* signifies a sustained sequence of tones, a drawn out series of notes—as in a musical strain.

The word *stress* derives from *strain* and also originally referred to both an applied force that contracts the body and to the relative emphasis placed upon a musical sound or spoken utterance. Thus, *stress* originally indicated yang centripetal energy. A stressed or accented syllable was actively voiced compared with an unaccented or unstressed syllable, which was unvoiced. In the heart, the stressed beat or force of contraction is the systolic beat, in which the blood is pumped from the ventricles to the lungs and the rest of the body. The unstressed heartbeat is the diastolic beat in which the ventricles relax and expand with incoming blood.

Stress has changed in meaning from indicating a strong, bright, active yang quality to indicating an oppressive, dark, passive, excessively yin quality. This transformation appears to have taken place gradually over many centuries as whole grains and vegetables were increasingly displaced in the traditional English diet by meat, poultry, and other overly yang foods in combination with sugar, spices, and other extreme yin foods. During the period between the decline of the traditional world and the rise of the modern world, as the proportion of yang foods in the diet increased, other *str* words developed that signified overcontraction. These words include *strangle, constrain, constrict, restrain, restrict,* and *astringent.* Still, *stress* in the sense of hardship was viewed until the late middle ages as an integral part of life to be overcome cheerfully and appreciated for strengthening the character, tempering the will, and developing qualities of endurance and understanding. Only in modern times has *stress* lost its original significance and come to mean almost exclusively a mentally, emotionally, or physically disruptive or disquieting force. We might say that *stress* has turned into his opposite, *distress,* from which it is now nearly indistinguishable.

Our preoccupation with stress today signifies that we are no longer in harmony with our environment. Stress is the yang impulse, the active tendency, the force of contraction that gives accent, color, and meaning to life. For many of us, life has become a burden. We are under constant stress. When we say that we can no longer cope with stress, we are saying that we can no longer cope with life because of a lack of basic health and vitality. For many people, modern life has lost its rhythm and melody. The technology that we have mobilized to eliminate stress from our life has often become a source of deep anxiety and resulted in a further loss of our human quality.

Our task today is to restore the rhythm to contemporary life, to create merry sounds in communion with nature, and to set our hearts to beating again.

14

Diet, Exercise, and the Heart

Modern civilization provides many benefits and conveniences. However, some material advances have resulted in a decline in our physical health and vitality. Over the last four centuries, hard physical labor has gradually disappeared from modern life. Today agriculture, transportation, and manufacturing are almost completely mechanized. Even simple household tasks like sweeping the floor, washing the dishes, and preparing food are performed with the aid of labor-saving devices. Our leisure time is also largely automated. Instead of playing among ourselves, we watch others play on television, at the movies, or in sports stadiums. Instead of making music together, we listen to music that is recorded.

Of course, there is nothing wrong in enjoying these forms of relaxation—in moderation. However, in many cases, the active side of our lives is undeveloped, and as a society we have become a nation of passive spectators rather than active participants. The overly refined and rich food that we eat every day has desensitized our bodies and minds so that we require ever more extreme stimuli—such as loud music, violent drama, and sexually explicit material—to stimulate and energize us.

PHYSICAL ACTIVITY AND THE HEALTHY HEART

Physical activity is the more yang side of life and encompasses hard manual labor, light to moderate activity, walking, dancing, cooking, cleaning house, various exercises, and relaxation techniques. In general, physical activity serves to contract the body, including the heart and the internal organs. Active people, for example, tend to weigh less than inactive ones, who are more expanded or yin. In an ordinary healthy person, vigorous activity contributes to the more efficient metabolism of absorbed nutrients. Ingested carbohydrates, fats, and protein are broken down more smoothly in the digestive tract, the intestines are more flexible and stronger blood quality is produced, and the cells and tissues will oxidize energy more effectively.

To understand this process, we need to look at the effects of physical activity on the healthy heart.[1] Normally, the heart at rest pumps about 5 to 6 quarts of blood per minute. At the peak of activity, the volume per minute will rise to about 25 quarts. Therefore, the amount of blood ejected by the ventricles with each stroke will also rise. For example, instead of two ounces a stroke, four ounces may be pumped. Similarly, the number of heartbeats per minute will climb to meet the increased demands of the cells and tissues for more freshly oxygenated blood. The blood supply to the working muscles increases several-fold, from about 20 percent up to 90 percent. The blood vessels in the activated muscles dilate, while those in the unactivated muscles and the internal organs contract.

Until the heart adjusts to the demands placed upon it, physical activity can be stressful. However, as conditioning develops over time, the added strain on the heart and circulatory system is compensated for by the body's more effective use of oxygen. Normally, the cells and tissues extract about 30 percent of the available oxygen from the blood. During periods of heavy physical activity this proportion can climb to 75 percent. The net result is a strengthening of the fibers in the heart muscle as the force of contraction develops. During periods of rest as well as activity, more blood is pumped with each heartbeat. The heartbeat rate itself also falls, and the arteries and other blood vessels of the body widen. Very active persons, for example, may have a resting heartbeat rate of 45 per minute compared with a normal 60 to 70, and their hearts may pump up to twice as much blood per beat as the average person.

Overall, physical activity reduces the strain on the cardiovascular system and makes the heart and other organs more flexible. In addition to experiencing weight loss, persons who engage in regular physical activity tend to have slightly lower blood pressure, and LDL cholesterol and triglyceride levels may also be a little lower.[2] When performed outdoors, physical activity contributes to our awareness and appreciation of the natural world. It also helps build self-confidence, increase tolerance to stress, and produce feelings of tranquility, thus contributing to our overall mental, emotional, and spiritual development as well.

PHYSICAL ACTIVITY AND THE UNHEALTHY HEART

Among individuals eating the modern diet, exercise and conditioning may produce some of these same positive effects. However, until the fundamental source of imbalance is corrected—the daily way of eating—these benefits will be partial or temporary. Negative results may also arise as a result of applying a yang force (physical activity) on a cardiovascular system already subjected to excessive yang factors such as meat, dairy food, poultry, and eggs. For example, the highest heart attack rate in the world is found in Eastern Finland among hardworking lumberjacks and farmers.[3] Some degree of animal food is appropriate for this cold northern climate, and vigorous physical activity generally helps to discharge the protein wastes and toxic byproducts of animal food consumption. However, the modern Finnish diet contains excessive amounts of saturated fat and cholesterol. Hard physical activity combines with this overly contracted diet to give the Finns the highest rate of coronary heart disease in the world.

In a body subjected to a high volume of animal food, increased physical activity generates high levels of urea, lactic acid, and other waste products. Produced during periods of exertion, these substances are absorbed by the muscle fibers and the blood.[4] As a result, the blood becomes more acidic; the intestines become clogged with fat, mucus, and accumulated protein wastes and stagnate; and the arterioles and other blood vessels may constrict even more, accelerating the atherosclerotic process. Thus, many persons who jog, work out, or engage in other vigorous exercise to strengthen their cardiovascular systems may actually be weakening their hearts if they continue to consume large amounts of animal food. The effect is similar to switching from butter to margarine to reduce cholesterol intake only to find that the margarine serves to redistribute cholesterol in the blood to the cells and tissues, thereby increasing the risk of heart disease. Thus, for someone with a more yin, overly expanded heart or high blood pressure, physical activity may present too much of a strain, leading to possible irregular heart rhythms and congestive heart failure.

When considering the appropriate level of physical activity, we must look at a balance of all the factors in our way of life, including our way of eating. Medical studies have generally approached the question of exercise within this larger perspective. The original Framingham Heart Study director, Thomas Dawber, M.D., noted, "The benefits of physical activity are related first primarily to survival after development of myocardial infarction rather than to diminished incidence of the disease."[5] William Kennel, M.D., a subsequent director of the project, further observed, "Physical exercise alone is not enough to counterbalance the incidence of other powerful atherogenic traits."[6] A study published in the *Journal of the American Medical Association* found that men who jogged regularly had seven times the estimated death rate from coronary heart disease while running than the nonrunning population had during more sedentary activities. The researchers concluded that "exercise contributes to sudden death in susceptible persons."[7] A *New England Journal of Medicine* study found that the risk of cardiac arrest during exercise was higher for both physically active and sedentary men, though overall the physically active men had less cardiac arrest during vigorous activity than the sedentary group.[8]

The results are clear: unless the diet is changed, physical activity will not significantly reduce the risk of heart disease and may even increase it. If the diet is changed, physical activity will have a beneficial effect on mind and body, contributing to improved functioning on all levels.

CHEWING AND OBESITY

Whenever anyone asks me to recommend a suitable form of exercise, I advise them to begin with chewing. Chewing utilizes all the muscles of the body and is the key to proper digestion. Thorough chewing releases an important enzyme in the mouth that begins to alkalinize foodstuffs and prevent their premature absorption into the blood. By contributing to the more efficient utilization of nutrients, chewing is like physical activity in that it increases the proportion of oxygen extracted from the blood. Thus, it is important to chew each mouthful very well, at least fifty times and up to a hundred or more, or until the food becomes liquified. Mahatma Gandhi, a life-long student of proper chewing, had a saying: "Drink your foods and chew your drinks." It is good advice. Food also tastes sweeter when it is thoroughly chewed and contributes to greater satisfaction of the meal. To condition the body, pressure-cooked brown rice and other whole cereal grains are excellent for beginning, intermediate, and advanced chewers. As your enjoyment of chewing develops, you may wish to add whole wheat berries, whole grain rye, or whole dried corn to the rice, in a proportion of about one part wheat, rye, or corn to four parts rice. These grains are especially chewy and are beneficial to novice as well as marathon chewers.

Provided our food is well chewed and thoroughly mixed with saliva, we may eat as much food in the Standard Macrobiotic Diet as we wish without danger of becoming overweight. Obesity is caused not only by eating improper food, especially refined flour, sugar, fat, other oily, greasy foods, animal protein, and excess liquid, but also by inadequate chewing and lack of physical activity. The intestines become sluggish from the repeated intake of meat, sugar, refined flour, chemicals, and other imbalanced items and lose the ability to absorb nutrients into the blood. For example, in Asia one reason people nowadays prefer white rice is that it does not require so much chewing as brown rice. White rice provides less energy and is not balanced nutritionally, and after years of eating it people's health and vitality decline, their ability to concentrate and chew diminishes, and overweight develops.

Thus, to compensate for poor-quality food, inadequate chewing, and stagnating intestines, people eat more and more. However, increased volume yields diminished returns and consequently an appetite that is never satisfied. Obesity is the result. Psychological factors arising from chaotic metabolism also enter into the process and reinforce cravings and compulsive behavior. When they exceed the body's normal and then its abnormal rate of discharge, excessive fat, protein, and refined carbohydrates begin to accumulate in the intestines, the thighs, the buttocks, and eventually around the inner organs, including the heart. Recommended body weights have generally been reduced in modern society during the last few decades but are still about 10 to 20 pounds higher than the weights of healthy persons in traditional societies, where heart disease, cancer, and other degenerative disorders are uncommon.

On the macrobiotic diet, most people experience weight loss during the first several months as accumulated excess from the past way of eating is discharged from the body, energy flow is restored, and the quality of the blood starts to change. As intestinal functioning improves, the weight usually begins to climb again, stabilizing at a level that is neither too thin nor too plump. When following the macrobiotic diet, there is no need for the generally healthy person to count calories, watch the waistline, or forgo delicious natural desserts. Simplicity, balance, and moderation are the key concepts. Even with good organic and natural-quality foods, it is preferable not to overeat. Ideally, we should leave the table slightly less than full. This is eating to our heart's content in both senses of the word.

TYPES OF PHYSICAL ACTIVITY

Physical activity is often classified as either static or dynamic. Static exercise, also known as isometric exercise, includes such activities as weight lifting or water skiing and involves strengthening certain muscles with little or no movement of the joints and bones. Dynamic exercise, also called aerobic exercise, includes such activities as running and swimming and involves the rhythmic, repetitive use of a large number of muscles as well as the joints and bones.

The medical profession discourages people with cardiovascular conditions from participating in static (isometric) exercise. Such exercise can result in excessive rise in blood pressure, irregular heartbeat, and temporarily diminished pumping capacity. Heart attacks and strokes commonly occur during periods of heavy isometric activity, such as snow shoveling, or after light isometric activity, such as lifting to the mouth a fork containing fatty food.

Dynamic (aerobic) exercise is generally recommended by doctors for conditioning the cardiovascular system, except for those who are at high risk for heart disease or who have suffered a heart attack or stroke. Dynamic exercise may help reduce the heart rate, improve blood circulation, and increase the diameter of the coronary arteries. For those with overactive or underactive hearts, aerobic exercise is potentially harmful unless accompanied by dietary modifications. There are many instances of both professional and amateur atheletes dying of heart attacks while conditioning.

For a healthy individual eating a well-balanced grain and vegetable diet, both isometric exercise, such as hard physical labor, and aerobic exercise, such as walking or running, are beneficial. So long as it does not produce exhaustion, such physical activity may be engaged in regularly. Within moderation, most exercise, static and dynamic, should present no strain on the healthy cardiovascular system and will strengthen the heart.

To promote better circulation of the blood and the body's natural flow of electromagnetic energy, direct contact with the elements of nature is advisable. Walking outdoors on the grass, soil, or sand, preferably barefoot, is excellent conditioning for the entire body. Swimming is ideally done in salt water whose alkalinity is beneficial to the bloodstream, though fresh water lakes or streams that are unpolluted are also suitable. Swimming in pools that contain chlorinated water and other chemicals should be kept to a minimum.

Cooking and preparing foods are also excellent aerobic disciplines. Cutting vegetables, washing grains and beans, carrying spring water, making tofu and seitan, kneading whole grain bread dough, and similar activities involve the use of a wide range of muscles, joints, and bones. Doing dishes, washing floors, and performing other household tasks are also excellent forms of physical activity and should be shared regularly by all family members. Outside, chopping wood, gardening, and scything are traditional activities that exercise all the body's different physiological systems. Any activity that can be performed in a calm, steady way with fluid or circular movements will help unify the body and mind, the self and the cosmos.

From a larger perspective, the distinction between static and dynamic exercise is not so important as the distinction between exercise that contributes to the smooth flow of electromagnetic energy through the body and exercise that does not. The most integrated activities are those that make use of the meridians and the points along them that harmonize electromagnetic currents throughout the body. When the energy flow along certain meridians is less than normal, physical stimulation is applied to supply energy or activate energy flow. When the energy flow is excessive, physical stimulation is applied to reduce energy and restore balance. The arts for supplying or reducing energy have been developed for thousands of years in all traditional cultures. In the East, these arts include acupuncture, moxibustion, shiatsu massage, palm healing, yoga, tai chi chuan, aikido, and other arts.

Many exercises that call for bending or stretching the body, neck, head, arms, and legs in certain ways give various effects to the energy flow along the meridians, freeing some areas from stagnation and supplying energy to compensate for deficiencies in others. Although not well understood today, these arts were originally designed in ancient times to harmonize the electromagnetic currents of the meridians, which naturally results in the smooth development of our physical, mental, and spiritual condition.

Yoga, tai chi, Dō-in, or other exercises that stimulate the energy pathways in the body are highly recommended. Often they have special techniques for strengthening particular organs and systems of the body, including the heart and circulatory system. When studying one of these arts, it is best to find an instructor who is eating macrobiotically and who thoroughly understands the principles of energy flow on which these systems were originally based. Proper breathing is also very important to harmonize the electromagnetic forces of Heaven and Earth as well as to strengthen the lungs and improve oxygen intake. Breathing methods are usually an integral part of the traditional arts.

DŌ-IN OR SELF-MASSAGE

Among the various arts to promote health and longevity, Dō-in or self-massage is the simplest and most basic. Dō-in can be practiced alone, in one's spare time, for as little as one minute to thirty minutes or more. Dō-in does not require any advanced knowledge of anatomy or acupressure points or any instruments, as do acupuncture and moxa, nor does it require another person to practice with, as do shiatsu and palm healing. Finally, Dō-in does not require any vigorous or unusual activity, which may be required from time to time with other physical training.

Dō-in uses the electromagnetic flow—the energy current running throughout the body—with simple, normal movements, including the use of meridians and several key pressure points. It also combines other principal functions of the body, such as breathing, chanting, and meditation. Part III includes some simple Dō-in postures, as well as several breathing, chanting, stretching, and walking exercises, that will especially strengthen the heart and circulatory system. A few minutes of Dō-in each day will help reduce tensions in mind and body and harmonize the whole condition.

HARMONIZING OUR PHYSICAL ENVIRONMENT

At the same time that we are stimulating the natural energy flow in ourselves, we should reduce our exposure to artificial electromagnetic energy that may change the atmospheric charge surrounding us, adversely affecting our mental and physical condition. We often notice a general fatigue, mental irritability, and unnatural metabolism as the result of electrical appliances, fluorescent lights, high voltage lines, or other artificial sources of electromagnetic radiation in our environment. Cooking on an electric range or in a microwave oven produces undesirable vibratory effects on our metabolism and should be avoided. Synthetic home furnishings and artificial building materials may prevent healthy relaxation.

Synthetic clothing, such as that made of nylon, polyester, and acrylic, impedes the regular flow of energy through the body. It is advisable not to wear these types of fabric directly next to the skin. Cotton undergarments are the ideal alternative, and as we gradually replace our wardrobe with all-natural clothing made of 100 percent cotton, linen, or silk, we begin to feel more comfortable. Use of synthetic sheets, blankets, and other furnishings should also be minimized, if possible. Metallic accessories, such as rings, pendants, and other jewelry, can transmit an electromagnetic charge and should therefore be kept to a minimum.

Free circulation of air and direct access to sunlight should be allowed in our homes, and the addition of several green plants in each room will help to stimulate deeper breathing by increasing the amount of available oxygen. Performing some quiet activity in a green environment is more beneficial to our lungs and heart than working outdoors in a polluted environment or indoors in a sterile one. Television, particularly color TV, and computer terminals are draining and should be used moderately to minimize radiation to the chest region. Long, hot baths or showers, which deplete the supply of minerals in the body, should also be minimized. In general, our physical environment should be open, happy, and free of any dark or heavy features.

When we increase our physical activity, eat a more centrally balanced diet, and center our thoughts and feelings, we naturally begin to reduce our reliance upon unnecessary technological comforts. Our physical and mental flexibility and our natural immunity to disease are restored, and our bodies adjust more easily to extremes of hot and cold, making us less dependent on central heating in winter and on air conditioning in summer.

Those of us who follow the macrobiotic way of life appreciate and continue to use some of the technological advances that modern civilization offers. However, we seek to reduce our dependence on excessive electronic or mechanical conveniences that may hinder the smooth exchange of energy between ourselves and our natural environment. We especially try to avoid those features of modern life that may contribute to the development of disease or make recovery from disease more difficult.

SPORTS AND THE SPIRIT OF PLAY

Modern sports help to develop many physical and mental skills and also teach us how to work together as a team or larger community. However, from a physiological standpoint, they have some serious drawbacks. With the exception of sports that require the even motion of all parts of the body, modern sports tend to create imbalance by emphasizing one side of the body or one basic kind of motion. For instance, football develops bending over forward motion to the neglect of expansive postures or backward movement. Baseball develops one arm, hand, and shoulder to the neglect of the other side. Over time, repeated motions in one half of the torso or one limb create imbalances in the body. Usually, the spine becomes twisted, affecting the nervous system in that area and straining various organs, including the heart. Running, golf, basketball, and other sports affect the spine in slightly different ways. Sports doctors and chiropractors can often tell an athlete's sport by which specific vertebrae are strained.[9] Finally, modern sports' increasing emphasis on performance, winning, and monetary compensation over team loyalty creates mental and psychological imbalances contributing further to physical instability and overall disharmony.

In traditional societies, organized sports were usually not necessary because people kept active by tending to the crops, walking for water or firewood, preparing home-cooked meals, cleaning house, playing with the children, and performing other daily tasks. Vigorous activities were an integral part of life. People ate simply and had no need to discharge excess consumption of animal food in nonviolent social rituals such as sports or violent rituals such as war.

Traditional people kept in top physical shape. On a simple diet of grains and vegetables, supplemented occasionally by small amounts of animal food, they regularly performed feats of strength and endurance that remain unmatched in the present day. Before the era of modern communications, for example, runners unified the land, transmitting news, carrying messages, and conducting business between regions. The runners were noted for their honesty, memory, and endurance. In the Americas, at the time of the Spanish arrival in the sixteenth century, word among the Indians traveled about 150 miles a day. It was not uncommon for a single runner to go this entire distance, though in some areas relays were used. The native peoples considered running a spiritual discipline. The men and women who ran lived very simply and on runs usually ate only roasted corn. Anthropologist Peter Nabokov, author of *Indian Running*, recounted in an interview the advice one traditional runner received from an old man in his community, "Young one, as you run, look to the mountain top. Keep your gaze fixed on that mountain, and you will feel the miles melt beneath your feet. Do this and in time you will feel as if you can leap over bushes, trees, and even the river."[10]

The Tarahumara Indians of Mexico preserve some of these early traditions today. *Raamuri*, their name for themselves, derives from a kickball game that involves running a hundred miles or more. The group contest involves bounding through mountain streams, scrambling over rocky ridges, and playing at night by the light of pitch-pine torches carried by the players. Women play a variation of the running game using hoops instead of a wooden ball.

Once, during the 1928 Olympics, held in Europe, two Tarahumara marathoners running for Mexico continued past the finish line because they had not understood that the race was only 26 miles long. In competition, however, the Tarahumaras usually did not fare so well. Commenting on the Indians' experience of modern conditions, Nabokov notes:

> Their normal metabolism could not make the adjustment from their normal diet of kovisiki, pinole or corn gruel to a training program of eggs, milk, and beefsteak. At home they shunned the fried foods of their Mexican neighbors, preferring roasted or boiled foods. Nor did they much like meat, sweets, or fat. Running in endless circles bored them. These races gave them bad dreams, they said. The cleated leather shoes required at Olympic meets did not conform to their splayed, bark-hard feet. The scrutiny of howling strangers contrasted with the support of backers and friends at home and the winding stretches of quiet mountain trails.[11]

Sports have a place in modern society, but they should be balanced to condition the body as a whole. Runners and walkers, for example, should occasionally go backward or sideways. Baseball players should try switchhitting and golfers should experiment with putting with the opposite hand. Meanwhile, a balanced diet will improve regular performance and play. For example, a Japanese professional baseball team recently changed its clubhouse diet and underwent a remarkable transformation. According to an April 15, 1984 *Parade Magazine* article:

> A Japanese baseball team climbed from the cellar to first place by switching to a macrobiotic diet. Beginning in October 1981, when he took over as manager of the Seibu Lions, Tatsuro Hirooka prescribed a dietary change for his players, who had finished in last place the previous season. Hirooka limited their meat intake and banned polished rice and sugar alto

gether. Instead, he said, his players would eat unpolished rice, tofu, fish and soybean milk. The following spring, he ordered them onto a vegetable and soy diet.

Hirooka told his men that meats and other "animal" foods increase an athlete's susceptibility to injuries. Natural foods, on the other hand, protect the body from sprains and dislocations and keep the mind clear.

The Lions took a lot of ribbing during the 1982 season. The manager of the Nippon-Ham Fighters—a team sponsored by a major meat company—called the Lions "the goat team" and sneered, "They are only eating weeds." But the Lions edged out the Ham Fighters for the Pacific League championship in what sportwriters called the "Vegetable vs. Meat War," and went on to beat the Chunichi Dragons in the Japan Series. Seibu again won the Pacific League championship and the Japan Series in 1983. Food for thought, isn't it?[12]

The same principles of variety and flexibility can be applied in the workplace, where physical imbalances commonly result from long hours spent sitting at a desk, typing, observing a video display terminal, or performing one kind of motion on an assembly line. Some kind of stretching, relaxation, and breathing exercises to balance the curvature of the spine, stimulate the flow of electromagnetic energy, and unify the mind and body are very helpful.

Vigorous physical activity is important to offset the sedentary nature of modern life. A person should be as active as his or her health allows without becoming tired or overworked. Along with proper diet and right thinking, balanced exercise is one of the three pillars of health. As our physical condition and our judgment improve, life becomes more enjoyable and infinitely amusing. Our work becomes our play, and our play becomes our work. From morning till night, we are tirelessly active to realize our endless dream.

As our health improves, all our activities express a natural balance of strength and gentleness, endurance and spontaneity, perseverance and flexibility. The distinctions between physical and mental, natural and artificial, and self and cosmos begin to dissolve. We experience action in inaction and rest in ceaseless activity. Eventually, harmonizing our hearts with the universal spirit, we become one with the eternal order of the universe.

15

The Artificial Heart and the Future of Humanity

Since the middle 1960s, the incidence of cardiovascular disease in modern society has steadily declined as people began to reduce their intake of saturated fat and cholesterol, cut back on smoking, and exercise more. These are healthy developments, and cardiologists are in the forefront of those in the medical profession encouraging dietary change. However, at the same time technological developments in heart disease treatment continue undiminished, threatening to eclipse this positive trend. For example, in a recent feature story in the *New York Times Magazine*, Harry Schwartz, a writer in residence at Columbia University's College of Physicians and Surgeons and a former member of the *Times'* editorial board, explained:

> Life-style changes have their limits. Many Americans refuse to be prudent. . . . So most medical attention is focused less on prevention than on cure. . . . Physicians today emphasize what Dr. Lewis Thomas has called "halfway technology" —expensive treatments for disease rather than effective prevention. That technology is now being rapidly developed on a dozen different fronts, in a kind of free-for-all funded by the Federal Government and private entrepreneurs. Both the cardiovascular CAT scan and the nuclear magnetic-resonance machines represent potential billion-dollar markets. Pharmaceutical companies are in fierce competition over new beta-blocker drugs. Three months after Barney Clark's opera-

tion [for implantation of an artificial heart], private investors poured $5 million into Kolff Medical. . . . The end result could well be a pill or some other medication that could protect people from atherosclerosis. . . .[1]

Actually, such an effort is already under way. Procter and Gamble has developed an artificial fat substitute called *sucrose polyester* (SPE) that can be consumed in place of saturated fats and that blocks absorption of cholesterol in the intestine. So far this product has only been tested on rats, not people.[2]

In the 1980s, cardiology remains the single largest specialty within medicine, accounting for about 10 percent of all surgeons and trained nurses. There are about 7,000 coronary care units in major hospitals around the country. Each year about 1.6 million heart and blood vessel operations and procedures are performed, including about 1,000 coronary bypass and open-heart surgery operations each day. In the 1960s, artificial pacemakers were introduced, and today a half million Americans have been fitted with these devices, which regulate the heart's electrical activity. The newer models have lithium batteries that last five years, and they can transmit data on heart rhythms by radio directly to the outside. After several years of mixed results, heart transplants are again popular. Though only several hundred transplants are done each year, their number is doubling every twelve months. The major drawback is lack of donors.

All these developments, culminating in the first test of the artificial heart, represent a triumph of modern technological civilization. However, from a larger historical perspective, they are part of a degenerating trend toward the increasing mechanization of life. At a recent conference in Asia on the future of humanity, a group of engineers and scientists gave a name to this general development: the Era of Bionization. They foresaw that it would begin in 1980, last into the next century, and be characterized by the widespread artificial manipulation and control of biological functions. For many years, technological intervention has been limited to the environment, the workplace, and the home. Now it is possible to intervene directly into the process of life itself, altering the biological quality of human beings and other forms of life. This approach is not entirely new. It has been practiced for many years as part of modern medicine. However, until now it has been limited to experimental work or to those who could afford it. In the future, these services will become universal, affordable by almost everyone who desires them.

For example, with the spread of degenerative diseases, modern medicine has developed surgical procedures in which an organ, part of an organ, or gland is removed and replaced with parts made from dacron, nylon, teflon, orlon, or some other artificial material or with organs from another person or animal. In an operation called *xenography,* a heart valve from a cow or pig is inserted into the human heart to replace diseased valves. A baboon heart has also been implanted in a human child in an experimental operation. Human heart, kidney, and liver transplants are becoming more common as well, and the availability of totally artificial organs, including the artificial heart, can be expected in the near future. Already many millions of people have had their bones and joints replaced with metal or plastic components, have received pacemakers to regulate their heartbeats, or go to a medical center from once to several times a week for kidney dialysis.

Until now, the removal or replacement of body parts has been restricted primarily to cases in which the original organ has become diseased. Now, however, some people are being encouraged to submit to surgery while they are healthy to prevent possible illness in the future. By the early 1990s, the artificial heart will be within the reach of the average consumer. Harry Schwartz writes:

> It seems all but certain that, within a decade or so, the medical profession will be deluged by demands for "prophylactic" artificial hearts. Today, some women who have a family history suggesting that they will contract breast cancer are seeking and receiving prophylactic mastectomies. Surely many men and women in their 40's and 50's who are beginning to show signs of heart disease will want to trade in their old hearts for a new model.[3]

According to traditional Far Eastern understanding, the heart is not just a physical organ monitoring blood circulation. It is also an energy center governing the flow of Heaven's and Earth's forces—including natural electromagnetic energy and other vibrational waves—throughout the body, especially through the heart, heart governor, triple heater, and small intestine meridians.

As we have seen, improper diet, especially excessive animal food, can obstruct and block these channels which supply or discharge energy throughout the body. When the heart or other natural organ is removed, the energy flowing through these channels and charging the various organs, tissues, and cells of the body, including the brain cells, becomes distorted or disrupted. Surgery, organ transplants, or organ implants that ignore these energy functions will sooner or later produce detrimental effects on the whole body, including the physical and psychological metabolism. In the case of minor surgery or the replacement of peripheral organs, the damage is comparatively moderate. However, in the case of major surgery or the replacement of a major organ, such as the heart, the damage is often severe. As a result of a lack of adaptability or disturbed energy circulation, the patient's period of survival is usually very limited.

Organ transplants and implants, moreover, may involve problems of a spiritual nature, which as we have seen are inseparable from physical problems. For example, after the initial euphoria about Barney Clark's artificial heart implant, it was reported that he suffered from serious depression and complained to psychiatrists that his "mind was shot" and he wanted to die. William Schroeder, the second artificial heart patient, also reportedly suffered from depression and other adverse mental and psychological effects following his operation.

It is a narrow, limited view of life and the natural world to deal with human organs only as physical, material substances. It is necessary that we also understand their role in maintaining life as a whole, contributing to physical, psychological, and spiritual harmony.

THE DECLINE OF THE FAMILY

As our health and judgment have deteriorated, the family has ceased to provide a home for many modern people. This trend will continue as long as technology continues to intervene directly in the process of life. Coupled with artificial contraception and the option of abortion, the process of giving birth is becoming rapidly automated, and babies are becoming consumer goods. Test-tube babies, artificial insemination, surrogate mothers, sperm bank fathers, and determination of the baby's sex in the womb through amniocentesis are gradually being introduced and are revolutionizing society's understanding of human life and the biological, ethical, and legal relations between parents and children. Even more highly refined procedures, including recombinant DNA, cloning, and superovulation techniques, lie around the corner.

These developments are producing an artificial species. When sperm and egg share no organic relationship, offspring will have no biological connection with their parents, grandparents, or ancestors. With the loss of this natural relationship comes a distortion of the species. Children of these processes may look like human beings, but they will not have passed through the natural evolutionary environment nor received a balanced charge from Heaven and Earth's forces. This new, weakened species will collapse very easily before the middle of the next century.

Meanwhile, normal human reproduction is becoming more difficult. Both men and women are rapidly losing their natural qualities. Impotence and infertility are vastly higher today than even fifty years ago. Prostate problems, weak sperm or none whatsoever, high blood pressure—all combine with the epidemic of women's reproductive problems (hysterectomies, ovarian cysts, chaotic menstruation, and breast cancer) to cause the diminishment of the natural human species.

At present the modern world is dominated by a nonhuman way of eating that has given rise to several competing races. These include the cow race, nourished on milk, ice cream, and other dairy products; the wolf race, which feeds on hamburger, steak, and other types of beef; the tiger race, brought up on pork, ham, and hot dogs; the fish race, which consumes too much seafood; the hawk race, bred on chicken, gravy, and other sticky, greasy foods; the monkey race, partial to fruits, especially from another climate zone and out of season, and raw foods; and the snake race, which consumes large amounts of eggs. Imbalanced ways of thinking result from longtime consumption of these extreme foods, including conforming herdlike behavior, aggressiveness and violence, stubbornness, deviousness, scattered and chaotic tendencies, and sly, sneaky behavior. The degeneration of the human race into competing subhuman animal races is the cause of the mistrust, fear, and violence we express toward one another. In the scientific study mentioned earlier, it was forecast that human life would end before the middle of the next century, not from nuclear war but from internal decline. To reverse this direction—to develop human consciousness, bringing out qualities of harmony, balance, and compassion—we must return to whole grains and vegetables as the center of our diet—the human food that has nourished our ancestors for thousands and thousands of years.

THE CHALLENGE OF COMPUTERS AND ROBOTS

At the social level, Bionization will be characterized by the replacement of human beings by a variety of machines. Computers are already performing many household, business, and educational activities. Their integration into daily life has proceeded with astonishing speed. While there is nothing inherently wrong with computers, in practice they tend to further shield modern people from the natural world around them.

If the 1980s is the decade of the personal computer, the 1990s may be the decade of the personal robot. There are now small models available that can vacuum, pick up after their master, patrol the neighborhood, walk the dog, pour drinks, regulate the microwave oven, deliver the mail, make phone calls, and perform other programmed tasks. There is HERO JR., for example, which was introduced to consumers during the Christmas 1984 season at a cost of about $500. According to the sales catalog:

> A very friendly robot, HERO JR. will fit right in with your family and into your home. He sings songs, plays games, tells nursery rhymes, recites poems, guards your home and he can even wake you in the morning. Without supervision or help, HERO JR. will explore his surroundings and will seek to remain near his human companions. . . . The traits comprising HERO JR.'s dynamic personality include: singing songs like "Daisy" and "America"; speaking preprogrammed English phrases; exploring and moving about, using his sensors to avoid most obstacles and seeking out humans; playing games such as "Cowboys and Robots," "Let's Count" and "Tickle Robot"; telling a nursery rhyme; and gabbing in "Roblish" (a robot gibberish that sounds like English). . . . HERO JR. also has

another human-like characteristic, it can go to sleep. This occurs randomly as part of his personality and allows the Robot to conserve battery power by keeping only critical circuits energized.[4]

In the future, robots may pose the single most important challenge to human beings. Unlike humans, robots do not get heart disease or cancer, demand pay raises or vacations, or require love and understanding. During the next twenty years, robots may take over many jobs in factories, companies, government, and the home. As human relations continue to degenerate, robots will eventually become available for a variety of surrogate personal functions. Given the breakdown of the family, alienation between the sexes, and reluctance to bring children into the nuclear age, robots may begin to provide satisfaction for people's emotional and even sexual needs. The first generation of robots will be able to replace husbands and wives in the living room, kitchen, and workshop. The second generation, which may look entirely human, talk, and express emotions, may replace them in the bedroom. Unlike real people, robots do not suffer from impotence or frigidity, nor do they argue or become frustrated. The *Boston Globe* recently ran a photograph in its entertainment section of a young woman at a nightclub dancing with the club's robot. This may be a sign of things to come.

Along with increased mechanization of the body, the coming era will witness more widespread control and manipulation of the mind—a development termed *Psychonization*. This process has already begun in schools, hospitals, and prisons with the routine administration of tranquilizers, sedatives, and other drugs to modify behavior. In the future, drugs and chemicals will be introduced to control common moods, feelings, perceptions, and possibly even beliefs and opinions. On a less recreational basis, synthetic hormones and other substances may be used to quell various forms of social unrest, such as riots, strikes, and political dissent. Subliminal advertising and suggestion, such as antishoplifting messages in department store Muzak, are already reportedly widespread.

In the last few years, genetic engineers have begun to experiment programming physical and psychological traits in and out of selected organisms. At the University of Pennsylvania, human growth hormones have been placed in mouse embryos. The mice grew twice as big as normal and passed their human genetic material to their offspring. In England, a "sheep-goat" has been produced combining characteristics of both species. These experiments are raising the issue of eugenics, the selective breeding of the human race. Instead of racial and ethnic traits as in the past, scientists now are beginning to use medical criteria such as a family history of apparent genetic immunity to heart disease, certain forms of cancer, and other degenerative disorders to justify artificial attempts to improve the human race.

In the short run, genetic manipulation might result in less disease and longer life, but over time unless the basic way of life is changed, including day to day way of eating, the same sicknesses will recur. Moreover, a society with standardized genes will be extremely susceptible to new, unforeseeable changes and influences in the environment. In the past, the wealth and diversity of different genetic strains have protected members of the same species from extinction during periods of unusual climate change and other factors.

In his article "Who Should Play God?" in the *East West Journal*, Jeremy Rifkin, author of *Algeny* and a critic of genetic engineering, asked:

"Who will make the decision as to what genes should be bred into and what genes should be eliminated from the germ life, the hereditary blueprint of the human species? . . . Are we wise enough and smart enough to design the blueprint for future generations, who might have to survive in environments radically different from the ones we're involved with now? . . . The Iroquois Indians, who were a very advanced civilization from whom we borrowed a lot of our ideas of democratic government, had a very interesting practice for decision-making. When the council of elders had to decide on a political course of action, they first had to trace their decision to several generations in the future and ask how will this decision affect them. . . . We have yet to embrace that kind of concept in Western civilization. We have to, for the survival of future generations of plants, animals, and human beings will depend on the decisions we make now."[5]

THE FUTURE OF HUMANITY

If these trends continue, human life as we know it will fundamentally change. At the beginning of the Industrial Revolution in the seventeenth century, philosopher Thomas Hobbes introduced the metaphor of life as a mechanical process. In the introduction to *Leviathan*, he wrote:

> For seeing life is but a motion of limbs, the beginning whereof is in some principal part within; why may we not say, that all Automata (Engines that move themselves by springs and wheels as doth a watch) have artificial life. For what is the Heart, but a Spring; and the Nerves, but so many Strings; and the joints, but so many Wheels, giving motion to the whole Body, such as was intended by the Artificer?[6]

The time is now approaching when it will become cheaper, quicker, and more efficient to replace diseased and even normal body parts with artificial ones rather than heal sickness or maintain regular human functioning. To ensure continued consumption, new model kidneys, livers, hearts, hands, feet, and ears will continually be introduced, offering more streamlined design, extra attachments, and better performance. In this way the Industrial Revolution will come to its logical end: the production, consumption, and planned obsolescence of our own bodies. Human life will become transformed into a machine. We will have lost our human hearts.

The question is, How are we to recover natural immunity to disease and natural survivability and regenerate the human species? Modern science is not the answer; its approach only advances our unnatural status. We must instead build up our original biological strength through natural methods. That means we should not use chemically synthesized food but rather organic, natural-quality, naturally processed whole foods. To maintain our human integrity we should use traditional human food such as whole cereal grains, vegetables, and beans, along with sea salt and sea vegetables to maintain our natural evolutionary inheritance. We should reduce as much as possible all unnatural factors such as tropical fruits in a temperate zone, canned, frozen, or radioactively treated food, and various artificial nonfoods.

Along with the change to a wholesome diet, we must become more physically active. We should take time and discipline ourselves to exercise so that natural energy can flow and be released. Some kind of exercise—running, playing ball, chopping wood—is necessary. As much as possible we should walk up stairs instead of taking the elevator, walk to work instead of driving, and play among ourselves rather than watch other people play.

Gradually, as we restore our diet and life-style, natural immune power—natural sustaining strength—will return. This is the only way the human species—men, women, and children—can be secure and create a harmonious future.

TWO MODELS OF THE FUTURE

In this book we look at the value of the macrobiotic approach in preventing and relieving heart disease and other circulatory disorders. The Framingham Heart Study found that the blood pressure and serum cholesterol levels of those following the macrobiotic approach are the lowest ever recorded in industrial society. They coincide almost exactly with those of the Tarahumaras, the only native community in North America entirely free of high blood pressure, heart attacks, stroke, and the other diseases of modern times (see Table 23).

The Tarahumaras have successfully resisted the trend among native cultures to assimilate the more destructive features of modern times, including the modern way of eating. In the same way, within modern society, the macrobiotic community appears to be the only group so far that has entirely reversed the trend toward

Table 23. COMPARISON OF AVERAGE AMERICAN, TARAHUMARA, AND MACROBIOTIC BLOOD VALUES

Social Group	Serum Cholesterol	Blood Pressure Men	Blood Pressure Women
Average American	220	120/80	120/80
Tarahumara Indian	125	111/73	110/73
Macrobiotic	126	110/61	101/58

degeneration. There are several vegetarian, semivegetarian, and holistic communities such as the Seventh Day Adventists, the Mormons, and others whose members have significantly less heart disease and cancer than do members of the society as a whole, but the incidence of serious illnesses among their members is still relatively high. While epidemiological studies of the macrobiotic community remain to be made, in my personal experience of over thirty years' teaching and counseling, I can say that I know of no one who has stayed faithfully on the diet and followed proper cooking techniques who has developed heart disease, cancer, or other degenerative illness.

Unlike the Tarahumaras, who have remained apart from modern civilization and preserved their traditional way of life, including their way of eating, the macrobiotic community has developed within modern society and has integrated a naturally balanced diet and life-style with those aspects of technology and industrialization that are beneficial. We drive cars, fly in planes, use computers, watch television, and make use of many other modern conveniences. However, we do so in a spirit of moderation, always balancing the time and energy we spend in these pursuits with walks in the woods, visits to the seashore, and other quiet periods of contemplation surrounded by just the sights and sounds of nature.

The gentle Tarahumara culture, which has existed for many centuries in Mexico, represents a sharp contrast to the fiery Aztec culture, which it has long survived. In the same way, the macrobiotic community offers a natural and peaceful alternative to the extreme way of life of modern society, which like Aztec society is turning in on itself and declining due to self-induced heart failure. The Tarahumara and the macrobiotic ways of life offer two healthy models. Between these two poles of North America—the Indians in the Southwest and the macrobiotics in the Northeast—the rest of the continent experiences varying degrees of biological degeneration from heart disease, cancer, mental illness, and loss of reproductive ability. The balanced, commonsense approach to life of these two communities offers the rest of North America, and the planet as a whole, a peaceful and healthy future and will ensure the continued evolution of humanity toward the highest possible biological and spiritual level for thousands of years to come.

PART II

A Guide to Different Cardiovascular Conditions

16

Getting Well

In Part I we looked at how to prevent heart disease. In this part of the book we shall discuss relieving the more common forms of cardiovascular illness with more natural methods. It is important for you to understand that the advice given in this section is educational, not medical. Illness is caused by our daily way of life, including our dietary practices. Unless we take full responsibility for our condition and, along with our families, initiate changes in our life-style and diet, there is little possibility for real improvement of our health. For this reason, we strongly recommend that everyone continue to study the relationship between health, diet, and life-style and especially learn proper cooking techniques. Even after years of macrobiotic practice, we continue to study and strive to keep our minds open to nature and the changing world around us. To recover and develop, we must realize that our health and happiness are entirely within our own hands and not in the hands of others, including macrobiotic counselors as well as medical doctors.

PROPER EVALUATION

When treating illness with dietary methods, it is important that the person's condition be properly classified as predominantly yin or yang or occasionally as a combination of both. Once the evaluation has been made, dietary recommendations can be specifically adjusted to alleviate the particular deficiency or excess.

In many cases, it will be readily apparent what the person's condition is. However, some symptoms, such as abnormal blood pressure or atherosclerosis, can arise from different causes. If there is any question concerning the origin of the underlying condition, it is advisable to see a qualified macrobiotic counselor or a medical doctor trained in the macrobiotic method. Otherwise, the dietary recommendations followed may be the opposite of what is needed. While in most cases the foods involved are balanced and will not cause harm, improvement may be unnecessarily delayed because the incorrect factor is emphasized. In the beginning, it is a good idea to seek experienced advice. Similarly, everyone is strongly encouraged to take macrobiotic cooking classes from experienced instructors. Books like ours can point you in a new direction, but until you have actually tasted the food and seen it prepared correctly, you will not have a standard against which to judge your own cooking. Most of the difficulties that people encounter when switching to the new diet stem from faulty cooking methods. No matter how experienced you may be in some other style of cooking, it is necessary to take a few introductory lessons in macrobiotic cooking. The proper use of salt, oil, and other seasonings can make the difference between a heart patient's getting well or remaining sick.

COOPERATING WITH MEDICAL PERSONNEL

It is often asked whether the heart patient interested in trying a dietary approach to his or her disease should continue seeking medical attention and taking medication. In general, while modern medicines can help relieve various symptoms, they may also have potentially harmful side effects.

For example, the *Journal of the American Medical Association*, recently published results of a major study showing that medication for high blood pressure is unlikely to prolong life and prevent cardiovascular disease and may even prove harmful. "Those tested with antihypertensive drugs had significantly higher coronary rates and total mortality than did those less intensively treated."[1] Meanwhile, the *New England Journal of Medicine* reported that antiarrhythmic drugs appear to have caused seizures and cardiac arrest in about 6 percent of patients sampled and that 20 to 30 percent of patients seemed to get worse.[2] Quinidine, the oldest and most commonly prescribed drug for irregular heartbeat, was especially singled out. Beta blockers, a new class of drugs that inhibit nervous impulses governing heart rate, have been associated with harmful side effects and premature death. One study found that heart patients taking placeboes had a 92 percent survival rate compared with a rate of 79 percent for heart attack victims who started taking the drug from 1 to 7.5 years after their attack.[3] Propranolol, the most common of the beta blockers, sold under the trade name Inderal, has been linked with fatigue, depression, impotence, lung disease, and heart failure.[4] Epinephrine injections, given to emergency heart patients, turned out to be more acid than believed and, according to the *New York Times*, contributed "to some deaths it was designed to prevent."[5] Streptokinase, an anticoagulant used to prevent blood clotting and hailed as a major advance when it was introduced in 1982, turned out to cause major bleeding in up to 10 percent of patients and to result in other complications.[6]

Heart surgery is also problematic, despite optimism regarding advances in open-heart techniques and the coronary bypass graft. A *Journal of the American Medical Association* study found that "psychosis after open-heart surgery is more common than anticipated and may be almost universal."[7] In 1983 the National Heart, Lung, and Blood Institute released results of a comprehensive ten-year study of coronary bypass results. Doctors found that there was no difference in the long-term mortality rate among heart patients who received this form of surgery and patients who underwent other forms of treatment.[8] "Whether the patients survived because of the operation or in spite of it is unknown. The major question now is not whether the operation can be done but whether it should be done," concluded the editorialist in *Circulation*, a professional heart research journal, in an earlier issue devoted to the bypass controversy.[9] Other bypass follow-up studies have shown that the operation contributes to increased plaque buildup in the new vessels as well as the older ones near the grafted area. "It may be concluded that atherosclerosis develops at an accelerated pace in vein grafts as compared with native coronary arteries," another study in *Circulation* concluded.[10] Researchers report that 20 to 30 percent of new grafts are blocked up after six months and another 30 percent become clogged in subsequent years.[11] About 50 percent of bypass patients suffer persistent or recurrent angina and 20 percent have future heart attacks.[12] Artificial pacemaker implantations have also been performed in excess. Dr. Bernard Lown, a noted cardiologist at Harvard Medical School, has estimated that 80 percent of the pacemakers currently being inserted are unnecessary.[13]

Such findings—and by the medical profession itself—reaffirm the wisdom of the Yellow Emperor's Classic. Twenty-five hundred years ago, the Chinese medical text noted: "To live against Yin and Yang which should be obeyed results from the internal resistance to the way of Heaven. Therefore, the sages will prevent disease rather than cure it, maintain order rather than correcting disorder, which is the ultimate principle of wisdom. To cure a disease with medicines or to correct a disorder is like digging a well when one already feels thirsty. . . ."[14]

Prevention is more sensible than cure, and even with most serious heart conditions it is not necessarily too late to correct the underlying imbalances that gave rise to the condition through diet rather than intervention in basic body metabolism. Adopting a high-fiber, low-fat, low-cholesterol diet is far simpler, effective, and healthy than having an illeubypass, an operation in which up to 7 feet of the small intestine is removed to reduce the amount of cholesterol in the blood.

On the other hand, modern medicine has made many positive advances in emergency treatment over the years, as well as in the control and relief of pain. In some cases it may be necessary to take advantage of the life-saving apparatus and techniques afforded by hospitals. For example, if a patient can no longer eat and is rapidly losing weight, it may be necessary to supply intravenous glucose injections until body metabolism is restored. Meanwhile, soft whole grains and mashed vegetables can be prepared and given to the patient in the hospital room until her or his appetite returns. Similarly, there may be situations in which surgery is advisable, as for certain congenital heart defects. Each case must be considered on its own merits.

In respect to medication, the general rule is to reduce reliance on pharmaceuticals slowly rather than all at once. Medicines that keep vital body functions going, such as certain hormone replacements or insulin, should be continued until improvements in health and vitality from the new way of eating are observed. Then, preferably under medical supervision, use of these medications may very slowly be tapered off over a period of from several months to several years as the condition naturally improves. If an essential organ has been replaced, use of the medication or hormone may need to be continued for a lifetime.

Another type of medication includes substances that affect or control bodily conditions such as blood pressure and heart rhythm. As improvement is observed because of the new way of eating, these medications also may be gradually reduced, usually over a period of from one to four months, and again under medical supervision if desired.

A third type of medication includes sedatives, tranquilizers, stimulants, and nutritional supplements. Examples are thorazine, sleeping pills, vitamin capsules, and mineral tablets. In most instances, use of these substances can be discontinued much sooner, usually within ten days to two months.

The time periods suggested above are only an average. Each case is unique. Until the blood quality starts to change through proper eating, the patient discontinuing medication needs to proceed slowly. Normally, it takes the blood plasma ten days to change in quality. Within this period, the patient may experience relief in digestive and respiratory functions as well as the easing of bodily pain. After about two weeks on the diet, circulatory and excretory changes are experienced, the emotions begin to change, and the patient will generally feel less depressed and less angry. Nervous functions are observed to improve after about a month, and thinking tends to become clearer and more focused. After about four months, the body's red blood cells have completely changed in quality, and the skin, bones, organs, and tissues begin to heal. At this time the person's relations with family and friends often become gentler, more respectful, and more loving. Nervous cells take three seasons or approximately nine months to alter in their functional ability, and afterward the person's view of life may become broader, more flexible, and more understanding. Total harmony can take three to seven years or more to achieve, at which time universal consciousness begins to develop. Once again, these averages are very general, and the actual time it will take to restore full health will vary with each person.

During the transition from the modern diet to the macrobiotic diet, the body begins to cleanse itself from the old way of eating and discharge accumulations of mucus, fat, and toxins. This may be accompanied by some abnormal physical reactions that may last from three to ten days and in some cases up to four months until the quality of blood is changed. These reactions may take the form of general fatigue, pains and aches, fever, chills, coughing, abnormal sweating and frequent urination, skin discharges, unusual body odors, diarrhea or constipation, decrease of sexual desire and vitality, temporary cessation of menstruation, mental irritability, or other possible transitory experiences. In most cases, these are transitory signs that the body is beginning to change itself. However, the rate of change and discharge may be too fast and may need to be slowed down to minimize discomfort. Occasionally, these symptoms may arise because of faulty understanding or practice, especially improper cooking, as well as a lack of variety and different quality of dishes, so if any of these signs arise, it is advisable to seek guidance from a qualified macrobiotic dietary or nutritional consultant or medical doctor trained in this approach.

In general, we advise people to keep their regular doctors and other therapists informed of their progress on the macrobiotic diet and to have periodic medical checks. Full medical records documenting the improved cardiovascular condition and restoration of other normal bodily functions can prove helpful to future medical and nutritional researchers. Ideally, the macrobiotic dietary or nutritional counselor and the medical doctor—who may sometimes be the same person—will work together to monitor the patient's condition. In this way, the best possible dietary recommendations and emergency medical relief are available.

OTHER DIETARY AND HOLISTIC METHODS

Over the last several years, the American Heart Association and other medical, nutritional, and educational organizations have issued broad dietary guidelines calling for substantial reductions in fat and sugar consumption and increases in the consumption of whole grains, vegetables, and fresh fruit. Several holistic health clinics and popular books on nutrition and heart disease are also moving in this direction. We welcome these efforts and would like to cooperate with all activities aimed at reducing heart disease through simple, safe, inexpensive methods.

As a result of increased public awareness of diet, exercise, and life-style, heart disease mortality has fallen in the United States during the last fifteen years. A 5, 10, or 20 percent reduction in heart attacks and strokes is a significant development, and all these organizations have played an important role in bringing about the change in thinking that led to the reduction.

But we still require maximum protection from cardiovascular illness. Despite the growing awareness of nutrition, the mechanism by which different foods and combinations of food give rise to different diseases is imperfectly understood. As we have seen in Part I, in addition to saturated fat and cholesterol, a variety of other dietary factors, such as sugar, spices, tropical fruits and vegetables, refined flour, and chemicalized foods, also contribute to heart disease, but their contribution is not so widely recognized. Some of the dietary advice currently offered heart patients by holistic heart clinics fails to take into account the three fundamentally different types of cardiovascular disease. For example, fresh salads and fruit may be beneficial to a heart attack patient with an overly yang condition, but these foods could be hazardous to someone with a serious heart condition caused by underlying yin factors. Opposite causes can give rise to similar symptoms, so not all patients with the same form of cardiovascular disease can be approached in the same way.

At the practical level, moreover, families, schools, hospitals, and other institutions lack adequate recipes to prepare meals low in fat, cholesterol, and sugar and high in complex carbohydrates and fiber. However well meaning, the menus now available often seem to be made by feeding raw data on nutrients into a computer. In many cases, the suggested meals have never actually been tried out by real people for an appropriate length of time.

The Framingham Heart Study found that the typical American family relies on about ten to twelve basic recipes to make up their weekly menu. These recipes taste good and are enjoyable, even if they are not healthy. For a family to change its way of eating, the new food must also be tasty and satisfying. Health food has a reputation for being good for you but unpalatable, and much of this reputation is deserved.

The macrobiotic recipes and menus presented in Part III are based on the living experience of countless people over many centuries. Many of these recipes have been handed down by our ancestors or are taken from traditional societies around the world where heart problems, cancer, and other degenerative disorders are rare. The recipes are eaten daily by hundreds of thousands of modern macrobiotic families across North America, Europe, and elsewhere and are delicious, wholesome, and satisfying.

PROPER PRACTICE

Many physical disorders reflect underlying emotional and spiritual imbalances, including ignorance, arrogance, prejudice, rigidity, and the tendency to accuse others without self-reflection. People suffering from such imbalances also become dependent on others, forgetting that the person really responsible in all cases is they themselves. To attain lasting health and happiness, we all need to develop a spirit of humility, modesty, and gratitude to nature, society, and our families if we are to recover from our problems. A happy, positive mind, cheerfulness, and a joyful mood also lead to future improvement. With the proper outlook, no obstacles are insurmountable, and we learn to embrace sickness and difficulty, as well as health and happiness, for what they have to teach us about ourselves and the marvelous order of the infinite universe.

17

Dietary Recommendations

To treat an overly yang, contracted heart or circulatory condition, we should first eliminate extreme foods of all kinds, especially those high in saturated fat and cholesterol such as red meat, eggs, and dairy products. The Standard Macrobiotic Diet should be observed, slightly emphasizing good-quality yin foods to bring the heart back into balance. For example, a person with a yang condition should eat food that is slightly lighter cooked, such as steamed and lightly boiled vegetables. Salads and raw vegetables are fine in moderate amounts. Occasionally, locally grown fruit and fruit juice are also suitable for this condition if taken in moderate volume. These are examples of good-quality yin foods. Less miso and less tamari soy sauce should also be used in soup, and the soup should have only a mild flavor. Wakame seaweed and some vegetables should also be included in the soup stock. Beans, especially azukis, chick-peas, and lentils, are also encouraged. Hard leafy green vegetables are an excellent source of fiber and very effective in helping the body discharge the excess fat that has accumulated in and around the heart, the blood vessels, the intestines, and elsewhere. A slight pungent taste in cooking, such as ginger, radish, daikon, scallions, or onions, will also help to melt accumulated fat. Depending on the individual case, fish and seafood should be minimized until the condition improves. Naturally sweetened desserts may be taken occasionally in small amounts.

For an overly yin condition in which the heart is swollen, weak, and beats irregularly, we have to eat the Standard Macrobiotic Diet, again eliminating such foods as red meat, dairy products, refined grains, artificial chemicals, and refined sugar. At the same time, more good-quality yang foods should be included. The cooking should be longer, and the grains eaten—50 to 60 percent of the daily intake of food by volume—should usually be pressure-cooked. Slightly roasted, burnt, or bitter-tasting food, even the bottom crusty part of pressure-cooked rice, is not to be ignored for this condition. Miso soup and tamari soy sauce broth can be a little stronger, and vegetables can be slightly crispier. Fish can be included as an occasional dish several times a week. When fish is eaten, the portions should be small, and a little grated ginger should be used as a garnish. Ginger helps us digest any oils that may be used in cooking, but cooking oil should be kept to a minimum. Whole grain and vegetable dishes should always be the principal food, even if fish is served with the meal. Depending on the individual case, raw salad, fruit, juice, and desserts, even naturally sweetened desserts, should be minimized for the initial period until the condition stabilizes. Traditional nonaromatic, nonstimulant herbal beverages may be taken to drink in comfortable amounts, but liquid intake should be moderate.

For heart disease caused by extremes of both yin and yang, a more central way of eating is recommended. Depending upon the individual case, consumption of supplementary foods such as fish, seafood, fruit, fresh salad, juice, and dessert may need to be reduced until the condition improves.

In addition to the regular foods in the Standard Macrobiotic Diet, special side dishes may need to be prepared. In the East, red millet has traditionally been believed to strengthen the heart. Corn, especially whole dried corn, possesses many of its qualities and is highly recommended for cardiovascular conditions. However, most of the corn commonly available today is hybrid and cannot provide energy and vitality. Furthermore, most commercial corn is also produced with large amounts of chemical fertilizers and pesticides. Original Indian corn is harder to locate but preserves the strengthening qualities of the traditional whole grain. It is available in some natural food stores and is known as open-pollinated or standard corn. Several organic seed companies stock small quantities of seeds for traditional varieties of corn for those who wish to grow them in their own gardens. Whenever possible, organic corn should be obtained for any of the corn recipes in Part III.

In Far Eastern medicine, the heart is correlated with a slightly bitter taste. Bitter-tasting vegetables such as watercress, mustard greens, dandelion greens, turnip greens, and burdock are especially stimulating to the heart and blood vessels. Lightly roasted sesame seeds and gomashio (roasted sesame salt) are also slightly bitter and are excellent for restoring elasticity to the heart and diseased arteries. It is interesting to note that digitalis, a drug commonly given to heart patients, is bitter.

Round, heart-shaped vegetables, such as fall and winter squashes, radishes, onions, rutabagas, and turnips, also have beneficial effects for the cardiovascular system. Guidelines for special dishes are listed in each section. Recipes and condiments using these ingredients are included in Part III.

In addition to dietary modifications, some cases of heart disease may require special attention, including external compresses or other treatments. Again, guidelines are provided in each case and methods of implementation are grouped together in Part III in the chapter on home cares. These remedies are inexpensive, easy to prepare, and if used properly totally safe. However, if unnecessarily applied, overused, or incorrectly administered, they may be slightly counterproductive. Their application will differ a little with each individual, and it is best to consult an experienced macrobiotic dietary or nutritional counselor or medical professional for guidance if there is any question about their use. Lifestyle suggestions, including recommendations for mental and physical exercises, may also be given in some instances and are further described in Part III.

In the case of heart patients who have had surgery, drug therapy, hormonal therapy, or previous nutritional counseling, the macrobiotic dietary guidelines may need further modification to balance the effects of the medical treatment as well as those of the underlying heart or vascular condition. Therefore, it is advisable for such a patient to consult a medical doctor, nutritional consultant, or other appropriate professional on how to adjust the macrobiotic diet to his or her unique medical situation and nutritional needs. Together with proper food preparation and cooking, it may be necessary to continue periodic medical checkups to monitor the patient's changing condition as these adjustments, which may include increased total food consumption, especially of protein, complex carbohydrates, minerals, vitamins, or saturated vegetable or animal fat, are implemented. Thus, the macrobiotic diet can be adjusted to compensate for the effects of prior or ongoing medical attention.

PERSONALITIES AT HIGH RISK

While every individual is unique, heart disease tends to develop among certain types of people.[1] Three of the most common personalities at high risk are described below, and a profile is also given of those with more healthy hearts. There are many gradations in between, but this discussion provides a useful overview. Dietary recommendations are provided for each type.

Overactive Heart (A More Yang Condition)

These people have high blood pressure and usually atherosclerosis, which has resulted in fatty deposits both in the coronary arteries or other blood vessels and fatty accumulations in and around the heart muscle itself. This group is susceptible to sudden massive heart attack or stroke, which may result in immediate death. Well-known examples from history include President Taft, Winston Churchill, and Leonid Brezhnev.

Constitutionally, people in this category are usually on the shorter side, squat, and have thick bones. The hands are large and the facial features tight or closely set. The ears are large and the lobes detached, the hands and tongue square, the body hair ample, and there is a tendency to baldness in men. Skin color is red or bright pink.

Socially these individuals are outgoing, verbal, practical, and blunt in their manner. The voice is strong, commanding, and often loud. Emotional determination, including outbursts, are frequent but grudges are rarely kept, as these persons by nature are generous and fair. Thinking is direct and intuitive but often stubborn. These people often brag that they have never missed a day of work in their lives and believe they can eat anything with impunity. Such persons thrive on challenges, have innate reservoirs of energy, and will persevere regardless of the obstacles.

In many ways, such people are very admirable. Their iron constitutions are inherited from hard-working parents, grandparents, and ancestors who ate plenty of whole grains and vegetables and who passed along their stamina and common sense to their descendants. However, if they stray from their ancestral heritage, particularly in their daily way of eating, the offspring can become insensitive to others and too self-assured to reflect on their own behavior and life-style—until it is too late. In addition to heart attack, these people are especially susceptible to appendicitis, hemorrhoids, kidney stones, hardening of the arteries and liver, menstrual cramps or hardened prostate, colon cancer, and hardening of the back muscles.

In combination with the regular intake of sugar, dairy products, excessive fluids, and often hard liquor, the excessive intake of saturated fat and cholesterol, particularly from beef, pork, and salted foods, commonly gives rise to this overactive heart condition. Weak kidneys, as shown by bags under the eyes from accumulating mucus, fat, or water, often result as well. Horizontal lines on the forehead show weakened intestines, and vertical lines between the eyebrows indicate hardening of the liver.

Dietary recommendations to help relieve this condition for an initial period of a few months are 50 to 60 percent whole cereal grains, especially brown rice, barley, and whole dried corn (avoid buckwheat); 5 to 10 percent light miso soup or tamari soy sauce broth, with vegetables, grains, beans, and often with sea vegetables; 25 to 30 percent seasonal vegetables, especially green leafy vegetables cooked in various styles and occasionally raw salads; and 5 to 10 percent beans, beans products such as tofu and tempeh, and sea vegetables. Consumption of fish and seafood should be limited until the condition improves, and all other animal food as well as alcohol, sugar, refined flour, and tobacco should be entirely discontinued. Naturally sweetened desserts and fresh locally grown fruit, primarily cooked or dried but sometimes raw, may be taken occasionally, two to three times a week. Regular beverages may include nonaromatic traditional herb beverages such as bancha tea or roasted barley and other grain teas. Quick pickles and light condiments may also be taken daily. Ginger compresses applied occasionally over the area of the kidneys will improve circulation of the blood and help eliminate excessive accumulations of fat and cholesterol. Fresh air will help strengthen the lungs and improve oxygen intake. Spending time in the high mountains or deep woods is beneficial to individuals with overactive hearts. The seashore, the desert, and hot climates in general are less comfortable until the condition of the heart stabilizes.

Underactive Heart (A More Yin Condition)

The second group suffers from a tendency toward low blood pressure (often following a long period of high blood pressure) and a generally weakened, congested heart. People in this category may suffer strokes or heart attacks but are much more likely to survive them than those in the first group. Tendencies toward lung and respiratory ailments, anemia, melancholy and depression, leukemia, and lymphoma or breast cancer may also be present. Prominent examples from the past include Woodrow Wilson and Jean-Paul Sartre.

People with underactive hearts are generally introverted by nature and to others appear shy, retiring, lacking in self-confidence, quiet, tired, and prone to illness. Constitutionally, they tend to have a thin stature, long hands, delicate bone structure, and light body hair. Their faces are often long and the features spread apart. The nose is usually long, the tongue and hands round, the ears small and with attached lobes, and the skin pale, white, purple, swollen, or watery. The voice is softer, often low, and may express sadness or sorrow. These people are idealistic, future-oriented, and often spiritually directed.

An underactive heart is caused primarily by excessive intake of sugar, sweets, soft drinks, tropical foods, juices, fruits, milk, yogurt, ice cream, salads, alcohol, coffee, medication and other drugs, vitamin pills, and other more relaxing substances, though a moderate amount of animal food is often eaten as well. To relieve this condition, the daily diet for an initial period of several months should consist of 50 to 60 percent whole cereal grains, especially brown rice, barley, buckwheat, and roasted corn; 5 to 10 percent thick miso soup or tamari soy sauce broth; 25 to 30 percent seasonal vegetables, with more root vegetables such as carrots and daikon white radish and more hard leafy greens such as kale and collards; and 5 to 10 percent beans, bean products, and sea vegetables. Fish may be eaten 2 to 3 times a week, but raw salads, fresh fruit, and naturally sweetened desserts should be limited until the condition improves. If cravings arise for something sweet, cooked fruit or dried fruit may occasionally be taken in small amounts. Beverages may include bancha tea, roasted brown rice tea, and occasionally mu tea.

Light to moderate physical activity, as well as chanting and breathing exercises, will help strengthen the weak hearts and lungs of people suffering from this condition. Warmer, drier environments such as sea or coastal regions or desert climates with strong clean air will be more therapeutic to this condition than wet, colder regions or higher altitudes.

Irregular Heart (A Combination of Excessively Yin and Yang Conditions)

The third group suffers from heart murmurs, disturbances in heart rhythms, or other abnormalities in coordination between the left and right sides of the heart. High blood pressure and atherosclerosis may also be present. These people are also susceptible to oily or dry skin, alternating diarrhea and constipation, diabetes, hypoglycemia, jaundice, and lung, pancreatic, or kidney cancer.

Constitutionally, the people in this group are medium in shape and size, bone structure, and facial features. There is often a cleft in the tip of the nose, and the lips may be swollen, especially the lower lip, showing intestinal disorders. A yellow or brown skin color may be present. These people are tense, nervous, excitable, talkative, impatient, giddy, and given to excessive laughter. Speech may be very glib, or there may be an impediment. Thinking is mercurial, erratic, and unfocused. On the one hand this can result in originality and innovation; on the other, in skepticism and fanatic behavior. These people often find it hard to make up their minds, to complete one activity before starting another, or to assume a comfortable position. They often drum their fingers, shake their legs, or blink their eyes excessively. Noted examples include Anwar Sadat and Peter Sellers.

Heart irregularities result from the overconsumption of extreme combinations of food on a regular basis. These may include meat and sugar, eggs and honey, chicken and mashed potatoes and gravy, fish and chips, cheese and wine, and various mineral and vitamin supplements.

To restore a healthy condition, the daily diet for an initial period of several months should include 50 to 60 percent whole cereal grains, especially brown rice, barley, millet, oats, and corn; 5 to 10 percent medium strength miso soup and tamari soy sauce broth; 25 to 30 percent various seasonal vegetables, including round vegetables, such as fall and winter squashes, cabbages, and onions, and sweet vegetables such as carrots and daikon; and 5 to 10 percent beans, bean products, and sea vegetables. Supplemental foods, including white-meat fish, salads, and naturally sweetened desserts, should be taken in moderation until the condition improves. Beverages may include natural nonaromatic herb teas such as bancha twig tea, roasted grain tea, or grain coffee.

A balance of mental and physical activities, including moderate exercise and meditation, will be helpful to correct this condition and restore a more regular, relaxed heart rhythm and coordination between the two chambers. Environmental extremes of all kinds should be avoided until the condition improves.

A Healthy Heart (A Balanced Condition)

In modern society, there is emerging a community of families and individuals who are reversing the trend toward biological degeneration and the development of heart disease, cancer, and other chronic disorders. Taking responsibility for their own health and well-being, these people are changing their way of life, including daily eating patterns. While there is no single body type or personality corresponding to this group, they share many characteristics. Constitutionally, people who develop healthy hearts may be drawn from among any of the three previous groups as well as from among the many gradations in between. They tend to be divided among (1) individuals in already generally good health who are intuitive or philosophical in outlook and who recognize quickly the nutritional, social, and spiritual benefits of a whole grain– and vegetable-based diet and (2) individuals who are seriously ill and who may have tried a variety of conventional and unconventional medical and dietary approaches without success.

Noted individuals who have changed to the macrobiotic way of life include Gloria Swanson, Bill Dufty, Terence Hill, John Denver, and Dirk Benedict.

As the daily way of eating is changed, various physical and mental improvements are experienced by both types of persons, and life in general becomes more orderly and harmonious. For those with serious illnesses, including heart ailments, relief of pain, a rise in energy and vitality, and the gradual disappearance of symptoms are generally felt during the first weeks of macrobiotic practice as the quality of the blood begins to change. In almost all cases, the heart rate stabilizes, blood pressure normalizes, and cholesterol levels diminish to levels of low to very low risk for heart attack and stroke. Those in good health also experience strengthening of circulatory and respiratory functions as well as better digestion and elimination.

Over time, the appearance subtly changes. The head gradually takes on a more round or oval shape, like a grain of rice or wheat. Excess weight is lost, the posture improves, and the body grows more flexible and supple, less susceptible to discomfort in extremes of hot and cold. As a whole, the facial features become more symmetrical and evenly developed. The eyes are clear and focused, the nose returns to average roundness, and the lips resume their natural shape, neither too swollen nor too recessed. The skin is clear, slightly shining, and slightly moist. The nails straighten and grow uncracked and unblemished. The hair is shiny, silky, and without split ends.

As the inner organs and outer physique begin to heal, the emotions begin to change, and the person's thinking becomes clearer and more focused, the attitude more peaceful and appreciative, and the bodily movements more graceful and smooth. Estrangements between parent and child, man and woman, employee and employer, and other divisions are often bridged as the individual examines his or her life and comes to accept full responsibility for the past. Difficulties and illnesses are appreciated both for disclosing an underlying imbalance and for providing the opportunity for change, growth, and understanding.

A more developed sense of social consciousness may arise as the effect of a sensible daily diet and more natural way of life on family affairs, public health, and the fate of the world is recognized. This may take the form of counseling and educational pursuits, food and agricultural projects, and activities to achieve world peace and world order.

Gradually, the person's view of life becomes broader, more flexible, and more understanding. Total harmony can take up to a decade or longer to achieve, after which time universal consciousness begins to develop. Having learned the secret of transmuting daily nourishment into health and vitality through proper food selection and cooking methods, these people can prevent the development of serious illness, guide others toward health and happiness, adjust to all climates and environments, and acquire the will and strength to realize their goals in life.

While the overall result of macrobiotics is to maximize personal health and consciousness, there are various ups and downs along the way. Persons practicing macrobiotics must be careful to take a middle way between too lax and too strict practice. Unless a modest attitude is continually cultivated, there is a tendency to become too conceptual, exclusive, and doctrinaire. However, macrobiotic people can guard against these excesses through self-reflection, prayer, and meditation so that they do not separate themselves from others but continually see everyone on this planet as brothers and sisters in the endless journey of life.

DIETARY GUIDELINES FOR RELIEVING CARDIOVASCULAR DISEASE

When properly applied, the macrobiotic diet can help to restore an excessively yin or yang condition to one of more natural balance. Table 24 summarizes the common types of heart disease discussed in Part II and classifies them under three different headings: a more yin condition, a more yang condition, or a combination of both. In some cases, such as abnormal blood pressure, irregular heartbeat, or stroke, similar conditions can be produced by opposite causes. Illnesses should be carefully evaluated to be certain which form is involved.

In the table, *regular* means suitable for daily use, *occasionally* means permissible for use two to three times a week, and *avoid, limit,* or *minimize* indicates not to use at all or very rarely. In addition to these general guidelines, the discussion of each specific

Table 24. DIETARY RECOMMENDATIONS FOR RELIEVING HEART DISEASE*

Kind of Food	1. More Yin Condition	2. Excess Yin and Yang Condition	3. More Yang Condition
General cooking	Slightly more salty, stronger cooking	Moderate cooking	Less salty, lighter cooking
Grains (50 to 60% of daily volume)	Brown rice, barley, corn, whole wheat, millet, buckwheat, regularly; oats, rye, occasionally; baked flour products occasionally; noodles/pasta occasionally	Brown rice, barley, whole wheat, corn, regularly; millet, buckwheat, oats, rye, occasionally; bread and baked flour products minimize; noodles/pasta occasionally	Brown rice, barley, corn, whole wheat, regularly; oats, rye, occasionally; millet, buckwheat, minimize; bread and baked flour products minimize; noodles/pasta occasionally
Soup (1 to 2 cups or bowls daily)	Slightly stronger flavor (slightly more miso, tamari soy sauce, or sea salt)	Moderate flavor	Milder flavor (less miso, tamari soy sauce, or sea salt)
Vegetables (25 to 30% daily volume)	All temperate-climate types daily but emphasize more root varieties, moderate amount of round ones, and less leafy greens; avoid raw salad; occasional boiled or pressed salad	All temperate-climate types daily but emphasize more round varieties; minimize raw salad; frequent boiled or pressed salad	All temperate-climate types daily but emphasize more leafy greens, round ones; less root ones; occasional raw salad; frequent boiled or pressed salad

*These guidelines are only for the initial period until the condition improves, approximately 1 to 2 months, depending upon the individual case.

Table 24 (continued)

Kind of Food	1. More Yin Condition	2. Excess Yin and Yang Condition	3. More Yang Condition
Beans and bean products (5% daily)	A little more strongly seasoned, use less regularly	Moderately seasoned and moderate volume	Lightly seasoned, use more regularly
Sea vegetables (5% daily volume)	Longer cooking, slightly thicker taste	Moderate cooking, medium taste	Quicker cooking, lighter taste
Pickles (small volume daily)	More longtime, stronger pickles	Either type in moderation	More shorttime, lighter pickles
Condiments (tiny volume daily)	Stronger use	Moderate use	Lighter use
Animal food	Occasional small volume of white-meat fish or seafood	Minimize fish or seafood	Avoid or minimize fish or seafood
Oil	Occasional use, dark sesame only; apply with brush as little as possible; consume no raw oil	Occasional use, dark sesame or corn oil only; apply with brush as little as possible; consume no raw oil	Regular use, sesame or corn oil only in moderation, consume no raw oil
Fruit/Dessert	Avoid or minimize; a few raisins or other dried and cooked fruit if cravings arise	Small amount of dried or cooked fruit (locally grown and seasonal) if craved or naturally sweetened dessert	Occasional dried, cooked, or raw fruit and naturally sweetened dessert

Table 24 *(continued)*

Kind of Food	1. More Yin Condition	2. Excess Yin and Yang Condition	3. More Yang Condition
Seeds and nuts	Occasional lightly roasted seeds; limit nuts and nut butters	Occasional lightly roasted seeds; a few nuts and nut butters	Occasional lightly roasted seeds; a few nuts and nut butters
Beverages	Longer cooked, thicker-tasting bancha or other traditional tea	Medium cooked, medium-tasting bancha or other traditional tea	Shorter cooked, lighter-tasting bancha or other traditional tea

condition also includes special dishes that may be prepared and included in the meal. The recipes for these special dishes, as well as the regular dishes, are gathered together in Part III.

For all forms of cardiovascular disease, all extremely imbalanced foods in the modern diet must be substantionally reduced. These include meat, poultry, eggs, milk, cheese, yogurt, and other dairy products; refined salt; sugar, honey, and other refined sweeteners; soft drinks, coffee, black tea, and other strong stimulants or aromatic beverages; refined oils of either animal or vegetable quality, mayonnaise, margarine (including soy margarine), and artificial dressings; all oily and greasy foods; spices, herbs, and ginseng; refined flour, white rice, and other polished grains; all foods containing chemicals, additives, and preservatives; tropical foods of all kinds, including tomatoes, potatoes, and eggplants (unless you live in a tropical area); all canned food, frozen food, artificially preserved foods, instant food, sprayed food, dyed food, and irradiated food; and all vitamins and supplements.

As the condition of health returns (usually after a period of one to two months, though it will depend on the individual case), a wider form of the Standard Macrobiotic Diet, as described in Part I, may be gradually adopted, including more fish and seafood, fresh salads, fruit, juices, and naturally sweetened desserts. This wider form of the diet, averaged and balanced for people in generally good health, may then be followed, with slight individual modifications now and then, for an indefinite period of time.

18

Abnormal Blood Pressure

The origin and development of abnormally high or low blood pressure was described in detail in Chapter 10, which should be reread thoroughly. Specific types of irregular blood pressure will be described below. Modern medicine generally treats this condition with a sodium (salt) restricted diet, weight loss programs, and a variety of drugs including diuretics, strong antihypertensive agents such as reserpine, vasodilators, and beta blockers. These medications are effective to some extent in controlling blood pressure and thus preventing serious complications such as stroke or heart attack, but they do not eliminate underlying causes and often have undesirable side effects. A balanced whole foods diet can usually relieve abnormal blood pressure without recourse to potentially harmful medications.

SYSTOLIC HYPERTENSION

In general hypertension (high blood pressure) takes two forms. The first, systolic hypertension (commonly called *benign atherosclerotic hypertension*) occurs most frequently in adults over fifty and involves the simple hardening of the larger arteries and generalized arteriosclerosis in the smaller arteries and vessels. In this form of hypertension, the systolic pressure rises, for example, from the upper normal average of 140 to 160, 180, 200, or more, while the diastolic pressure falls to 60, 50, or even lower. Though generally considered mild, as its name implies, this form of high blood pressure can lead to congestive heart failure or coronary heart disease.

This is a more yang form of disorder, caused primarily by excessive intake of animal food, refined salt, and hard baked flour products. To relieve this condition, meat, poultry, eggs, and dairy foods should generally be avoided, as well as sugar, spices, white flour, foods of tropical origin, coffee and other stimulants, alcohol, and other excessive yin items. Cooking should be on the lighter side, with less unrefined sea salt used in seasoning. In addition to the basic dietary recommendations listed under Column 3 in Table 24 for conditions arising from a more yang source, there are a few special dishes that are beneficial for this condition. They include a small side dish of daikon and kombu boiled together, boiled salad, steamed greens, and for an initial period of a few weeks a little grated daikon with a taste of tamari soy sauce two or three times a week to help discharge accumulated fats and toxins from the body.

Except for scrubbing the whole body once or twice daily with a towel that has been immersed in hot water, there are no specific home cares for this condition. The scrubbing will help strengthen circulation. Moderate exercise may be engaged in, but vigorous exercise should be avoided. Breathing exercises and meditation may also be helpful to this condition.

If properly followed, these guidelines should lower the blood pressure to normal within about three to four months.

DIASTOLIC HYPERTENSION

In this form of high blood pressure, both systolic and diastolic pressures rise to abnormally high levels—200/125, for instance. This condition is potentially very serious, for it puts an additional burden on the left ventricle, which must pump blood to the whole body against increased pressure. Under the increased workload, the heart muscle will initially thicken, but ultimately it is in danger of failing, leading to congestive heart failure or left heart failure. The arterial walls are also stressed, a condition that may lead to stroke. This form of high blood pressure can weaken the kidneys;

it may also result from kidney disorders. This form of abnormal blood pressure is often referred to as *essential hypertension*, and in modern society it is a very common condition.

Like systolic hypertension, diastolic hypertension results from excessive consumption of animal food, high in fat and cholesterol, but contributing to the rise of diastolic pressure is the chronic overconsumption of sugar, sweets, milk, and other light dairy products; oily and greasy foods; juices and fruits; tropical foods; alcohol; spices; and other overly expansive substances on the yin end of the food spectrum. Of course, almost everyone on the modern diet, including those with benign atherosclerotic hypertension, eats both extreme yin and yang foods. However, proportionately, people with diastolic hypertension eat more sugary, liquid, juicy, and raw items.

To relieve this condition, a more centrally balanced form of the Standard Macrobiotic Diet is recommended. Column 2 of Table 24 should be followed for basic guidelines in the selection and preparation of food during the initial period. Special dishes include steamed greens consumed regularly, dried daikon and kombu cooked together regularly, and vegetables cooked *nishime* style (see Chapter 32, "Recipes") occasionally. Scrubbing the whole body with a hot squeezed towel will help promote even blood circulation. Long, hot baths and showers should be avoided to minimize the loss of minerals from the body. Moderate physical activity, breathing exercises, and meditation or similar practice may be very beneficial for this condition. If the diet is properly implemented, improvement should be substantial within three to four months, though of course the new way of eating, relaxed somewhat after normal health returns, needs to be followed to prevent blood pressure from elevating again.

RENAL HYPERTENSION

This form of abnormally high blood pressure is associated with kidney disease. Reduced blood flow in the kidneys may result from kidney stones, hardened arteries or blood clots in the kidneys, chronic infection, or chronic inflammation in that region.

Like diastolic hypertension, which it sometimes causes, renal hypertension is produced by a combination of excessively yin and excessively yang factors. In many kidney disorders, dairy food is a primary factor, especially heavy cheese intake, together with mucus- and fat-forming foods such as other types of animal food, sugar, and refined flour. Cold foods, such as ice cream and icy beverages, are also often involved, especially in the case of kidney stones and kidney failure.

To relieve this condition, a more centrally balanced form of the Standard Macrobiotic Diet should be implemented. The dietary guidelines in the middle column of Table 24 may be supplemented often with the following special dishes: azuki beans cooked with kombu, dandelion greens and roots, and lotus root cooked with other vegetables. A hot, wet towel applied to the region of the kidneys will help relieve pain. If this application is too weak, a ginger compress may be administered. Moderate exercise and other physical, mental, and emotional activities may be engaged in.

PHEOCHROMOCYTOMA HYPERTENSION

This form of high blood pressure results from a tumor in the adrenal glands, causing the production of large amounts of the hormone epinephrine, which elevates blood pressure dangerously. Like renal hypertension, it results primarily from the consumption of hard dairy food, such as cheese, and the consumption of eggs in combination with other animal fat. Dietary practice is similar as for renal hypertension.

ADRENOCORTICAL ADENOMA HYPERTENSION

This is another form of tumor that affects the adrenals and can result in abnormal retention of salt and water in the body, leading to high blood pressure. Again, dairy foods and egg fat are chiefly responsible, though in this case the dairy food is usually more soft varieties such as cottage cheese and yogurt. The more centrally balanced diet described under renal hypertension may also be followed to relieve this condition.

HYPERTENSION OF PREGNANCY

About a quarter-million American women a year suffer from complications of high blood pressure during pregnancy, often resulting in loss of their unborn babies. The first, more yang form of this disorder is called *preeclampsia* or *eclampsia* and involves kidney malfunction. The body retains excessive amounts of water, producing edema or swelling, and excess protein is excreted in the urine. This condition often requires careful medical attention because it can lead to convulsions and even death. It is caused principally by the excessive consumption of animal food, including dairy food, as well as excessively salty food, sugar, and other yin factors. To ease this condition, follow the nutritional guidelines in Column 3 of Table 24. In addition, the following special dishes may be prepared often: boiled leafy green vegetables, boiled salad, steamed greens, much less salty-tasting food in general, dishes minimizing oil, and good-quality bean or bean product dishes as a source of protein.

The second form of hypertension that can occur during pregnancy is common essential hypertension. This condition usually was present before conception and often results in a rise in blood pressure during the last few months of pregnancy. It is usually not so serious as eclampsia. In form, it is more yin in origin and can be relieved by following the suggestions noted above under diastolic hypertension.

CUSHING'S SYNDROME

An overactive pituitary gland (a gland at the base of the brain) may suddenly result in increased adrenal activity, leading to seriously high blood pressure. This condition is called *Cushing's Syndrome* and appears to be caused by the intake of spices or other strong stimulants, such as coffee, aromatic drinks, cola beverages, alcohol, chocolate, carob, sugar, and tropical fruits and vegetables. To relieve this condition, which is excessively yin in origin, follow the guidelines in Column 1 of Table 24. On the whole, for a period of a few weeks, the food should be slightly more yang to balance the excessively yin condition. Special dishes may include frequent nishime-style vegetable dishes, a dish consisting of squash, azuki beans, and kombu cooked together, round vegetables such as cabbages, onions, or squashes prepared boiled or steamed, regular good-quality complex carbohydrates such as found in whole grains, and proper minerals such as those in sea vegetables. Kombu is particularly good and may be included in other dishes as well as cooked with other sea vegetables in small amounts daily. Needless to say, after the condition is improved, the scope of the macrobiotic diet may be broadened.

LOW BLOOD PRESSURE

Low blood pressure is known medically as *hypotension* and may take two forms. The most common form is the end result of high blood pressure, when an overburdened heart becomes so enlarged and swollen that it finally begins to give out and blood pressure falls from dramatically high levels to low ones. This is the more yin form of low blood pressure and results from extreme consumption of all kinds of food, but especially a lack of good-quality salt and minerals. Sugar, sweets, fruit, juices, soda, and other extreme yin foods have usually been consumed in high amounts, giving rise to the initial high blood pressure. A slightly more yang style of macrobiotic cooking should be adopted to relieve this condition. The nutritional recommendations in Column 1 of Table 24 may be observed for the initial period until improvement is experienced. Good-quality sea salt and minerals are essential to overcoming this condition, and sea vegetables, especially kombu, may be emphasized in the daily diet.

The other form of low blood pressure results from an overly yang condition. The heart is simply too constricted to move very much as a result of long-term consumption of too much salty food, too much baked food, and too much heavy, long-cooked-down food. Salt intake should be minimized and large amounts of hard, green leafy vegetables emphasized. Follow the nutritional guidelines in Column 3 of Table 24 to overcome this type of low blood pressure.

19

Coronary Disease
and Heart Attack

Atherosclerosis, the underlying cause of coronary heart disease, was described at length in Chapter 10. Before proceeding, please review this chapter and earlier discussions of the role of saturated fat and cholesterol in the formation of coronary heart disease, the most lethal form of degenerative illness in modern society (see Figure 19).

In general, coronary heart disease is caused by longtime consumption of excessively yang animal foods, including meat, eggs, poultry, dairy food, and to a lesser extent fish and seafood, especially the more fatty varieties. Other fatty and oily foods and refined white flour are also primary causes, while sugar, other refined sweets, fruit and juices, tropical foods, coffee and other stimulants, alcohol, spices, drugs and medications are secondary factors that can enhance the atherosclerotic process.

The coronary bypass is the most common form of major surgery in the United States today. In this operation, a vein from the leg or occasionally the arm is transplanted and attached to the aorta and the affected coronary artery or arteries past the point of obstruction, thus detouring the clogged areas. The terms *double* or *triple bypass* refer to the number of clogged arteries that are detoured in the operation. While this operation can restore more normal blood circulation to the heart's internal circuit, its effects are usually not very long lasting. Within six months of surgery, about 20 to 30 percent of vein grafts are obstructed by new plaque buildup or blood clots. Meanwhile, above the site of the bypass, the

Figure 19. The Coronary Arteries (shaded areas show
atherosclerotic plaque)

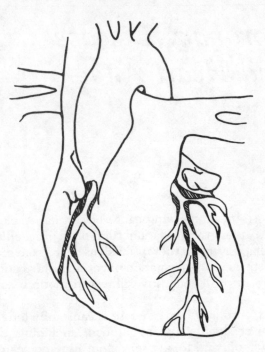

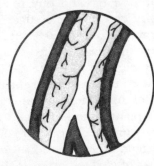

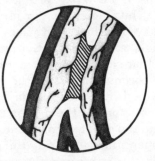

Narrowed
coronary artery

Blocked
coronary artery

rate of atherosclerosis is accelerated, resulting in faster deposit of fat and cholesterol in other regions. Within cardiology, the bypass operation is very controversial, and as noted earlier recent studies show that most bypasses are unnecessary and do not result in longer survival than other means of treatment.

In a few life-threatening cases, surgery may be necessary for coronary heart disease, but to permanently recover from this disease, the daily way of eating must be changed. Only then can the atherosclerotic condition that gave rise to the obstructions be halted, and in most cases it can be reversed. Over time, on a balanced whole foods diet, the arteries will become more flexible, blood quality will improve, and accumulated deposits of fat and cholesterol will naturally be discharged through normal body channels. To relieve the development of coronary heart disease, follow the dietary guidelines in Column 3 of Table 24. Special dishes may include miso soup daily, steamed greens daily, boiled daikon and kombu cooked together often, and a small volume of grated daikon eaten occasionally to help discharge accumulations of fat and cholesterol. Scrubbing the whole body with a hot, squeezed towel will also help circulation. The peripheral parts of the hands and feet may be massaged frequently. Dō-in exercises and occasionally shiatsu massage are also beneficial. Walking is good exercise for coronary conditions, and other light exercise, especially breathing exercises, may prove very helpful. Strenuous exercise and activities should be avoided.

ANGINA PECTORIS

Angina pectoris is a form of coronary atherosclerotic disease in which tightness, a smothering sensation, or pain is experienced in the chest. It is usually accompanied by shortness of breath, pounding of the heart, light perspiration, and feelings of alarm. Angina usually is felt when the level of activity reaches a certain plateau: The same number of stairs are climbed before pain is felt, or so many blocks can be walked before shortness of breath results. Because the coronary arteries are blocked, the flow of blood is impeded and the heart's performance is at a low level. Beyond a certain threshold, not enough oxygen is available to carry on normal activities, and an attack of angina results. In most cases, for anginal pain to be experienced the opening of the coronary artery or arteries must be obstructed at least 70 percent by plaque. Angina often comes after a large meal and is often a precursor to myocardial infarction (heart attack).

Modern medicine treats angina with a variety of drugs and chemical substances that reduce the amount of oxygen needed by the heart and thus raise the threshold at which symptoms appear. These include nitroglycerine, which dilates the veins and immediately lowers the strain on the heart; isosobide, which has a similar effect to nitroglycerine but is several times longer-lasting in its potency; beta blockers, which block sympathetic nerve tissue in the heart, regulating heart rate; and calcium-blocking drugs that impede the movement of calcium ions in the tissue, controlling one form of angina.

Angina pectoris represents an advanced degeneration of the coronary vessels. The initial form it takes, stable angina, brings about pain and shortness of breath at the same level of activity. Eventually, this gives way to unstable angina, at which time symptoms appear at progressively lower levels of activity. Compared with coronary heart disease without angina, the presence of angina usually indicates that the person has consumed substantially more animal food high in saturated fat and dietary cholesterol, along with refined salt and dairy food, especially cheese. Regular coronary heart disease also results from the consumption of large amounts of animal fat, but the fat is often more unsaturated in quality, and proportionately less salt and more soft dairy foods such as milk and butter are usually consumed.

There is a rarer form called *Prinzmetal angina* or *variant angina* in which chest pain and shortness of breath are experienced without any apparent relation to level of activity. These symptoms often appear at rest or even sleeping at night, unlike regular angina, which is always relieved when a certain threshold of inactivity is reached. This form of angina is associated with coronary spasm as well as atherosclerosis. It arises from a combination of excessively yin and excessively yang factors. In addition to heavy animal food, large amounts of spices, sugar, fruit, juice, coffee, alcohol, stimulants, chocolate, or tropical food are usually involved in bringing on this more chaotic condition. Emotional factors are also often involved, stimulating hormones that cause the vessels to constrict or go into spasm.

Regular angina pectoris can be relieved by following the dietary guidelines for coronary heart disease. Prinzmetal angina can be eased by adopting a more central form of the diet described in Column 2 of Table 24.

MYOCARDIAL INFARCTION

This is the common medical term for heart attack and usually follows an advanced stage of coronary heart disease or angina pectoris. An infarct is an area of dead tissue that results when blood supply is cut off to a specific region and it does not get enough oxygen or other nutrients to remain alive. An infarct in the brain constitutes one kind of stroke. Infarcts may also occur in the liver, kidneys, or other organs. In the heart, it most commonly occurs in the left ventricle, which is the major chamber pumping blood to the body as a whole.

A heart attack is usually the result of a coronary atheroma that obstructs an artery, shutting off the flow of blood completely. It may also result, however, from a blood clot, a hemorrhage, an abscess, or a coronary spasm. Depending on the location and the strength of the collateral blood vessels that take over and fill in for obstructed ones, a myocardial infarction may be mild, severe, or lethal. Complications include irregular heart rhythms, including ventricular fibrillation, the major cause of sudden death; heart block and conductive malfunctions; congestive heart failure; shock; and infection. Most heart attack patients are hospitalized in modern coronary care units and treated with rest, drugs, and surgery, depending on the nature and severity of the attack.

The macrobiotic nutritional approach to heart attack is similar to the general dietary guidelines for coronary heart disease and angina pectoris noted above. Massage of the inside end of the little finger on each hand can help stimulate the heart meridian. This form of therapy is often practiced in modern Coronary Pulmonary Resuscitation (CPR), though it is an ancient Oriental technique. Except in life-threatening cases, surgery is not highly recommended, though other forms of medical attention may be required. In cases not needing emergency medical intervention, the heart can be strengthened by providing every day strong miso soup cooked with daikon and other vegetables and a cup of ume-sho-kuzu drink twice a day, with several hours in between cupfuls, for three days. For general vitality, genuine brown rice cream can be given to the heart attack patient once or more each day. The feet and hands should be kept warm at all times, while the forehead should be cool. Rest, good food, and self-reflection are the three keys to recovering from a heart attack. Once the way of life has been changed, normal health and vitality will gradually return, and level of activity may be gradually increased. Light physical exercise, especially walking, is recommended.

20

Stroke

Stroke or cerebral vascular disease results from diminished blood flow to some part of the brain (see Figures 20 and 21). It is usually caused by an atherosclerotic blood clot in one of the cerebral arteries or a rupture of a blood vessel wall. In addition to a thrombus or hemorrhage, a stroke may be produced by an embolus or blood clot that forms in the aorta, heart, or other region, breaks off, and travels to the brain. Pressure on the blood vessels in the skull, as from a tumor, can also produce a seizure. A stroke can be mild, severe, or fatal. Among those who survive, some degree of speech loss, motor function loss, or paralysis often results.

CEREBRAL THROMBOSIS

This type of stroke, also known as an *atherothrombic brain infarction* or *thrombic stroke,* is the most common variety and is similar to a myocardial infarction. In a cerebral thrombosis, however, atherosclerotic plaque, instead of obstructing the coronary arteries, develops in the arterial branches to the head, narrowing and ultimately occluding the blood vessels supplying oxygen, nourishment, and electric impulses to an area of the brain. Depending on the site and severity of the attack, a cerebral thrombosis can be transient or permanent, leading to varying degrees of disability. In general, strokes of all kinds are slightly more yin in origin than heart attacks, arising from a combination of excessively expansive

271

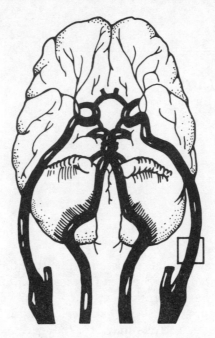

Figure 20. Blood Circulation to the Brain

as well as excessively contractive foods. The blood circulation to the head is accelerated by the overconsumption of sugar, sweets, spices, coffee and other stimulants, soft drinks, fruit, juices, liquid in general, alcohol, drugs, and some medication, in addition to meat, poultry, eggs, dairy food, and salty food.

While strokes arise from a combination of overly yin and overly yang substances, the location of the occlusion indicates in each specific case the predominant type of food giving rise to the disease. Infarctions in the middle cerebral artery, causing paralysis and sensory loss on the opposite side of the body as well as loss of vision, speech, and comprehension, usually arise from both extremes. Infarctions in the anterior cerebral artery are more yin in origin, arising from relatively more sugar, oily and greasy food, liquids, and stimulants, while those in the posterior cerebral artery are more yang, produced by such foods as eggs and hard cheese. Infarctions in the brain stem, resulting in difficulties in swallowing, tongue paralysis, loss of sensation on one side of the face and opposite side of the body, and lack of coordination, can result from

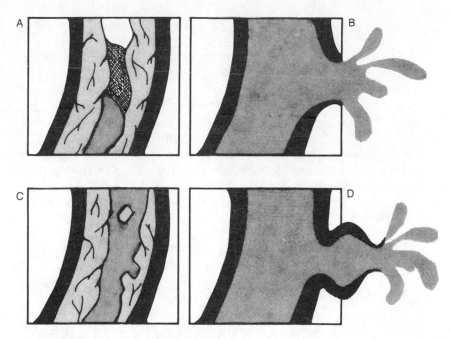

Figure 21. Major Causes of Stroke

A. Thrombus   C. Embolism
B. Hemorrhage   D. Aneurysm (ruptured)

either extreme yin or extreme yang factors, depending on exactly where in the brain stem the thrombosis is located. Infarctions in the upper brain stem usually involve a combination of less extreme foodstuffs than those in the base of the brain stem, which may result in paralysis to both sides of the body. In general, blockages in the arteries servicing the left side of the brain result in tissue death in the left brain region and disability in the right side of the body. Left side seizures commonly result in speech impairment and may be classified as more yin in origin. Blockages in the arteries servicing the right side of the brain result in tissue death in the right brain region and disability in the left side of the body. Right side seizures often result in loss of spatial orientation and may be classified as more yang in origin. Strokes arising in the back part of the head, affecting vision, are more yang, while those in the front part of the head, governing motor function, are more yin. Strokes on the top surface are generally more yin and those on lateral (side) surfaces are usually more a combination of extreme yin and extreme yang factors.

For stroke, a more central form of the Standard Macrobiotic Diet should be followed, slightly emphasizing good-quality yang foods, especially sea vegetables, which should be frequently used even in small volume, to strengthen arterial walls and help discharge accumulated deposits of fat and cholesterol. Good-quality unrefined vegetable oil is also important to give flexibility to arteries. However, it should be taken only in very small amounts, since excessive oil is usually one of the primary causes of the original condition. The dietary guidelines in Column 1 of Table 24 may be observed, except for strokes involving more yang factors, in which case Column 2 may be followed. Among special dishes the following are very beneficial: nishime-style vegetables cooked regularly, dried daikon, carrots, and kombu cooked together often, and genuine brown rice cream with umeboshi plums. In addition, a small volume of the following condiments may be taken often: tekka, umeboshi plums, and shio kombu.

If the person is experiencing a high fever from stroke, a tofu plaster may be applied repeatedly on the head over the area affected. This home care has been traditionally used in the Orient to help reduce high fever and stabilize the condition. Rest is essential for recuperating stroke victims, so it is better not to exercise or engage in anything but light activity. Light breathing exercises may also be beneficial.

CEREBRAL HEMORRHAGE

The other major type of stroke is called a *cerebral hemorrhage* and arises when an artery ruptures and blood discharges into the brain tissue or over the brain surface. This form of stroke usually arises from severely high blood pressure, which causes the artery to burst. Bleeding into the brain tissue can result in serious disability, loss of consciousness, and death. Bleeding over the surface of the brain is usually less severe and may result in temporary loss of consciousness and strong headaches but less disability.

Cerebral hemorrhage can take two forms. The first is called *primary intracerebral hemorrhage*. Its incidence is especially high among black people in the South, most of whom have high blood pressure. A primary intracerebral hemorrhage usually involves sudden strong headaches, nausea, and vomiting, followed by loss of consciousness and often death. The second type of cerebral hemorrhage is called a *subarachnoid hemorrhage* and results from rupture of an aneurysm in a part of the brain called the *Circle of Willis*. Symptoms are similar to the first type, though pain in the head may be more intense. Subarachnoid hemorrhage often leads to sudden death; about 50 percent of victims die before reaching the hospital.

Cerebral hemorrhage is caused by a combination of excessive yin and yang factors but compared with cerebral thrombosis is more yin. Overconsumption of extremely expansive foods, especially alcohol, coffee, fruit juice, soft drinks, and other liquids, sends blood rushing to the head. On top of long-term animal food consumption, which hardens the arteries, yin intake creates the conditions for a rupture as blood pressure rises and the heart is forced to pump harder to provide oxygen to the brain and other tissues. In the case of primary intracerebral hemorrhage, milk and dairy food are usually major factors. The modern black diet, high in pork fat, oily and greasy foods, herbs and spices, and sugar, often leads to high blood pressure and turbulent blood flow. Subarachnoid hemorrhage is even more yin in origin, arising from excessive intake of such substances as fruit juice, stimulants, sugar, oil, and alcohol. To prevent and deal with these forms of stroke, observe the dietary guidelines in Column 1 of Table 24 and the special dishes for stroke described above under cerebral thrombosis. The same home cares and exercise recommendations also apply.

21

Heart Failure and Cardiomyopathy

Heart failure, or the impairment of the pumping function of either ventricle, may result from any type of heart disease. It is not a specific illness but is often the end result of other circulatory disorders, including high blood pressure, atherosclerosis, heart attack, or stroke. Often excess fluid accumulates in the pumping chamber, in which case congestive heart failure results. Depending upon the extent of loss of contractive power, heart failure may be relatively mild, serious, or fatal.

Heart failure is classified into several forms. The most common type is left heart failure, in which the left ventricle becomes overburdened from hardening of the arteries or high blood pressure and the lungs become congested with blood. Because of this excess fluid, breathing is impaired and shortness of breath, gasping, and panting usually result. This condition may also be caused by rheumatic heart disease, which affects the proper functioning of the heart valves.

Right heart failure may result from lung diseases such as tuberculosis, pulmonary hypertension, valve disorders on the right side of the heart, or congestion in the legs, liver, or other regions and organs of the body. When the right ventricle becomes weak, blood backs up in the veins. As fluid leaks out to the tissues, gravity propels it to the lower extremities, resulting in progressive swelling in the ankles, feet, legs, thighs, and abdomen.

Since heart failure can be caused by a wide variety of circulatory problems, there is no single set of dietary recommendations for this condition. In many cases, it is caused by both excessive yin and excessive yang factors, in which case a more moderate macrobiotic diet may be followed. For proper dietary guidance, the underlying condition must be properly evaluated.

In general, for a weak, overly expanded heart, in addition to the regular standard diet, special dishes such as koi koku (carp and burdock soup) are strengthening, as is fried rice. Ranshio (a raw egg mixed with a little tamari soy sauce; see Chapter 34, "Home Cares") is also traditionally used in the Far East to stimulate circulation and strengthen the heart. This may be taken slowly, once a day, for no more than three days. Egg oil, obtained by pan-frying (without cooking oil) an egg down to a charcoallike consistency and squeezing out the oil, may also be taken in small quantities for a few days to strengthen the heart.

CARDIOMYOPATHY

Cardiomyopathy is a disease of the heart muscle and an increasingly common degenerative condition among modern people. It involves the abnormal enlargement of one of the ventricles or the heart cavity as a whole, leading to a variety of progressive complications, including shortness of breath, chest pain, irregular heartbeat, development of thrombi or emboli, and sudden death. It is generally considered terminal by modern medicine, though drugs are usually administered to slow its effects. Many heart patients seeking heart transplants have cardiomyopathy, such as Dr. Barney Clark, the recipient of the first artificial heart.

The more common form of this illness is called *congestive cardiomyopathy* and involves swelling and stretching of the entire heart (see Figure 22). Fibrous tissue begins to replace normal muscle cells, ventricular contraction weakens, and congestive heart failure usually results.

The other major form is called *hypertrophic cardiomyopathy* and usually involves the enlargement of the left ventricular muscle, though occasionally the right one is involved. This condition occurs most frequently in teenagers and young adults.

Both types of cardiomyopathy are caused by excessive yin and excessive yang dietary factors taken in combination, especially foods high in saturated fat and cholesterol, such as meat, oily and

Figure 22. Congestive Cardiomyopathy

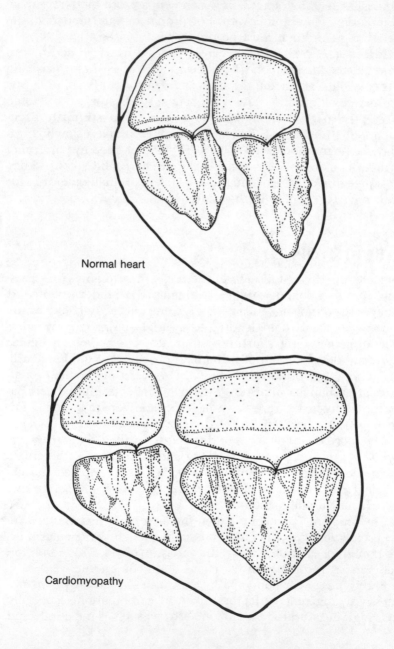

Normal heart

Cardiomyopathy

greasy food, and salty food, combined with unsaturated fats, sugar, candy bars, sweets, dairy food, and occasionally alcohol. In the body, most of these substances are converted into fat, which proceeds to enter the heart muscle and develops into layers of fat, enlarging and weakening the heart.

Hypertrophic cardiomyopathy results from proportionately more extreme yin food among these imbalanced items, especially such items as potatoes, fried foods, sugar, chocolate, and other sweets. For both types of cardiomyopathy, a more central macrobiotic way of eating should be followed. It is very important that whole cereal grains be the focal point of each meal and that miso soup be taken every day, along with hard green leafy vegetables. A small volume of good-quality unrefined vegetable oil may be used occasionally for sautéed vegetables. Consumption of all baked flour products, fruits, and juices should be reduced for several months until the condition improves. The special dishes mentioned above for heart failure, such as koi koku soup, fried rice, miso soup, and daikon and daikon tops cooked and seasoned lightly with miso or tamari soy sauce are helpful. Drinks such as ranshio and egg oil may also be beneficial to strengthen the heart in general, but only when taken for a few days. Cardiomyopathy is in most cases reversible with proper dietary practice, so that a heart transplant should be carefully considered to determine whether it is necessary. However, each particular case must be evaluated on its own, and in more serious instances existing medical attention needs to be continued until the condition stabilizes.

22

Irregular Heartbeats

Irregular heartbeats—or cardiac arrhythmias, as they are also known—may arise if the heart's electrical generator, the sinoatrial node, fails to function properly or if it discharges too much or not often enough. The atrioventricular node, which receives impulses from the sinoatrial node and conducts a charge to the ventricles, may also perform incorrectly, leading to a condition known as heart block.

The most common types of irregular heartbeat include *paroxysmal tachycardia,* in which the heart suddenly starts beating rapidly—up to 200 to 300 times a minute—leading to possible congestive heart failure; *persistent bradycardia,* in which the heartbeat drops to 60 or below, resulting in possible fainting or dizziness; *atrial fibrillation* or flutter, in which the atria enlarge, beat rapidly and often chaotically, leading to possible heart failure; and *ventricular fibrillation* or standstill, in which the ventricles stop beating and begin to twitch erratically, leading to sudden death in minutes unless there is emergency intervention. *Atrioventricular block,* resulting from a failure of cells in the AV node to conduct, can cause the heartbeat to slow or stop entirely. Electrical impulses can also be blocked if one or more bundle-branches leading from the AV node to the ventricles become impaired. The medical treatment for more serious cases of irregular heartbeat is implantation of an artificial pacemaker in the heart to regulate electrical activity.

Cardiac arrhythmias can arise from congenital defects caused largely by the mother's diet during pregnancy, from dysfunctions arising in infancy, or from present improper eating patterns. In general, all irregular heartbeats arise from a combination of excessively yin and excessively yang factors. While the overall way of eating is usually imbalanced, stimulants such as coffee, black tea, cola, and chocolate, as well as excessive sugar, fruits, juices, drugs, chemicals, and alcohol, can contribute to irregularity, especially to rapid heartbeat. Emotional factors and stress are also often involved.

In many cases, a regular heartbeat can be completely recovered by following life-style adjustments, including a change in the daily way of eating. In other cases, some improvement can be obtained. Depending on the case, this may take from about six months to two years or more. For the initial period, the nutritional guidelines in Column 2 of Table 24 may be followed to help relieve irregular heartbeats or heart block, emphasizing proportionately more yang factors such as more root vegetables; longer, slower cooking; and a little higher percentage of whole grains. Overall, the diet should be centrally balanced, with just a mild salt (sea salt, miso, or tamari soy sauce) taste to cooking.

For a heartbeat that is abnormally high, ranshio (a raw egg mixed with a little tamari soy sauce; Chapter 34, "Home Cares") may be taken once a day for no more than three days. This will slow down the heart. Similarly, a little egg oil may be consumed. This is made by pan-frying an egg (without using cooking oil) in a skillet until it is cooked down to almost charcoal in appearance and squeezing out the oil. Fried rice and koi koku (carp and burdock soup) are also good for strengthening the heart and may be taken occasionally in small amounts.

23

Valve Disorders

The heart has four sets of valves: (1) *the tricuspid valve,* which connects the right atrium and right ventricle; (2) *the pulmonic valve,* which connects the right ventricle and pulmonary artery; (3) *the mitral valve,* which connects the left atrium and left ventricle; and (4) *the aortic valve,* which connects the left ventricle and aorta. When the valves become infected, inflamed, or otherwise fail to perform properly, blood may back up or leak, producing a variety of complications, including abnormal heart sounds, heart murmurs, and in some cases heart failure. Depending upon the condition, these can range from mild to serious.

Valve disorders take two primary forms: *stenosis,* or narrowing, in which the valves do not open completely; and *regurgitation,* or loosening, in which the valves do not meet and close properly (see Figure 23). The major types of valve diseases are classified as follows:

Aortic Regurgitation, in which up to half the blood ejected during pumping returns to the left ventricle during diastole, or the filling phase of the cycle. To make room for the leaking blood, the left ventricle enlarges and thickens, leading in some cases to congestive heart failure.

Aortic Stenosis, in which the left ventricle must work harder to pump blood through a narrowed aortic valve. As blood pressure backs up in the lungs, shortness of breath can result, leading eventually to left heart failure. This condition often worsens in middle age and without surgery can be potentially fatal.

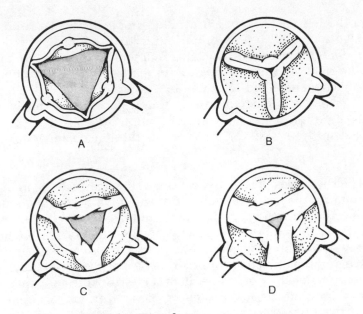

Figure 23. Valve Disorders

A. Normal open valve   C. Stenotic opened valve
B. Normal closed valve   D. Insufficiently closed valve

Mitral Regurgitation involves blood leaking back from the left ventricle to left atrium as the result of a weakened mitral valve. At one time this was the most prevalent form of rheumatic heart disease. It can also be caused by tendon and muscle disorders or calcification of the area around the valve. During pumping, a large volume of blood goes back into the left atrium instead of into the aorta. As a result the left ventricle can increase in size to pump more blood from the atrium or the left atrium can expand tremendously to accommodate the backward flow of blood.

Mitral Stenosis, in which blood entering the left ventricle is impeded by a narrowed valve, leading to fluid backing up in the lungs and right side of the heart. In serious cases, this can lead to heart failure. Rheumatic fever is usually the cause of this condition.

Mitral Valve Prolapse or Barlow's Syndrome involves the dislocation of one of the cusps or leaflets of the mitral valve during contraction in the atrium. A small volume of blood may leak back from the left ventricle to left atrium, producing a characteristic clicking sound but usually requiring no treatment.

Pulmonic Stenosis, in which the pulmonic valve narrows, causing the right ventricle to expand tremendously. This condition is usually congenital and is treated by surgery.

Tricuspid Malfunctions are extremely uncommon, though occasionally they arise as a result of complications when blood is backed up from valvular disorders in the left chambers of the heart.

The rhythmic opening and closing of the heart valves produce the sound of the heartbeat. A heart murmur is any irregular sound produced during the pumping cycle and may be perceived with a stethoscope as short or long, loud or soft, high- or low-pitched, or may exhibit other qualities. Murmurs can also arise as a result of structural malfunctions in other vessels of the circulatory system or functional abnormalities in other parts of the body that put added strain on the heart, such as high fever, anemia, and an overactive thyroid condition.

As a whole, valve disorders develop during the fetal or the infant stages as a result of underconsumption of the proper amount of complex carbohydrates or overconsumption of excessively yin substances on the part of the mother or child. These yin substances include such foods and beverages as sugar, chocolate, honey and other sweets, fruit, fruit juice, tropical foods, chemicalized and artificial foods, and drugs and medications. Mineral depletion results, causing looseness of the valves or eventual narrowing when scar tissue or calcification results from fever or infection.

Depending upon the individual case, valve diseases may be difficult to recover from completely, especially if they are congenital. However, the person's condition definitely can be improved by eating well, in most cases making surgery unnecessary.

For the initial period, a slightly more yang but centrally balanced macrobiotic diet should be followed (Column 1 in Table 24). Sweets, fruit, juices, stimulants, and all aromatic substances should be avoided or limited until the condition improves. In addition to various dishes within the Standard Macrobiotic Diet, sautéed vegetables, especially cabbages, onions, and carrots, may be taken often. A small side dish of hiziki or arame sea vegetable may be prepared frequently with a little oil and with a slight taste of tamari soy sauce. Miso soup should also be consumed regularly and will help to strengthen the valves and restore balance between the affected chambers of the heart.

24

Rheumatic, Pulmonary, and Infectious Heart Disease

Prior to World War II, which brought an epidemic of coronary heart disease, most heart disease resulted from rheumatic fever, pulmonary heart disease, or a variety of diseases that affected the linings of the heart. While the symptoms of these disorders can be controlled by penicillin and other antibiotics and are no longer common in modern society, they are rampant in many other parts of the world where the modern diet is in the process of being adopted.

RHEUMATIC FEVER AND RHEUMATIC HEART DISEASE

Rheumatic fever, developing from a streptococcal throat infection, can lead to heart valve deformities, such as mitral stenosis, resulting in serious impairment of the heart's pumping cycle and possible heart failure. Rhematic fever is usually a childhood affliction, affecting boys and girls in elementary school or in their early to middle teens. Symptoms include fever, progressive aches and pains in the joints, and inflammation in various organs and regions of the body. It most commonly occurs from late fall to early spring.

Rheumatic carditis is another form of rheumatic disease in which the layers of the heart, including the endocardium covering the heart valves, become inflamed. As a result, the aortic and mitral valves can become deformed, seriously affecting the normal flow of blood into and out of the left heart chambers. In acute conditions, death can result. In the United States today, about 14,000 fatalities occur every year from rheumatic heart disease.

Both types of rheumatic disorders arise from a combination of excessive yin and excessive yang dietary factors. In addition to eggs and foods made from eggs such as egg salad, which medical studies have shown to be a common source of streptococcal infection, rheumatic fever results from overconsumption of animal food in conjunction with sugar, chocolate, and other sweets; tropical fruits and juices; soft drinks, especially cold beverages; and other imbalanced fare.

To relieve rheumatic fever, a more centrally balanced way of eating should be adopted (see Column 2 of Table 24) for an initial period. Good miso soup, with brown rice or barley cooked in it, may be taken regularly for this condition. All animal food, including fish and seafood, as well as fruit, juices, and raw food, should be avoided for several days or until the condition improves.

In case of acute rheumatic carditis, medical attention is needed. In less serious cases and for ordinary rheumatic fever, balanced daily food, proper home care, and rest and relaxation should help relieve the condition. In the Far East, rheumatic and other high fevers have traditionally been reduced by applying a carp plaster. To prepare, crush and mash a whole, live carp. Wrap the crushed fish in a thick towel and apply to the chest, front and back. During this application, the fever should decrease rapidly. The body temperature should be checked every 5 to 7 minutes, and when it falls to just slightly above normal, the carp plaster should be removed. In the event that the carp has just been killed to make this plaster, one teaspoon of fresh carp blood may be taken orally before giving the plaster.

PULMONARY HEART DISEASE

Pulmonary heart disease, also known as *chronic cor pulmonale*, results from a variety of lung disorders, which lead to the obstruction of blood flow from the right side of the heart. Pulmonary hypertension commonly results: The blood pressure in the pulmonary artery and its branches rises from a normal 10 to 12 to 40, 60, 80, 100, or more. Lung or heart failure, or the formation of blood clots or emboli in the pulmonary vessels, is often the result.

Pulmonary heart disease usually arises from the long-term consumption of an imbalanced diet emphasizing excessively yin factors. These include such items as ice cream, icy beverages, sugar, chocolate, sweets, cheese, milk, butter, tropical foods, fruits, juices, and other cold, expansive substances. To relieve this condition, a more yang form of the macrobiotic diet should be followed for the initial period. In addition to the foods listed in Column 1 of Table 24, special dishes may include regular nishime-style vegetables, such as carrots, carrot tops, lotus root, and kombu cooked together; frequent but small amounts of kinpura-style burdock or lotus root; regular, good-quality miso soup; a small amount of shio kombu condiment; and ume-sho-kuzu drink twice a day for about three days. A mustard plaster, applied on the front of the chest until the skin becomes hot and red, may be administered once a day for about three to four days. Light breathing exercises are also good for strengthening the lungs and pulmonary vessels.

INFECTIOUS HEART DISEASE

The layers of the heart can become infected or inflamed as a result of pneumonia, polio, measles, chicken pox, appendicitis, meningitis, and other viral- or bacterial-induced disorders (see Figure 24). The most common forms of infectious heart disease include *pericarditis,* in which the protective outer covering of the heart becomes infected or inflamed; *myocarditis,* in which the heart muscle is affected; and *infectious endocarditis,* in which the surface lining of the heart is weakened.

Like rheumatic fever, infectious heart disease is produced by a combination of extreme factors, especially dairy food in combination with oily, fatty food, alcohol, soft drinks, and other extreme yin factors. To relieve infectious heart disorders, a more centrally balanced macrobiotic diet should be followed until the condition improves. Observe the nutritional guidelines in Column 2 of Table 24. In addition, all baked flour goods should be minimized, since they can produce mucus, enhancing the original condition. Special dishes may include steamed daikon and daikon tops with a

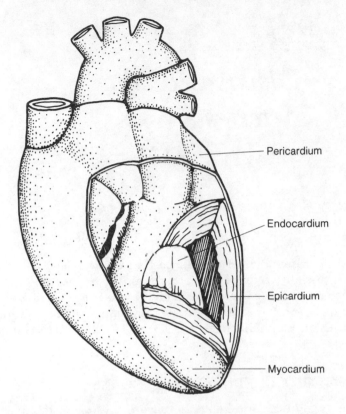

Figure 24. Layers of the Heart

slight taste of tamari soy sauce or miso taste, dried daikon cooked with carrots and kombu with a slight taste of tamari soy sauce or miso, and ume-sho-kuzu beverage once or twice a day for about three days. A leafy green vegetable compress applied to the chest may also help ease this condition in the beginning. For acute cases of infectious endocarditis, which arise suddenly and are immediately life-threatening, medical attention should be sought.

25

Diseases of the Arteries

The peripheral arteries transporting blood away from the heart are the site of circulatory disorders in many people in modern society. The blood vessels affected include the aorta and arterial branches to the arms, legs, and abdominal cavity. The principal forms of peripheral artery disease will be considered one by one.

ARTERIOSCLEROSIS OBLITERANS

This condition, also known as *chronic occlusive arterial disease*, involves atherosclerotic blockage of the arteries to the lower extremities. It is similiar to a myocardial infarction in the heart or a stroke in the brain. Because there are abundant smaller blood vessels in the legs and feet, collateral arteries often develop to keep the blood flowing around the obstruction. However, circulation is weaker than usual, and pains and cramps in the muscles frequently result. This discomfort is known as *intermittent claudication* and is often felt in the calf, thigh, hip, buttock, or lower part of the leg. Relief is usually experienced when the leg is raised or the level of activity reduced, just as attacks of angina pectoris are eased by reduced activity. In serious cases of arteriosclerosis obliterans, the obstructed area may become ulcerated and gangrenous, in which case it may have to be amputated. Persons with diabetes are especially susceptible to loss of a limb from this cause. Modern medicine has no essential treatment for this condition, except to ease the pain and to recommend reduced smoking, which is strongly associated with its increased incidence. A surgical process called *revascularization* in which a vein or synthetic artery is inserted to bypass the obstructed vessel is sometimes performed. However, a majority of grafts have been found to clog up again within five years.

Chronic occlusive arterial disease, like other forms of atherosclerosis, is caused primarily by the consumption of foods high in saturated fat and cholesterol, such as meat, eggs, dairy food of any kind, and fatty and oily foods in combination with sugar and sweets, heavy use of refined flour products, fruit and juices, and refined polyunsaturated oil.

In most cases, obstruction of the peripheral arteries can be reversed by adopting a more centrally balanced macrobiotic diet. For the first several months dietary extremes of both kinds should be avoided or minimized. Daily food preparation should follow Column 2 of Table 24. In addition, special dishes may include proportionately more leafy green vegetables such as broccoli, kale, cabbage, Chinese cabbage, and mustard greens, either boiled or water-sautéed; the frequent consumption of moderate amounts of sea vegetable dishes, especially kombu or wakame in soup, vegetable dishes, or salad; and the moderate use of salt, tamari soy sauce, or miso in seasoning. For a while, it is better not to use any oil in cooking or to minimize its use until the condition improves.

A hot water compress is often beneficial to this condition to relieve pains and cramps in the legs or feet. To apply, place a hot, squeezed towel on the affected area for five minutes, followed by a towel immersed in cold water on the same area for five minutes. Repeat several times. Moderate exercise, such as walking, may be beneficial, but extreme or strenuous activities should be avoided.

ACUTE THROMBOSIS OR EMBOLISM

When a peripheral artery becomes clogged with a blood clot (thrombus) or a blood clot breaks off from a distant area and becomes lodged in a smaller vessel (embolus), a serious, potentially life-threatening condition develops. Collateral blood vessels do not have time to take over for the obstructed artery, and the person may suddenly experience excruciating pain, cold, numbness, and paralysis in the area affected. For less serious cases, modern medicine prescribes anticoagulant drugs to prevent blood clots from forming. Surgery is performed in more serious cases to prevent gangrene from developing, which would require amputation.

Like arteriosclerosis obliterans, discussed above, thrombotic and embolic conditions are caused by the long-term consumption of excessively yang fare in combination with some forms of extreme yin fare. In the case of acute thrombosis and embolism, excessive intake of salt—through the consumption of organic tissue salts in animal food, salty cooking, highly salted convenience foods, or the habit of salting everything at the table—is often present.

The initial dietary recommendations for this condition are the same as those for arteriosclerosis obliterans. In addition, special dishes can include 1 tablespoon of grated daikon with a touch of tamari soy sauce, once daily for several days; and a small, regular side dish of daikon, daikon tops, and kombu cooked together with a light tamari soy sauce or a taste of miso. Application of alternating hot and cold towels, as discussed previously, is also beneficial.

ANEURYSM

An aneurysm occurs when part of an arterial wall weakens and balloons out into the surrounding tissue. Over time, because of the force of pressure exerted by the circulating blood, the sac enlarges and may rupture, leading to hemorrhaging and potentially fatal complications. An aneurysm most frequently occurs in the lower part of the aorta below the beginning of the arteries leading to the kidneys. However, it may occur in any branch of the arterial system. A related condition, *dissecting aneurysm,* occurs when the sac balloons into the artery itself, creating a false pathway for incoming blood and possibly blocking connecting vessels.

Like the peripheral artery diseases discussed above, this condition is caused primarily by underlying atherosclerotic complications resulting from long-term consumption of imbalanced yin and yang food. Regular aneurysm arises more from heavy fat combined with some form of extreme yin, while dissecting aneurysm involves proportionately more strong yin, such as sugar, chocolate, honey, sweets, spices, stimulants, drugs, and chemicals.

For both conditions, a more centrally balanced macrobiotic diet should be observed for the first several months. The guidelines in Column 2 of Table 24 may be followed, and these special dishes may be consumed: nishime-style root vegetables cooked every day with kombu; dried, shredded daikon boiled with carrots, lotus root, and kombu; well-cooked hiziki; and kinpura-style root vegetables. Miso soup and other sea vegetables are also very beneficial for strengthening the blood quality and healing injured blood vessels.

Externally, a tofu plaster may be applied over the area from which the blood is coming up (see Chapter 34, "Home Cares" for details). Leave on a few hours or until the tofu becomes warm. Take off and rest several hours, and then put on a new tofu plaster, repeating the procedure. Tofu plasters may be applied for two to three days, after which relief is usually experienced.

BUERGER'S DISEASE

This condition, also known as *thromboangitis obliterans,* is an inflammatory disorder of the circulatory and nervous systems that occurs only in smokers. The toes or fingers turn blue or cold, ulcerate, and become very painful. Eventually, larger arteries in the knees and thighs may be affected, in severe cases leading to amputation. Women rarely suffer from this condition, and most men affected are 45 or younger. Symptoms cease when smoking is stopped.

While tobacco symptomatizes pain and discomfort, the underlying cause of this disorder is the consumption of heavy animal foods—especially fatty, greasy, oily foods high in saturated fat, protein, and cholesterol—along with excessive salt consumption, including the consumption of foods treated with salt and salt-cured foods. Spices and stimulants often contribute to this disorder.

To relieve this condition, smoking should be stopped immediately and a slightly more yin form of the Standard Macrobiotic Diet practiced. In addition to the overall nutritional guidelines in Column 3 of Table 24 (page 255), special dishes to be used include the daily consumption of miso soup with wakame and green leafy vegetables; and the frequent consumption of leafy vegetables cooked or taken frequently in salads such as celery, lettuce, cabbage, Chinese cabbage, scallions, and radish. All animal food, including fish and seafood, should be discontinued for a few weeks or until the condition is improved.

RAYNAUD'S PHENOMENON

In this condition, the fingers and toes turn pale, numb, and cold as a result of emotional stress or a moderately cold environment. Spasms in the smaller arteries of the hands and feet drain blood into the veins, causing oxygen depletion in the extremities. This condition affects primarily young women and is rarely serious. Sometimes tiny sores and cracks appear, but the condition does not spread beyond the base of the fingers or toes. Two related conditions include *acrocynanosis,* in which the hands and feet are chronically blue and cold, and *livedo reticularis,* in which a motley pattern appears on the skin from the contraction of arterioles beneath the skin. Both these conditions also arise mostly in young women. In all three cases, vigorous massage of the hands or feet usually restores circulation.

Just as Buerger's Disease is an overly contracted, yang condition, so Raynaud's Phenomenon is an overly expanded, yin condition. Men and women are affected respectively because of constitutional factors—relatively more yang, centripetal energy manifested in men and more yin, centrifugal energy in women— as well as day-to-day dietary habits emphasizing one force over the other. In general, women consume much less animal food and proportionately more fruits, sweets, and liquids than men. In the case of Raynaud's Phenomenon and acrocyanosis, extreme yin in the form of sugar, chocolate, honey, soft drinks, stimulants, aromatic beverages such as mint tea, ice cream, light dairy food, icy cold beverages, and tropical foods are some of the foods that can constrict the small arteries in the hands and feet, leading to blueness and numbness.

To relieve these two conditions, a slightly more yang form of the Standard Macrobiotic Diet should be followed. In addition to observing the nutritional guidelines in Column 1 of Table 24 until the condition improves, hot miso soup should be taken frequently, as well as ume-sho-bancha tea or sho-bancha with a little grated ginger added to increase circulation.

The third condition, livedo reticularis, is caused more by a combination of extreme yin and extreme yang factors. Following the dietary recommendations in Column 2 for an initial period should prove beneficial. Miso soup with wakame and tofu may be taken often to help restore balance to the circulatory system.

Immersing the hands and feet in hot ginger water or placing hot, squeezed towels immersed in ginger water (see instructions for preparing a ginger compress in Chapter 34, "Home Cares") on the affected area should help restore circulation in all three instances. Intestinal weakness usually precedes or accompanies poor blood flow. A ginger compress applied to the intestinal region once a day for three days will be very helpful. Dō-in hand massage may also help restore normal circulation.

26

Diseases of the Veins

The veins are blood vessels that carry returning blood to the heart and lungs. They are thinner, more flexible, and under less pressure than arteries and except in cases of bypass surgery, when a vein from the leg is grafted onto a coronary artery, are not susceptible to atherosclerosis. However, veins are subject to swelling, inflammation, and partial or complete obstruction by a clot or embolus.

VARICOSE VEINS

Varicosity occurs when superficial veins, most commonly in the legs, swell. Blood can stagnate and back up in the lower extremities. Sometimes tiredness and heaviness are felt, but usually the condition is not uncomfortable. Both men and women may be affected. Varicose veins often present a cosmetic problem for women, who sometimes resort to drug treatment or even surgery.

In the past, many people believed that varicose veins were produced by excessive standing, overweight, tight clothing, pregnancy, or hereditary factors, but these are no longer considered by the medical profession to be primary causes. One survey found that in North America, 44 percent of women and 19 percent of men between 30 and 40 years of age, 54 percent and 23 percent respectively between 40 and 50, and 64 percent and 42 percent respectively over 60 have varicose veins.[1] In contrast, varicosity is very rare in traditional societies where the modern diet has not yet been adopted. For example, in Tanzania, 1.8 percent of women and 1.1 percent of men have varicose veins.[2]

In origin, varicose veins arise from a combination of extreme yin and extreme yang foods and beverages, especially dairy foods like cheese and eggs and hard, saturated fat like steak, hamburger, and chicken. Salty foods also contribute to this condition, as do sugar, chocolate, honey, and more excessively yin items usually eaten in combination with fatty substances.

To relieve this condition, a more centrally balanced macrobiotic diet should be followed for the first several months. The nutritional guidelines in Column 2 of Table 24 should be observed, with the salty taste being light to moderate. Special considerations include the regular intake of miso soup; the regular preparation of an azuki bean dish of any kind; the frequent consumption of nishime-style vegetables, especially daikon, carrots, lotus root, and kombu cooked together; and the consumption of sautéed vegetables or fried rice two or three times a week to provide the slight amount of oil needed for this condition. Immersing a towel in hot water, squeezing it out, and applying it to the varicose area for about five minutes, then following with a cold towel, will also be beneficial. Alternate hot and cold applications several times and repeat every day for a short period until relief is experienced.

PHLEBITIS

Phlebitis occurs when a blood clot develops in a vein and partially or completely impedes the flow of blood back toward the heart. It is also called *venous thrombosis, thrombophlebitis,* and *phlebothrombosis.* Phlebitis may occur in many regions of the body, though it is most common in the legs. Frequently, a part of the clot will break off and travel to the lungs, where it can lodge in the pulmonary vessels, leading to lung or heart failure (see Figure 25). In the United States, 50,000 people die from pulmonary embolism arising from phlebitis every year.

Modern medicine controls phlebitis primarily with anticoagulant drugs such as warfarin or heparin, which stop clotting. However, the underlying cause of this form of venous disease is excessive consumption of imbalanced foods. Recent medical studies in Africa have associated the development of deep vein throm-

Figure 25. Pulmonary Embolism

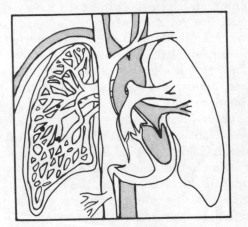

Black dots indicate blood clots
that have drifted from blood
vessels and lodged in the lungs.

bosis and pulmonary embolism with the low intake of dietary fiber.[3] In a clinical trial in Britain, phlebitis patients given diets higher in fiber experienced substantially reduced incidence of both disorders as well.[4]

Compared with the arteries, which are more yang in structure and function, the veins are yin and more susceptible to vascular disease caused by the consumption of extreme yin foods and beverages. In the case of phlebitis, potatoes, tomatoes, and other foods that originally came from the tropics and though grown here have not yet fully adapted to a temperate environment have often been regularly taken. However, clotting is a more yang process, showing that a high intake of meat and dairy food high in saturated fat and cholesterol, as well as an overabundance of refined salt, have usually been consumed over a long period of time as well.

To relieve phlebitis, all extreme foods in the modern diet need to be discontinued and a more moderate, centrally balanced macrobiotic diet adopted. The guidelines in Column 2 of Table 24 may be observed for the initial period. Special dishes include regular miso soup; dried daikon cooked together with carrots, lotus root, and kombu; and hard green leafy vegetables, steamed or water-sautéed, including daikon greens, carrot tops, mustard greens, and dandelion greens. The hot and cold water application mentioned above in connection with varicose veins may also be applied to the affected region.

27

Congenital Heart Disease

During the nine months of pregnancy, the developing embryonic heart is very sensitive to imbalances in the mother's diet and way of life. A wide variety of congenital abnormalities, resulting from nutritional imbalances and other factors such as emotional upset to the mother, affect this organ. According to the Centers for Disease Control in Atlanta, two of the more common congenital malformations—ventricular septal defect (VSD) and patent ductus arteriosus (PDA)—have increased substantially in recent years: The incidence of VSD doubled and that of PDA tripled between 1970 and 1976. These increases have continued into the 1980s, with both rising 38 percent between 1976 and 1980. Altogether about 25,000 babies are born with heart defects each year, of which about one-quarter die. Birth defects of all kinds have doubled during the past twenty-five years. In the 1950s, 2 percent of American babies were born with defects, compared with 4 percent in 1983.[1] In addition to improper diet, environmental pollution, increased smoking on the part of women, and the emotional impact of the decline of the modern family unit appear to be contributing factors.

Congenital heart defects can result when the mother's diet is deficient in minerals, complex carbohydrates, and other nutrients that produce a more contractive effect, or when a proper balance of fats, protein, and minerals, which gives elasticity to the motion of the heart, is lacking (see Figures 26 and 27). Often, the mother has overconsumed simple sugars, such as those in fruit, fruit juice, soft

300

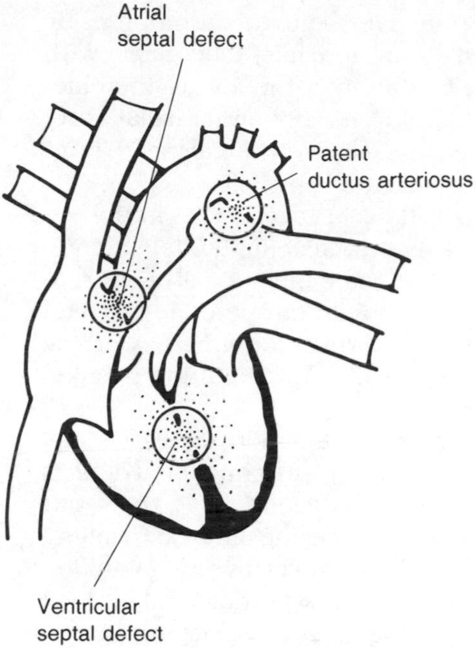

Atrial
septal defect

Patent
ductus arteriosus

Ventricular
septal defect

Figure 26.

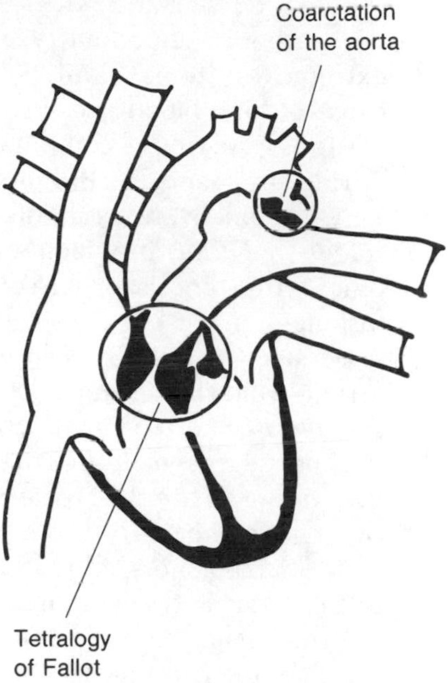

Coarctation
of the aorta

Tetralogy
of Fallot

Figure 27.

Congenital Heart Defects

drinks, and concentrated sweeteners, as well as liquids, drugs, medications, and other more expansive items. The consumption of such excessive yin foods and beverages can cause the tissues that separate the various sections of the heart—tissues that normally close completely in the womb or shortly after birth—to close only partially, leaving an opening. Incomplete fusion may occur in the tissues that divide the lower chambers of the heart *(ventricular septal defect)*, the upper chambers *(atrial septal defect)*, or those that divide the aorta and pulmonary artery *(patent ductus arteriosus)*.

Other common congenital abnormalities include *valve stenosis* and *atresia*, in which the heart valves are abnormally narrowed or closed entirely; *coarctation of the aorta*, in which a portion of the great artery leading away from the heart narrows severely; and *endocardial fibroelastosis*, in which the inner lining of the heart is unusually thickened. Congenital valve disorders may arise from rheumatic fever and generally involve the overconsumption by the mother of eggs, poultry, and other more fatty foods along with extreme yin items. Similarly, coarctation of the aorta—the chief cause of high blood pressure in children—and endocardial fibroelastosis arise from a combination of excessively imbalanced items during pregnancy or the nursing period.

Occasionally, several defects will occur together, as in the *tetrology of Fallot*, in which a large ventricular septal defect combines with stenosis, or narrowing, of the pulmonic valve. In rare instances, major blood vessels can become transposed in the fetal stage, and the baby is born with the aorta and pulmonary artery arising from the wrong side of the heart. This condition is called *transposition of the great arteries.*

The degree of impairment of heart function varies widely, depending on the type of defect. In many cases, congenital defects prevent the heart from pumping blood efficiently, and the result is chronic shortness of breath, coughing, pooling of blood, swelling of the liver, and accumulation of fluid, especially in the ankles. Another major complication occurs when a portion of the blood is prevented from passing through the lungs and exchanging carbon dioxide for oxygen. The blue color of this unoxygenated blood becomes visible through the baby's skin and is especially noticeable in the nail beds. Blue discoloration of the skin is known as *cyanosis*, and in very severe cases, the tips of the fingers become clubbed as a result of a lack of oxygen. Chronic fainting spells also occur. Normally, the baby's hand grasp should be strong and tight. The strength of the grasp reflex corresponds to the contracting power of the heart. If the grasp reflex is not strong, the heart is generally weak as a result of the mother's overconsumption of more yin foods and beverages during pregnancy.

The primary medical approach to congenital heart defects is corrective surgery. In some cases, especially those that are immediately life-threatening, this is necessary. However, in many cases, congenital defects are not immediately threatening and complications do not arise until middle age. While constitutional disorders of all kinds are difficult to correct completely, the Standard Macrobiotic Diet, when properly followed by the breastfeeding mother and by the child in the formative years, can help restore or improve the heart to a more normal function while strengthening the person's condition as a whole. This is especially true when the defect is the result of improper fusion of the heart tissues. Complex carbohydrates, especially those in whole cereal grains such as brown rice, aid in the establishment of a natural contracting process, as do foods rich in minerals, such as sea vegetables and hard, fibrous leafy greens. The proper use of seasonings and condiments is also very important, though only small amounts are needed. Foods such as fruits, raw foods, fats and oils, fluids, and other items that cause tissue expansion are best kept under proper control during the recovery process, either in the diet of the nursing mother or that of the child.

Mothers breastfeeding children with congenital heart defects can follow the general dietary guidelines in Column 1 of Table 24. Carp and burdock soup (koi koku) and mochi are especially beneficial to nursing mothers and will help to strengthen the circulatory condition of mother and child. A good-quality yin product is amasake, a fermented sweet rice beverage that may be taken in liquid form or solidified with kuzu to make puddings and other mildly sweet dishes. General dietary recommendations for infants and small children follow below. These may be observed for both healthy children and those with congenital heart defects or other disorders. However, in the case of existing heart conditions or other serious illness, dietary modifications may need to be made, depending upon the individual case. It is recommended that an experienced macrobiotic dietary or nutritional counselor or medical associate be consulted regarding these adjustments and home cares that may occasionally be needed.

BABY FOOD RECOMMENDATIONS

Our diet should change in accordance with the development of our teeth. The ideal food for the human infant is mother's milk, and all the baby's nourishment should come from this source for the first six to ten months. At that time, the quantity of breastmilk can gradually be decreased over the next six months while soft foods, containing practically no salt, are introduced and proportionately increased. Mother's milk should usually be stopped around the time the first molars appear (usually 12 to 14 months), and the baby's diet by then should consist mostly of soft, mashed foods.

Harder foods should be introduced around the time the first molars appear and their proportion gradually increase over the next year. By the age of 20 to 24 months, softly mashed foods should be replaced entirely by harder foods and comprise the mainstay of the diet.

At the beginning of the third year, a child can receive one-third to one-fourth the amount of salt used by an adult, depending upon its health. A child's intake of salt should continue to be less than an adult's until about the seventh or eighth year.

At age four, the Standard Macrobiotic Diet may be introduced, along with mild sea salt, miso, and other seasonings, including ginger. Different tastes appeal to us at different periods of our development. A natural sweet taste is particularly appealing to babies and children. In general, the following dietary recommendations may be followed:

Whole Grains

Cereal grain milk can be introduced after 8 months to 1 year as the baby's main food. The grain milk may also be given earlier to the baby as a replacement for mother's milk if the mother cannot breastfeed. Brown rice is the principal ingredient in cereal grain milk, and its nutrients come very close to mother's milk. To simulate the sweet taste of mother's milk and provide enough protein and fat for the baby's growth, sweet rice, which contains more of these factors, can be included, as can barley or other whole grains.

The cereal grain milk should be in the form of a soft, whole grain porridge consisting of 4 parts brown rice (preferably short-grain), 3 parts sweet brown rice, and 1 part barley. The cereal is preferably cooked with a piece of kombu, although this sea vegetable does not always have to be eaten. Millet and oats can be included from time to time. However, buckwheat, wheat, and rye are usually not given.

The cereal may be prepared by pressure-cooking or boiling. To pressure-cook, soak the grains overnight or for 24 hours if the weather is very cold. Pressure-cook with five times more water than grain (using the soaking water as well). Cook for about 1½ hours or until the cereal is soft and creamy in consistency. Use a medium-low flame after the grain comes to pressure. To boil, soak the cereals in the same way and boil with ten times more water until one-half the original volume of water remains. When the cereal comes to a boil, turn the flame to medium low and simmer.

When preparing grain milk cereal for a newborn or very small baby, place the cooked mixture into a cheesecloth sack and strain it to remove the bran. It can then be sweetened by adding 1 teaspoon of barley malt or rice syrup to 1 cup of grain milk. Heat the sweetened mixture and simmer several minutes before use.

When preparing the grain milk for an older baby, put the mixture into a suribachi or a hand food mill after it has finished cooking and mash it very thoroughly. Do not use a blender or electric device for grinding. After mashing the mixture, add a small amount of barley malt or rice syrup.

Once the grain milk has achieved the proper taste and consistency, heat the mixture to about body temperature and put it into a baby bottle. Cereal grain milk can be stored in a glass jar and reheated before subsequent feedings.

If either of the above cereal grain milks do not flow smoothly through the nipple, they can be further diluted with water and strained several times through cheesecloth. You may also enlarge the opening of the nipple with a large darning needle. Sterilize the tip of the needle by holding it over a flame before using it to enlarge the opening. Among nipples, special orthodontic nipples are preferred, as these tend to foster the natural development of the teeth and jaws.

The ingredients and proportions of the grain milk can be varied slightly, depending on the age and needs of the baby. Grain milk can also be used as one of the first soft foods that a baby is given once foods other than breast milk are introduced. In general, a more watery grain milk is recommended for younger babies, while older infants can receive a firmer mixture. Depending on the age of the baby, the proportion of water to cereal can range from 10:1 to 7:1 to 3:1.

Sesame seeds may be added to the grain milk if desired. The seeds should be well roasted and thoroughly crushed in a suribachi before being added. About 5 to 10 percent crushed seeds can be cooked along with the grains.

Babies may also be given special rice cream from time to time. To prepare, pressure-cook brown rice with 3 to 6 parts water and a 1-inch piece of kombu for at least two hours. (Do not add salt.) Squeeze the cooked rice and liquid through a piece of sanitized cheesecloth into a bowl. Put this thick liquid into a baby bottle, diluting and straining again if necessary. On occasion, the rice can be roasted prior to pressure-cooking.

Be careful to avoid giving babies ready-to-eat creamy cereals or porridges made with flour products.

Soup

Soup, especially broth, can be introduced after five months. The contents may include vegetables that have been mashed until creamy. No salt, miso, or tamari soy sauce should be added before the baby is ten months old. Thereafter, a slightly salty taste may be used for flavoring. However, if the baby's stool is green or if the baby experiences digestive troubles, a salty taste should be used only in small amounts and only for a short period.

Vegetables

In addition to grain milk, very young babies can be given the juice from cooked vegetables. To prepare, bring vegetables such as carrots, squash, cabbage, broccoli, or corn to a boil. A 1-inch piece of soaked kombu may be added. Simmer the ingredients over a low flame for thirty to forty-five minutes. Strain the liquid from cooking the vegetables through sanitized cheesecloth. Place in a bottle and give to the baby. Whole vegetables may be introduced after the baby is five to seven months old, usually when teeth come in and grains have been given for one month. When introducing vegetables to children, start with sweet vegetables such as carrots, cabbage, winter squash, onions, daikon, and Chinese cabbage. These may be boiled or steamed and should be well cooked and thoroughly mashed. Because it is usually difficult for children to eat greens, parents should make a special effort to see that they are eaten. Sweet greens such as kale and broccoli are generally preferred over slightly bitter-tasting greens such as watercress and mustard greens. Very mild seasoning may be added to vegetables after ten months to encourage the appetite. When baby's teeth start coming in, a raw carrot may be given as a toy to stimulate teething.

Beans

Naturally processed soy milk may be given to babies as a supplement to cereal grain milk. To prepare, soak about 3 cups of soybeans overnight, strain, and discard the soaking water. Grind the beans in an electric blender (this is one of the rare instances in which an electric device is used in macrobiotic cooking). Or if you have time and patience, a hand food mill can be used. Add about 6 quarts of water and a 1-inch piece of kombu to the bean mash and bring to a boil. Reduce flame to low and simmer for about five minutes. Stir continuously to prevent burning. Sprinkle cold water on the mash to stop the bubbling and bring gently to a boil again. Sprinkle cold water on the mash once more and again bring to a boil. (Don't cover the mash, as it will bubble over the top of the pot.) Place a cotton cloth or cheesecloth in a strainer and pour the liquid—the soy milk—through the strainer and into a bowl. Fold the corners of the cloth together to form a sack and squeeze out the remaining liquid. (The pulp, known as okara, can be saved and used in other dishes.) Put the soy milk in a bottle and feed to the baby. If the soy milk does not flow smoothly, dilute it with water and strain through a cheesecloth until the desired consistency is obtained. Soy milk is usually very sweet, but if additional sweetener is desired, barley malt or rice syrup can be added, as in the grain milk recipe. Soy milk can be stored and reheated to body temperature prior to use.

Whole beans can be introduced after eight months, but only small amounts of azuki beans, lentils, or chick-peas, cooked well with kombu and mashed thoroughly, are recommended. Other beans such as kidney beans, whole soybeans, and navy beans can also be served occasionally, provided they are cooked until very soft and mashed thoroughly. Beans may be seasoned with a tiny amount of sea salt or tamari soy sauce or sweetened with squash, barley malt, or rice syrup.

Sea Vegetables

Kombu is generally cooked with cereal grain milk but taken out after cooking. If mashed until very soft, a tiny amount of kombu may be given to babies, as well as a touch of nori or a taste of hiziki and arame. Generally, seaweeds can be introduced as a separate side dish after the child is one and a half to two years old.

Seasoning

No salt, miso, or tamari soy sauce should be given babies before they are ten months old. After that age, a slightly salty taste may be used for flavoring. At the beginning of the third year, a child can receive from one-third to one-fourth the amount of salt used by an adult. Seasoning can gradually be increased until age seven or eight, when it can be the same as older children and adults. During this time, children's and adult's food may be cooked together but before the final seasoning is added, the children's portion can be taken out and served separately. Dishes may also be seasoned minimally and additional seasoning added by adults at the table in the form of gomashio and other condiments. Generally, young children should not be given very much tempeh, seitan, tofu, and other foods high in salt or sodium. Moderate volumes, prepared very softly, may be given from time to time.

Animal Food

Until age four, infants ideally should not have any animal food, including fish, except in special cases where the child is weak, slightly anemic, or lacks energy. Then give about 1 tablespoon of white-meat fish or seafood that has been well boiled with vegetables and mashed. At age four, if desired, a small amount of white-meat fish or seafood may be included from time to time for enjoyment.

Fruit

Fruit may occasionally be given to babies and infants. Temperate-climate fruit, in season, can be introduced in small amounts—

about 1 tablespoon, cooked and mashed—after one and a half to two years of age. However, in some special cases, cooked apples or apple juice may be used temporarily as an adjustment for some conditions.

Pickles

Pickles that are traditionally made, quick and light in aging and seasoning can be introduced after the child is about five years of age.

Beverages

Daily drinks may include spring or well water (preferably boiled and cooled), bancha twig tea, cereal grain tea, apple juice (warm or hot), and amasake (which has been boiled with two times as much water and cooled).

For further information on baby and childhood nutrition and health, please refer to our book *Macrobiotic Pregnancy and Care of the Newborn,* or contact a qualified macrobiotic counselor.

28

Case Histories

The following personal accounts are of real men, women, and young people who have relieved or are currently relieving heart and circulatory disorders by using the dietary approach and other methods presented in this book. Many of these people have sought guidance from me in recent years and after restoring their health and vitality have gone on to become teachers or dietary and nutritional counselors. Some stories are drawn from case histories published by the East West Foundation and *East West Journal*. Others have been especially prepared for this volume. While these accounts are largely anecdotal, with varying degrees of medical documentation, we hope that they will encourage heart disease researchers to conduct case-control studies to measure the effectiveness of the macrobiotic approach and to propose modifications of the approach in light of evolving clinical experience. Through the Kushi Foundation, we would like to cooperate in these investigations, as we are now cooperating with various medical schools, hospitals, and community institutions in a variety of other fields. I am very grateful to all those who have shared their accounts in these pages and hope their experience will inspire and instruct others.

CARDIOVASCULAR CONDITION

After World War II, Jack Saunders went to work in the aircraft industry as an engineer and designer. He was based for a while in

California, where Chuck Yeager and other experimental pilots broke the sound barrier. In the 1960s, he began working at the General Electric plant in Lynn, Massachusetts, designing jet engines. Following routine company medical examinations, doctors at GE told him that he had the beginnings of a potentially serious heart condition. On the basis of his electrocardiogram (EKG), one physician later explained that he had had a "silent heart attack." While symptoms are not experienced, this condition can result in permanent damage to the heart and lead to more serious attacks in the future.

Saunders was introduced to macrobiotics in 1971 through a member of a yoga group who had read George Ohsawa and William Dufty's book, *You Are All Sanpaku*. After reading the book himself, Saunders began to cook macrobiotically and to attend my lectures in Boston.

"At this time I was very tense," Saunders recalls, "and often found it difficult to deal with people in stressful situations. After eating macrobiotically for only a few weeks, I relaxed quite remarkably and found I was much more effective in handling difficult situations with people. Shortly after I began the diet, I was instrumental in securing a contract which is still providing a good deal of the work for my company in Lynn. I have found this has become typical, and I really think my diet has aided me in dealing with customers and business."

After Saunders adopted the macrobiotic approach, his cardiovascular condition quickly disappeared. In a series of medical tests at GE in 1974, doctors reported that his heart was in good shape. "Slight [EKG] changes noted in 1972 and 1974 compared to tracings in 1964–1969 are indicative that sometime in the past he had an old anterior-septal myocardial infarction. The present EKG compared to 1972 is stable and there is no indication of a current problem," his medical records state.

Colleagues at GE at first found Saunders' diet unusual, but this never caused him any disruption at work. "I have noticed friends and colleagues my age having various health difficulties, ranging from mild to severe. And without exception, they eat and live in a chaotic fashion, ignoring natural foods and life-style. Even so, I feel that natural foods are not enough; without the guiding principles of yin and yang, natural foods alone cannot insure good health."

In addition to eating well, Saunders engages in some intense physical activity daily to activate his entire cardiovascular system. In addition to jogging and swimming, he is an avid mountain climber and has gone off on climbing expeditions all over the world. In 1984, he received an important assignment from GE to head up a major contract with Japanese industrialists, which took him to Japan.

"On my previous diet, I was not able to deal as well with people or to reconcile various differences between people. Macrobiotics has not only changed my physical health," he concludes, "it has changed my entire life."

Source: Jack Saunders, "Case History," in Michio Kushi, *Cancer and Heart Disease* (Tokyo: Japan Publications, 1982); medical records; and interview with Alex Jack, December 1983.

HEART ATTACK

Win Donovan was trying to remove a large stone from a sewer line when he suffered a heart attack. Like most people who suffer heart attacks, Donovan's life was radically changed by the devastating blow. Unlike most people whose hearts abruptly stop, however, Donovan says the event changed his life for the better.

On April 27, 1978, Win Donovan was building a house not far from his own home in Worthington, a small town in western Massachusetts. The thirty-eight-year-old contractor owned his own construction firm, and at this time, two years before mortgage rates shot up, business was good. In fact, work had been good for the past several years, and Donovan was doing less and less of the tough, physical labor that he had been accustomed to doing before the books were so black. This day was different, however, and Donovan was working hard.

As he struggled with the large rock, he suddenly felt nauseated. A swelling sensation gripped his chest. The swelling changed to pain, which spread from his heart to the rest of his chest and neck. His left arm hurt, and he began to sweat profusely. Donovan had been a volunteer ambulance driver in Worthington and recognized the symptoms. He was scared, but he did not panic.

A friend was standing nearby, and Donovan asked him to accompany him to the nearest hospital. They both jumped into

Donovan's truck, with Donovan behind the wheel. Soon, the pain grew intolerable and he turned the driving over to his friend. Donovan passed out before reaching the emergency room.

Donovan's heart attack did not come as a great surprise. Although he had not been sick for a day during the first thirty-five years of his life, his health had been declining for some time. By 1975, three years before his heart gave out, he had begun to experience some serious problems. That year, he contracted pneumonia, which left him with pleurisy. He also suffered from extreme kidney trouble. From 1976 until 1978, Donovan had four severe kidney attacks, all of which left him hospitalized and unconscious for days at a time. Meanwhile, his cholesterol level hovered at a dangerously high 358 mg. Once it had reached 395 mg. Most Americans have cholesterol levels at about 220, and anything above 250 is regarded as in the high-risk range for heart attack or stroke. Both his parents had had heart attacks within the previous three years, and his wife's father had died of a myocardial infarction, so Donovan was familiar with the disease.

Donovan had not paid any attention to his way of eating for most of his first three and a half decades. His family raised potatoes and beef, and when growing up he had worked with cattle on his uncle's farm. He took his strong constitution and active, outdoor way of life for granted and consumed large amounts of animal food, especially eggs, baloney, and cheese. Eating at home was usually on the run. The family had bought a microwave oven to streamline cooking even more but had not had time to use it. Donovan also smoked and drank heavily. "After I first got sick," he later recalled, "I was forced to change from hard whiskey to schnappes, coffee brandy, aspirin, and sweet-tasting ladies' drinks."

Doctors could not figure out what exactly was wrong with Donovan. According to his physician, Dr. William Shevin, who now practices in Putnam, Connecticut, Donovan had a disease "something on the order of lupus." With all the complications, Shevin says that Donovan was very, very ill. "It's hard to quantify how close anyone is to death," states Shevin, "but Win Donovan was a very sick man."

Donovan was also examined at the Lahey Clinic in Boston, and it was finally decided that he should take antibiotics, cortisone tablets called Prednisone, and diuretics. Nothing worked, however, and Donovan continued to have kidney attacks and recurring pleurisy pain throughout his chest.

While Donovan's health was rapidly declining, his younger brother, Greg, kept telling him about the macrobiotic approach to health. "I didn't really listen to him," Donovan remembers. "You know how it is with younger brothers."

After a while, however, Donovan started listening and made major changes in his diet. However, his practice was haphazard, he didn't take any cooking lessons, and he says that he had no real understanding of what he was putting in his mouth.

He had been trying to improve his diet for several months when his heart attack came in early April 1978. When Donovan regained consciousness in the hospital after the attack, his doctors had some bad news. The physicians told him that he would have to make immediate arrangements for a kidney dialysis machine, into which he would have to "plug himself" a couple of times per week to go on living. "A kidney machine is temporary," explains Donovan. "You stay with it until you can find a kidney donor for doctors to do a transplant. Donated kidneys last about four years. The doctors told me that I was very lucky to have six brothers and sisters as potential donors."

However, even with new kidneys, Donovan's heart probably would not be strong enough to survive. "The doctors told me not to make any long-range plans, like taking on any additional debts, because I was not going to be living much longer to pay them off," he recalls. Shortly thereafter, Donovan made his decision. "It was either decide to take macrobiotics seriously, or take out more life insurance and drive my car off a cliff. Deep inside somewhere I knew that I wasn't going to die. I guess what upset me most was one of the doctors there who kept saying 'thirty-eight-year-old man, drinks, smokes, typical, typical.' I wanted to live just to show he was wrong."

Later that summer, Donovan had another examination with Dr. Shevin. Donovan told Shevin that he had decided to either take another examination with the Lahey Clinic or meet with me. At that time, I was teaching at the East West Foundation's annual summer program, which was held at that time at Amherst College in Amherst, Massachusetts, not far from Donovan's hometown. Shevin, who was familiar with macrobiotics, did not discourage

Donovan from going to the Lahey Clinic, but he did encourage him to see me.

"At that point Donovan had decided to take better care of himself," recalls Shevin. "He decided to eat better-quality food, cut out smoking and drinking, and seek a higher quality of life. So I encouraged him to do that."

That August, Donovan and his wife went to Amherst but discovered that my consultations were filled. Instead, they saw Michael Rossoff, who had been teaching macrobiotics for nearly ten years and had an acupuncture practice with a medical doctor in Rockville, Maryland. When Rossoff saw Donovan, he did not pull any punches. "Michael told me that I was entirely to blame for my condition," Donovan looks back. "I had been soaking up sympathy from friends and relatives and everyone was telling me I was too young for this terrible thing to happen. Michael, however, told me that health and sickness were my responsibility and it was up to me to change my way of life."

Rossoff recommended the Standard Macrobiotic Diet, which Donovan says he finally began to understand for the first time, and some specific recommendations for Donovan's condition. "He was frightened enough to make dramatic changes in his life," Rossoff recalls, "and his wife was very supportive. That helped him change."

Donovan did not have to wait long to see changes in his condition. "After about a week, I stopped taking all medication," he says. "I was drinking daikon radish tea, and that worked as well if not better than the diuretic pills I was taking for my high blood pressure. The other pills I just stopped." The pain in his chest, which he had been experiencing regularly, vanished. He stopped having kidney attacks and has not had one since.

Three years of kidney and pleurisy attacks, a heart attack, and weeks in the hospital left Donovan weakened and lethargic. However, within weeks after starting the macrobiotic diet, his strength quickly returned; he began looking again for work.

Donovan returned to see Dr. Shevin shortly thereafter for an examination. "There was a remarkable change in him," says Shevin. "He was still discharging some protein through the urine, but that was a far secondary problem in comparison to the other major improvements he had made." Shevin recalls that all other signs in

Donovan's examination were normal, including pulse rate and blood pressure, both of which were dangerously elevated before Donovan changed his eating habits.

In September 1980, Donovan had his blood cholesterol level checked at the Beacon Medical Laboratories in Boston. It was 200 mg, a drop of nearly 200 mg from what it had been two years prior to his starting the macrobiotic diet. During this time, Donovan had taken no medication and engaged in no therapy; he had only changed his daily way of eating. His weight fell from 210 pounds to 150, and he felt healthier than before. Once, he tried to cash a money order, using his driver's license as identification. The license bore a photograph of Donovan taken three years earlier. The storekeeper looked at him and refused to cash the money order.

In 1980, Donovan ran into Ken Burns, a macrobiotics teacher in Boston who was conducting a wild foods foraging class. "We argued over the identification of a tree," Donovan remembers. "That impressed me. Until then I had changed my way of eating and felt better, but had not really wanted to study the philosophy of macrobiotics. I came to Boston to study with Ken and remodeled his house."

Donovan's understanding continued to grow, but he maintained the fiercely independent New England streak with which he had been born. Although the Standard Macrobiotic Diet does not recommend the consumption of ginseng and other strong herbs except for limited medicinal purposes, Donovan decided to experiment for himself. One year he found wild ginseng growing in the woods and consumed twelve roots in a month's time. Ginseng is an extremely yang substance and has a powerful contractive effect on the body. As a result, the blood circulation in Donovan's legs was so reduced that he couldn't sleep or urinate. "I became so tight that drinking a couple fifths of Jim Beam whiskey had no effect. I just couldn't loosen up after taking the ginseng." Finally, gangrene set in and he had to have one of his big toes cut off. It was a costly lesson.

Since then Donovan has been more careful. Today he and his wife are planning classes in macrobiotic cooking and homebuilding. The Donovans' two children, a twenty-one-year-old daughter and a seventeen-year-old son are also practicing macrobiotics. The daughter recently had a natural home birth. Two of Donovan's sisters are also practicing the new way of eating "pretty seriously," and his parents' diet has also substantially improved as a result of their son's experience.

Donovan's advice for other heart patients is to go slow and eat as widely as their condition permits. "In my experience grains are much more yang, more energizing than meat. Heart patients and others with circulatory problems are usually pretty active. Once their condition has stabilized, I recommend that they eat salads, fruit, occasional fish." Donovan also says that when he smoked cigarettes regularly, he noticed pain in his feet. When he tried switching to natural tobacco that did not contain sugar, chemicals, and other additives, he said he felt no pain.

Donovan's approach to contracting has also changed. "I used to build about six ranch houses a year. You just throw them together and they go up pretty quick. Now, I'm building timber frame houses, the kind they used to build three hundred years ago. They're better houses and there's a lot more challenge in it." Donovan wants to design a house aimed at improving people's health. He also has ideas for developing an air-envelope, solar power kit that people could assemble themselves or with the aid of a small contractor. He calls his dream house, which incorporates more natural principles, the North South East West House.

According to one of his former doctors, Win Donovan should be dead by now or on his second donated kidney. He is living proof that a serious heart attack can be overcome with natural methods and that a person can learn from past mistakes and go on to help and inspire others. When asked what the fundamental difference is between the Win Donovan of the past and Win Donovan now, he points to his heart and smiles, "I'm happier today."

Sources: This account is adapted from an article by Tom Monte, "Curing Heart Disease without the Knife: Win Donovan," *East West Journal* (November 1980), 38–39; updated by Alex Jack in an interview with Win Donovan, January 1984.

HIGH BLOOD PRESSURE

In 1976, after twenty-six years in the Marine Corps, Fletcher So-journer retired and went to work at Hahnumann Hospital Medical College in Philadelphia in an administrative capacity. In the service, the forty-three-year-old Sojourner had always had a clean bill of health and felt in good condition. One day, while carrying a sphygmomanometer, a device for measuring blood pressure in the arteries, to the emergency room, a doctor decided to test it out because it had just been repaired. " 'We'll use you,' the doctor told me," Sojourner later recalled. "As he started to check my blood pressure, his eyes got a little larger and he told me I'd better go see my personal physician."

That afternoon at the employee clinic, Fletcher made an appointment with a doctor who was an internationally known authority on hypertension. The doctor took his blood pressure, which was moderately elevated—145/114—and asked Sojourner whether he would be willing to go on a test drug called Endepromide. Sojourner agreed and went on the drug for a year, but the FDA revoked the drug's use and the doctor stopped it. During this time, Sojourner's blood pressure had dropped to the 130s/90s range. For the next two years he was put on Cellequin, which was also pulled off the market because of its harmful side effects, and he then took Hyperton and two diuretics.

Meanwhile, his wife had started eating macrobiotically to help relieve her hypoglycemia and encouraged Fletcher to change his basic way of eating. "I was an original skeptic," he admits. "I had had some rice and vegetables when I was stationed in the Far East, but I continued to cook my steak, drink Manhattans and martinis and that kind of thing." Nevertheless, Sojourner agreed to accompany his wife to an East West Foundation lecture and dinner in Philadelphia. Denny Waxman, the director, said that it was very hard to heal an illness without the support of a spouse or family. "I said to my wife, 'Let's go for it,' so I changed completely."

Fletcher immediately started to notice a weight reduction on the new diet, losing about 2 pounds a week. Within three months, he had lost 45 pounds and his weight stabilized at a trim 170 pounds. Sojourner says he felt so good that he wanted to stop his antihypertensive medication immediately, but Denny Waxman told him to wait a few more weeks. After six weeks of eating macrobiotic food, Sojourner stopped taking all drugs and went back to his doctor for a checkup. To his surprise, the doctor found that Sojourner's blood pressure had dropped to 122/72, well within the normal range, in less than two months.

Initially, Fletcher's doctors had never discussed diet with him other than to tell him to watch his intake of salt and to use a salt substitute. However, Sojourner says his physician at the medical college was so impressed with the results that he invited him to speak about diet in one of his classes.

At the time of his retirement from the Marine Corps, Sojourner was not very active or athletic. Now he jogs five miles a day and notices a general increase in his vitality. "My energy level has increased immeasurably. My stamina is phenomenal. Friends are very inquisitive. They see me running at lunch hour and wonder why they can't do the same thing. But they can't give up their meat or martinis."

In 1983, just turned fifty, Fletcher gave up his job at the hospital to open an East West Center in Ocean City, New Jersey, and teach macrobiotic cooking and philosophy with his wife. Not bad for a retired marine who was supposed to spend the rest of his life on experimental drugs.

Source: Interview with Fletcher Sojourner by Alex Jack, June 1983.

IRREGULAR HEARTBEAT AND HYPERTENSION

Mildred Christensen looked and acted older than her sixty-eight years. For many years she had been plagued by serious illnesses and had had several operations. In addition to an irregular heartbeat, heart palpitations, and high blood pressure, she suffered from arthritis, constant kidney and bladder infections, female disorders, loss of hearing, and was overweight. For fourteen years she had been on heart medication, including a digitalis-like drug, Inderal, and Motrin and Interon. In 1981, doctors told her that she had diabetes. Each day she took a total of eleven pills, one for each of her various ailments.

A native Kansan, Mildred had lived all her life in the small town of Concordia. Over the years her four sons and daughter had become accustomed to their mother's worsening condition and, though she was not bedridden, considered her somewhat of an invalid. Her husband, with whom she had run a tire store in Concordia, had recently died, and her children were concerned about the effect his passing would have on her condition.

Meanwhile, in Pittsburgh, Ivona Kemp, Mildred's daughter, was going through her own ordeal with breast cancer and had become involved with the macrobiotic approach to health. She had made so much progress in her own case that she wanted to see whether the diet might be of some help to her mother. In July 1982, Mrs. Christensen agreed to come for a visit to Pittsburgh. "She arrived at the airport so crippled from arthritis in her hips and knees that she could barely walk," Ivona later recalled, "and it was necessary to have an airline employee take Mother from the arrival gate to the front of the building in an electric cart. She appeared to be in worse health than a few months previously."

On the second day of her visit, Mrs. Christensen told her daughter that she would be returning to Kansas because she hadn't brought her walker and was in too much pain to stay. Ivona persuaded her to stay and told her she had a new diet that might help her condition. "I fixed her a plate exactly like mine and set it in front of her. She looked at the brown rice and sort of turned up her nose. She kept pulling out this diet a doctor had given her since discovering that she was diabetic. It called for a piece of lean meat, raw salad, and baked potato or steamed vegetables. 'This is what I'm supposed to eat. I don't think I should eat brown rice. It has too many carbohydrates.' I said, 'Mother, trust me,' but she wasn't very trusting the first few days."

Besides cooking macrobiotically prepared meals, Ivona gave her mother hot ginger compresses to help relieve the pain in her joints. Although she still did not like the rice at first, Mrs. Christensen decided to stay for the rest of her visit and continue eating her daughter's food. "One morning after she had been with me a couple of weeks," Ivona relates, "she announced that she felt better than she had in years! Well, I knew then that the corner of resistance had been turned. She studied those macrobiotic books zealously from then on. As she felt more energetic, she helped with the cooking and began to offer suggestions on my menus."

Mildred's two-week visit stretched into three and then four weeks. By then she was feeling so much better that she cut her arthritis medicine in half. One day she decided to accompany Ivona and her granddaughter to the Pittsburgh Zoo. "She walked the complete length of the zoo. It was unbelievable. I haven't seen her walk that far for twenty years," Ivona recalls.

In August, she had a consultation with macrobiotics teacher

Michael Rossoff, who was visiting Pittsburgh, and he further refined her diet, recommending special dishes of squash, azuki beans, and kombu cooked together, as well as sweet rice cooked with brown rice and sesame seeds. Shortly thereafter, Mrs. Christensen returned home with a new lease on life. Her bags were packed with several months' supply of macrobiotic food items that she felt she might not be able to find in a small Midwest town and a variety of cookbooks.

Back home, Mildred kept in touch with Ivona by phone, as they always had. "What a surprise to answer the phone in mid-week and hear mother's excited voice saying, 'You can't imagine what wonderful news I have. This morning when I woke up, my ear was on my watch and I could actually hear it tick. Why, I haven't been able to hear anything in that ear for at least six years!' "

At first her local doctor was skeptical of the new way of eating, but when her blood sugar count quickly returned to normal, he discontinued her oral insulin. As her weight lowered, as her blood pressure dropped from 190/110 to 135/70, and as the general improvement in her health became apparent, her physician reduced her heart medication from three pills daily to two, then to one, and told her to keep on with whatever she was eating as her condition had so much improved.

In January 1983, after six months on the diet, Mrs. Christensen went to Florida for a vacation and saw her daughter again. "With excited anticipation, I waited for her flight to arrive," says Ivona. "When she entered the gate, I was taken back. Here was my mother of years ago! She had lost a great deal of excess weight, walked with a spring in her step, had a happy smile on her face, and her eyes just glowed with health. Even her white hair had changed to a soft gray color."

By April, Mrs. Christenson was entirely off drugs, and she felt better than she had in decades. She could walk long distances for the first time in years. She started gardening again and worked in one of her son's orchards for five weeks. For longer distances, she got a bicycle, and she was active enough to organize a Bible study group at a senior citizens' center where she lived. "I can do whatever I want to now," Mildred smiles. "I believe she has indeed found what eluded Ponce de Leon," concludes Ivona, "—the eternal Fountain of Youth."

Both Mrs. Christensen and her daughter went on to study at

the Kushi Institute and are now writing a book together on their experiences.

Sources: Ivona Kemp, "Senior Citizens on Macrobiotics," *Macromuse* (February/March 1983), 13, 30; and interview with Mildred Christensen and Ivona Kemp by Alex Jack, June 1983.

IRREGULAR HEARTBEAT

Lori O'Neil's general condition was never very good. From childhood she had suffered constant fatigue, chronic throat and ear infections, anemia, and occasional mononucleosis. In November 1976, while living in Ann Arbor, Michigan, she began to develop extreme weakness and dizziness. "I began to feel my heart pounding in my chest," she recalls. "The heartbeat was irregular, with no pattern, often extremely rapid and pounding hard. For four months I was unable to work, as I was almost completely bedridden. I was given several medications, tranquilizers, and pain pills for palpitations, insomnia, and headaches."

Norpace kept the heartbeat close to normal, but the high dosage she was taking began to cause side effects: constipation, anxiety, and insomnia. She still felt very weak and dizzy.

In April 1977, she returned to work for three hours daily, doing mostly desk work because of the fatigue. By September of that year, her condition had not improved at all. While sitting in the waiting room at the University of Michigan Hospital one day, she spoke with an older woman, who told her how switching to a vegetarian diet and taking vitamin supplements had cured her of many ailments, including a partially paralyzed arm.

"I knew that my diet was not very good," Lori says, looking back, "so I was willing to try natural foods to improve my condition. I began by cutting all preservatives, chemicals, meat, and sugar from my diet. I began eating whole grain breads instead of white. I began to eat large amounts of fruits, vegetables, yogurt, and nuts, to use honey instead of sugar, and to take multivitamin tablets."

Five months later, in February 1978, she still had shown no improvement. Many times she tried to decrease the amount of medication she was taking for irregular heartbeat, but she could not do it. With any decrease in medication, the discomfort of the irregular heartbeat became unbearable.

That month she started following the macrobiotic diet and way of life, eating daily whole grains and brown rice, locally grown vegetables, beans, sea vegetables, miso or tamari soup, and occasionally cooked fruits as desserts. She stopped using dairy products, honey, nuts (except on rare occasions), and vitamins.

"Basically, the principle of macrobiotics is to eat organic, locally grown foods, as was traditional in most cultures for more than 5,000 years, while making minor adjustments to compensate for seasonal change and present condition. Somewhere in our civilization's past this simple approach to physical and mental health and happiness was lost—I was now recovering it again! The macrobiotic diet brought these results: within two or three weeks, my insomnia ended; I began to feel very refreshed in the morning upon awaking. I began to get up earlier and also to go to sleep earlier at night."

Her mental attitude also improved, and she began to feel generally happier. After about one month on the new diet, her heart began to beat less irregularly, and she reduced her dosage of Norpace by one-half. "My heart continued to grow stronger," she relates, "and after two months of macrobiotics I stopped taking all medication. At this time my heart was still 'skipping' occasionally, but this would not make me feel as light-headed, dizzy, or fatigued as before. Also, the pounding feeling in my chest with skipped beats was greatly reduced."

During the next six weeks, after stopping medication, she began to feel stronger very quickly. She felt much more energetic, and the palpitations were few. She began to exercise much more, as it was springtime, and spend more time outdoors. Lori was no longer held back by any symptoms. With friends, she was able to keep up in any sport or activity.

Lori describes her condition since then as one of continuous improvement. Any palpitations she has experienced have been minor and infrequent. She has also overcome other difficulties and experienced additional benefits since starting macrobiotics. "I used to be a quiet type of person, uncomfortable with strangers, even withdrawn, and always tried to avoid social get-togethers, strangers, and meeting new people. Now I love being with people, am more confident and comfortable with all people, and welcome making new friends."

She says that she has learned that mind and body cannot be separated. They are one and are affected by what we eat and drink daily. "I am now responsible for my own health, and I feel this is the way it was intended to be. I will continue to study macrobiotics and to adjust my diet according to my condition, to keep myself in the greatest possible state of health, both physically and mentally."

Source: Lori O'Neil, "Case History," in Michio Kushi, *Cancer and Heart Disease* (Tokyo: Japan Publications, 1982), 173–74.

ELEVATED LIPID LEVELS

Peter Klein had been plagued with illness from childhood, starting with an early reaction to cow's milk, the development of allergies, and the onset of severe asthma at the age of three. From then on he had difficulty breathing and frequently stayed up all night until he discovered that if he rocked back and forth in bed, he would eventually pass out. But he never knew whether he would wake up or suffocate, and when he did wake up, he knew there would be another night of struggle.

After three episodes of severe upper respiratory infection, the last being a case of pneumonia, he was hospitalized and placed in an oxygen tent for several months. After this, he went to a home for asthmatics in Denver. For the first time in life, he was free to play baseball, football, and basketball, and his condition improved. However, when he returned home, he still had an occasional attack until he moved to New Orleans to go to medical school.

When her son entered medical school, Peter's mother discovered that she had type IV hyperlipidemia, a blood disorder characterized by excess fat and oil (lipids) and associated with a higher risk of heart attack and stroke. Her doctor put her on a drug, Atronoid S. As soon as Peter found out about his mother's condition, he ran a test showing that he also had type IV hyperlipidemia, a condition that often runs in the same family. He also found that his uric acid count was 13.5 (normal is about 6). Hyperuricemia is usually a precursor of gout, and his elevated blood sugar level of 110 was a possible precursor of diabetes. Afterward, Peter's brother was tested and found to have a uric acid count of about 11. The brother decided to go on drug therapy, but Peter decided he was not going to take any drugs, especially the one recommended for him, since he knew one out of a thousand people who took it developed leukemia, the disease from which his father died.

"I concluded that I must be putting something into my body that was causing me to have an abnormal chemistry and decided to figure out how to get myself back in balance," Peter later recalled. "I decided to start by giving up animal foods, because their high protein content is converted to purine, which eventually shows up as uric acid. Animal foods such as dairy products and eggs are also high in the things that elevate the lipid level. I also started to eliminate sugar and sweets, since they often compromise the pancreas."

To pay his way through medical school, Peter had to work as many as thirty-nine hours a week and did not have much time to study beyond the required curriculum. Even though he had some idea of the foods he had to give up, he did not know what to eat and how to prepare it. The medical literature on nutrition was of little help, since he could not find diets that excluded animal food and sugar, while the recommended substitutes were usually highly processed or synthetic foods.

"During medical school I began to see more and more how the intake of certain substances contributed to illness and degeneration. It was easy to see how alcohol contributed to liver disease, pancreatitis and gastrointestinal problems, and how diets high in animal foods, dairy foods, and eggs contributed to cardiovascular disease, as did obesity in general. It was also obvious that sugar could lead to the development of hypoglycemia and mild maturity-onset diabetes, with related cardiovascular problems, heart attacks, strokes, blindness, impotence, and amputations. I also saw how smoking and air pollution led to lung disease, and from my personal experience realized how milk and orange juice led to mucus deposits that contributed to difficulty in breathing and asthma. I also saw how stress and the rapid pace of life led to tension and possible hypertension, and how quick decisions based on poor judgment led to frequent accidents and mistakes."

From working with many sick people, Peter saw how difficult it was to help them once their sickness had become acute, and he came to the conclusion that it would be much better to prevent illness than to try to treat it once it developed. After completing his internship in Los Angeles, he started his psychiatry residency and took a job working at an emergency room on weekends. It was there that he treated an architect who introduced him to the East West Center in Los Angeles in 1974.

Following an introductory lecture, Peter (now Dr. Klein) sat down to a macrobiotically prepared meal that began with miso soup and included grains and vegetables. "I enjoyed the food and the company of the people I met," he says, looking back. "As I chewed my food, I began to think that this was something I should have started long ago. The meals got better and better as my sensitivity to taste increased, and I soon realized that I was doing something that could lead to a change in my health and well-being.

"Eating macrobiotically has done a lot for me. It helped bring my cholesterol level down to normal, and I now feel that the quality of my blood will continue to improve, along with the condition of my blood vessels and my condition in general. I no longer worry about the degeneration of my blood vessels, a worry that plagued me when I found out that I had type IV hyperlipidemia.

"My blood pressure has dropped from 140/90 to 107/70 and my pulse rate, once 80 to 100, now is between 42 and 66. The macrobiotic diet also helped lower my blood sugar level to normal; thus I stopped worrying about diabetes, with its degeneration of the small arteries; 'blindness'; impotence; strokes; heart attacks; amputations; and nerve losses. Macrobiotics has also helped me with fears of gout, with its associated arthritis, possible kidney stones, and renal problems."

Over the last decade, Peter Klein, M.D., has helped other people make positive changes in their way of life and has been active in the macrobiotic community in the Washington, D.C., area, where he practices psychiatry. In his own practice he has emphasized group therapy and the importance of the support, encouragement, and nurturance that a family and friends provide. In the future he says he hopes to study more deeply the relationship of diet and behavior and cooperate with an increasing number of young macrobiotic physicians who are now graduating from medical school.

Source: Peter Klein, M.D., "Case History," in Michio Kushi,

Cancer and Heart Disease (Tokyo: Japan Publications, 1982), 189–91; and telephone interview with Alex Jack, March 29, 1984.

VARICOSE VEINS

Since high school, Patricia Goodwin had been feeling pain from arthritis, later diagnosed as a "tendency toward rheumatoid arthritis" by her doctor in Lynn, Massachusetts, in 1971. The stiffness was present in almost every joint in her body, but especially the hands, shoulders, and back. Such daily tasks as carrying books, reaching, or bending were uncomfortable. At times no movement was necessary to bring a dull, persistent ache to her back. The doctor took X-rays and prescribed Darvon and aspirin three times a day. The medication did not help, and after a couple of weeks she discontinued it.

Another problem Pat had was varicose veins, which like arthritis ran in the family and were considered to be inherited and therefore impossible to cure. The pain from them consisted of a tenderness and throbbing in the swollen veins, sometimes sharp enough to make walking difficult. Pat foresaw having to have operations and take drugs for this condition in the future.

In 1974, she began working as a waitress at the Seventh Inn Restaurant, a macrobiotic restaurant in Boston. Originally it was just a job, but after a couple of months she became curious about the macrobiotic diet that everyone who worked or ate there seemed to be enjoying. However, she did not appreciably change her way of eating, which at the time included the usual modern volume of meat and sugar, until she met her husband. "He was macrobiotic and when he asked me if I could cook, I said yes (though I could not) and I became macrobiotic immediately," she now confesses.

After just a few months on the diet, her arthritic condition began to improve. She forgot about the constant pain and stiffness of arthritis until one day she ate some cheese and drank some wine. "Right away I felt the old, familiar pain in my back. I then realized that the pain I had lived with for so long, not only had disappeared, but most certainly had been caused by my imbalanced eating."

Like the arthritis, the varicose veins began quickly to disappear. Only one of the swollen veins remained, and it was always the largest. But she never felt any pain or throbbing from it, as before, and never had any trouble walking. Within a few years, it disappeared entirely, too. When Pat became pregnant in 1982, she feared that the varicosity might return, since it is common among pregnant women, but it didn't and of her pregnancy she says she had a "very easy time."

Source: Patricia M. Goodwin, "Case History," in *Macrobiotic Case Histories*, No. 5 (Boston: East West Foundation, (Spring 1978), 14–15; and interview with Alex Jack, March, 1984.

THROMBOSIS

Pat Murray wasn't aware of any physical problems in her life until her first pregnancy in 1958 when she developed a hard, red lump in a vein in her right thigh. Her doctor suggested she simply ignore it. During the pregnancy, she gained a great deal of weight —40 or 50 pounds—and the baby was born with a condition that involved having a great deal of water in the head. Pat's symptoms cleared up after the delivery, and the lump disappeared.

In 1964, halfway through her second pregnancy, the same lump appeared again on the thigh, and the prenatal clinic advised her to ignore it. Toward the end of the pregnancy, however, the vein between the lump and the calf appeared very prominently. When she brought this to the doctor's attention, he advised her to stay off her feet. As the delivery approached, more lumps appeared, and they became very painful. Doctors at St. Vincent Hospital in New York examined her leg and told her she had a potentially serious condition, and when the prenatal clinic checked again, she was told she had thrombosis. The medical personnel told her that the blood circulation had virtually stopped in that area of the thigh, causing the pain. Pat was put in bed with her feet raised three feet higher than her head, and she received heat treatments on the leg.

The doctors told her that if a blood clot became loosed from the leg, it could become lodged in the heart or brain, which could prove fatal. During the entire pregnancy, she was put on a high protein diet by the prenatal clinic, consisting of about 90 percent meat, fish, and eggs, with little fat and little carbohydrate. "The effect of this diet was that I became very thin by the end of the pregnancy," Pat relates. "I stayed off the leg, and then after the birth, I was back in the hospital where I asked if a change in diet might help the condition. They said no, but had me see a specialist in New York. This was no help at all. I decided then, in 1965, to seek a cure for myself."

At the time, Dr. Frank Jarvis had written a popular health food book recommending apple cider vinegar for dissolving lumps of this sort. Pat tried his remedy and some of the pain did go away. She returned for a medical checkup and asked if diet could help. Once again the doctors told her no and recommended surgical removal of the vein if it became worse.

In 1969, Pat heard me lecturing on the application of yin and yang to achieve balance through the macrobiotic diet. Pat began to make further dietary changes, giving up meat and sugar. From 1958 to 1970 she had followed Adelle Davis's diet and had become considerably overweight. "The basic principle of Adelle Davis's diet seemed to be if a little is good for you, then more is better. So I was very big and quite watery."

In 1970 she heard me speak again and resolved to come to Boston to study macrobiotics. Within one week, the pain caused by the thrombosis disappeared. "I began eating grains and vegetables and I immediately experienced an improvement in the condition of the vein, as well as a greatly improved mental and spiritual condition," Pat explains. "My personality at the time had been very extreme in emotional terms. As I continued eating this way and working hard for six months, I noticed the vein improve, as well as an increased tendency toward less extreme actions and feelings. Now I've lost the excess weight and the vein has gone down and, in fact, it never hurts."

Pat has gone on to become a senior macrobiotic counselor. In addition to directing the East West Center in Newburyport, Massachusetts, she has opened a natural foods store, Corn Mother, cooked for and advised numerous cancer patients, and at the current time is counseling at a macrobiotic center in Los Angeles.

Source: Pat Murray, "Case History," in *Case History Report,* Vol. 1, No. 2 (Boston: East West Foundation, Winter 1976), 3–4.

CONGENITAL HEART DEFECT

Three weeks after Jessica Brown's birth on March 15, 1975, doctors discovered that she had pyloric stenosis, an abnormal narrowing in the opening leading from the lower stomach to the duodenum. Physicians near her home town of Tunbridge, Vermont, also found that she had a small hole between the upper chambers of her heart, a congenital condition known as atrial septal defect.

Jessica's parents, David and Debby Brown, had been vegetarians for about two years and were shocked by their daughter's heart condition. Doctors told them that Jessica would require open-heart surgery before age five to close the hole before serious complications developed.

Debby, who had been reading about macrobiotics since she was eighteen, felt that it was time to make more fundamental dietary changes. A close friend of the family was attending my lectures in Boston and helped convince them to give it a try. So, shortly after Jessica's original diagnosis, mother and father gradually began eating macrobiotically, eliminating dairy food and substantially reducing fish and other animal food consumption. Jessica, nursed by her mother, was thus essentially brought up on whole grains and vegetables from birth.

Just before her second birthday, I met Jessica and helped the family further adjust and modify their diet. "Michio told us to especially avoid fruits," Debby looks back. "He said that in two years, the murmur resulting from the congenital defect would be gone. He said there was nothing to worry about so long as we all ate well."

In 1979, when Jessica was four, the Browns took their daughter back to the same doctor who made the initial diagnosis. "He sat her up, listened very carefully to her heart, and couldn't hear anything unusual," Debby relates. "Then he laid her down, listened, and couldn't hear anything. Then he turned her over, listened very intently, and still couldn't hear anything. We were all very relieved. Michio's prediction was just right."

Since then, Jessica has been in perfect health. Now, at age nine, she is bright, active, and cheerful, and her parents are grateful that she did not have to have surgery.

An interesting postscript to this story involves Virginia Brown,

Jessica's grandmother, a registered nurse in Tunbridge. In August 1978, only a few months after David, Debby, and Jessica started macrobiotics, Virginia was diagnosed with Stage IV malignant melanoma, a deadly form of cancer that affects the moles on the skin and spreads rapidly through the body. David and Debby convinced Virginia to try a macrobiotic dietary approach, and she went on to completely restore her health after doctors told her that her condition was terminal. Her case history is included in *The Cancer-Prevention Diet* and is the subject of a new book to be published by Japan Publications.

Thus, little Jessica's strengthened heart has already helped save the life of her grandmother. This story of family unity and cooperation across three generations will inspire many other families to regain their health and happiness and attain peace of mind and heart.

Source: Interview with Debby Brown by Alex Jack, April 21, 1984.

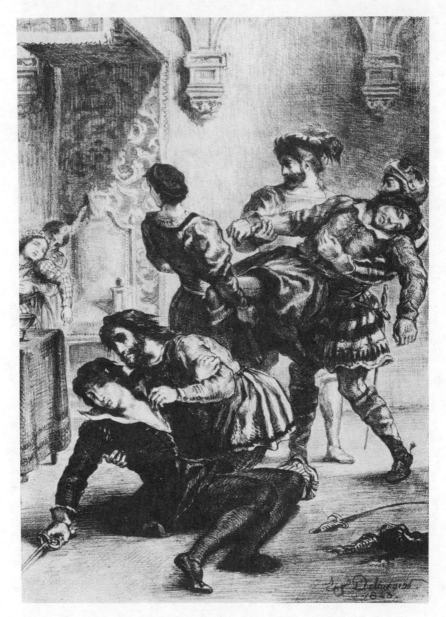

Figure 28. "Now cracks a noble heart."

29

The Tragical Case History of Prince Hamlet

Now cracks a noble heart.
—Horatio

The story of Hamlet is a tragic case history of psychologically induced heart disease. While the instrument of death in Act 5 is a thrust to the breast with the poisoned tip of a rapier, the sweet prince's noble heart is already sundered by the conflicting emotions within him. Just prior to the climactic swordplay, he confides to Horatio,

> Thou wouldst not think how ill all's here about my
> heart . . .[1]

All the other protagonists in the play also die or suffer from pierced hearts. Polonius, Laertes, and Claudius die with sword thrusts to the breast. Ophelia is drowned trying to put out the dying embers of a broken heart. Gertrude, the Queen mother, succumbs to the poisoned cup, but her heart has already been "cleft in twain" by Hamlet, who has turned upon her for marrying Claudius so suddenly after her husband's death. Even Elder Hamlet, we learn from the Ghost, has died from a poison that has commingled with his blood and stopped his heart from beating. Madness, real and feigned, is a theme in the drama, but the disorders of the mind are subordinate to a more profound spiritual sickness in the human breast.

Throughout the play, we find internal evidence for some of the environmental and dietary factors that led to the tragic downfall of a prince, a royal family, and a state. Polonius, the platitudinous Lord Chamberlain, betrays a nutritional source for his superficial, incomplete, and overly refined observations:

> 'Tis too much prov'd, that with devotion's visage
> And pious action we do sugar o'er
> The devil himself.[2]

In the scene where Hamlet debates whether to slay his murderous uncle at prayer, he describes Claudius as "full of bread." By this he means that the usurping king is completely given over to sensory indulgence. We may be certain that it is not a reference to the wholesome dark bread of the Scandinavian countryside, but to the same rich "funeral bak'd meats [that] did coldly furnish forth the marriage tables" when Claudius and Gertrude married in unseemly haste after Elder Hamlet's death.[3] Baked-meats were pies made of meat and spices and comprised a large part of the royal diet.

The Queen's dietary habits are not described, but it is probably safe to assume that she didn't do her own cooking. As a weak-willed mother and wife—"frailty, thy name is woman"—she evidently suffered from weak kidneys, probably brought about by too many sweets, fruits, and beverages.[4] She also appears to have eaten too much dairy food. Her son describes her as "feed[ing]" on "this fair mountain" and "batten[ing] on this moor"—images that bring to mind a cow grazing. In admonishing her, Hamlet further exclaims that her "sense is apoplex'd."[5] While this is metaphorical, high blood pressure and a propensity for stroke are indicated at the physical level.

Hamlet's "adder-fanged" friends, Rosencrantz and Guildenstern, attempt to betray him and "pluck out the heart of [his] mystery."[6] Typically obsequious courtiers, they also had too yin a diet—undoubtedly too much Danish pastry. At one point, Hamlet compares them to nuts that an ape (the king, Claudius) keeps in the corner of his mouth.

Many of Hamlet's dietary allusions are, like this one, said tongue in cheek. When Polonius says he will entertain the players "according to their desert," Hamlet quips, "Use every man after his desert, and who shall 'scape whipping?"[7] However, Hamlet is profoundly aware of the central importance of food in human development. In the scene in which he discusses the art of playwrighting and acting with the players, he commends their performance as "an excellent play, well digested in the scenes."[8] He goes on to approve of the lack of "sallets [salads] in the lines to make the matter savoury" and compares the composition to more nourishing fare that is "as wholesome as [naturally] sweet."[9] This passage is usually taken to embody Shakespeare's own philosophy of art and drama. The metaphor indicates that he disapproves of highly seasoned and spicy writing and novelty in acting. All the exotic side dishes of human experience may be found in Shakespeare's plays, but his clear, simple direct style and language are grounded in durable whole cereal grains, clear sparkling water, and the salty wit of the earth. All else is excess. He is the consummate poet of tradition, moderation, and common sense, taking age-old stories and truths and serving them up in a refreshing and original way.

In the scene where Claudius inquires about the fate of Polonius, Hamlet enlarges upon the theme of food as the evolutionary mode by which one species changes into another:

KING: *Now, Hamlet, where's Polonius?*
HAMLET: *At supper.*
KING: *At supper? Where?*
HAMLET: *Not where he eats, but where he is eaten. A
    certain convocation of politic worms are e'en at
    him. Your worm is your only emperor for diet* . . .[10]

This biological insight reminds us of the Taittireeya Upanishad,

From food are born all creatures; they live upon food, they are dissolved in food. Food is the chief of all things, the universal medicine. . . . I am this world and I eat this world. Who knows this, knows.[11]

Hamlet is also well schooled in physiognomy and medical philosophy and is aware of his own heart rhythms. When he first sees the Ghost, he exclaims:

> *My fate cries out*
> *And makes each petty artire [artery] in this body*
> *As hardy as the Nemean lion's nerve.* [12]

When the command to avenge his father's death is given, Hamlet swears vengeance with a reference to the heart.

> *Hold, hold, my heart,*
> *And you, my sinews, grow not instant old,*
> *But bear me stiffly up. . . .* [13]

We learn from the Ghost that the murder took place in an orchard. This disclosure allows us to understand more fully Elder Hamlet's character and glimpse some of the underlying biological dynamics of the play. By all accounts, the Elder Hamlet was a strong, energetic monarch. His son compares his looks to Hyperion (the Sun), his eyes to Mars, and his brow to Jupiter. From this description, we may conclude that Elder Hamlet was very yang, and even as a Ghost his commanding presence is felt. The physical differences between Elder Hamlet and his brother, Claudius, are contrasted in the scene where Hamlet shows their pictures to his mother. In contrast to the noble features and bearing of the father, the physiognomy of the uncle is weak and ailing. He is referred to as ulcerous, corrupt, infected, "a mildew'd ear." [14]

The source of Elder Hamlet's power and strength was evidently very yang food, including large amounts of meat pies, dried fish, and dairy food, as was customary in Scandinavia at that time as well as today. To balance this heavy animal food, the king was evidently in the habit of eating lighter, more relaxing fruits. Thus, he was napping in the orchard, probably after lunch, when Claudius attacked him. The Ghost's account of his death demonstrates an advanced awareness of his own cardiovascular system, as well as familiarity with dairy processing:

> *That swift as quicksilver it [the poison] courses through*
> *The natural gates and alleys of the body,*

And with a sudden vigour it doth posset
And curd, like eager droppings into milk
The thin and wholesome blood. . . .[15]

The effect of the poison on the bloodstream was not unlike the atherosclerotic development of a thrombus, or blood clot, but in this case the process was rapidly speeded up, from many years to a few minutes.

Unlike his brother, Claudius was weak in temperament and resolve. He undoubtedly also ate too much meat and dairy products, but he did not counterbalance this with fruit, as did Elder Hamlet. Like many sedentary people, Claudius turned to alcohol. His drinking problem is alluded to throughout the play. Whenever possible he reaches for his "draught of Rhenish." These alcoholic binges repel Hamlet, who expresses disgust at his uncle's rouses and wassails and refers to him as "the bloat King."[16] In the chapel scene, Hamlet forebears to slay him at prayer and vows to wait until Claudius is "drunk asleep, or in his rage."[17] At prayer, meanwhile, the remorseful king makes oblique reference to his atherosclerotic will,

Bow, stubborn knees; and heart with strings of steel,
Be soft as sinews of the new-born babe.[18]

To Elder Hamlet's extreme yang, Claudius represents extreme yin. Two brothers of the same stock, they mutually attract and repel each other. Just as meat and sugar are too volatile and explosive to coexist harmoniously within the human body on a regular basis, the two brothers collide, and their mutually exclusive ways of life lead to the degeneration of the body politic.

Hamlet's own constitution, personality, and way of eating is much more balanced and flexible than either his father's or uncle's. His "knotted locks" indicate that he inherited his father's curls, a sign of constitutional strength, but in his own words Hamlet is "not Hercules." He is neither as muscular nor as energetic as his father. Hamlet's philosophical bent, scholarly vocation, and wry wit show a highly developed mental nature. However, by temperament he is not aloof, withdrawn, or otherwise excessively yin. He also was an accomplished fencer, dressed fashionably, looked forward to governing the state, and to Ophelia pressed his suit aggressively.

Hamlet's naturally balanced ("sweet") disposition, gentle wit, and well-developed mental and physical activities indicate that he ate primarily grains and vegetables. Of course, as the son of the king, he was brought up on the rich fare of the palace, but he did not indulge in the excesses of either his father or his uncle. As a student in Wittenberg, Hamlet apparently came to enjoy the dark bread of the medieval German countryside and other traditional fare that was more nourishing than what was available at home.

A good sign of all-around health is the condition of the liver, which is sensitive to extremes of meat, sugar, and alcohol. It is also the seat of anger, rage, and revenge. In a telling passage, Hamlet compares his own liver to a dove's, a bird proverbial for its gentleness:

> But I am pigeon-liver'd and lack gall
> To make oppression bitter . . .[19]

Hamlet's inaction—his lack of anger and will to carry out the revenge—is the dramatic theme of the play. It is the problem that has perplexed generations of viewers and critics and, in T.S. Eliot's words, made *Hamlet* "the 'Mona Lisa' of literature." Why does Hamlet procrastinate in avenging his father's death? Why does he not immediately carry out the vow he has made to the Ghost? Why does he compel the poor spirit to return from the dead to his mother's chamber "to whet thy almost blunted purpose"? What is he waiting for?

The answer, of course, is very simple. Hamlet is constitutionally unable to slay another human being, even in retaliation for horrendous crimes. He has eaten grains and vegetables for most of his life and, by nature, has become very peaceful and forgiving. He recognizes that vengeance is just, but he also understands that there is a higher law. He abhors the prevalent code of "an eye for an eye." Moreover, he sees that a potential for excess and imbalance is in us all and that he will inevitably become corrupted by taking up arms. The Viking code of vengeance is anathema to him and he instinctively rejects it, along with the predatory way of life and way of eating from which it springs. Thus is set in motion an age-old dilemma: Should he observe ties of blood and loyalty or follow the promptings of his own heart?

After initially promising to obey the Ghost's command, Hamlet discovers that he is constitutionally and temperamentally unsuited to carry it out. Moreover, on further reflection, he wonders whether the Ghost is really "a spirit of health or goblin damn'd" leading him on to folly.[20] Hamlet must have proof that Claudius is really guilty. Thus he devises the play within a play to force his uncle's hand by recreating the murder scene. As the drama unfolds, Hamlet meditates on the relation of head and heart:

> . . . *Blest are those*
> *Whose blood and judgment are so well commeddled*
> *That they are not a pipe for Fortune's finger*
> *To sound what stop she please. Give me that man*
> *That is not passion's slave, and I will wear him*
> *In my heart's core, ay, in my heart of heart . . .*[21]

The struggle within Hamlet's breast between reason and passion, god and beast, nobility and baseness, forgiveness and revenge, and other pairs of complementary and antagonistic qualities is the universal field of experience on which we all contend. Even as he steels himself for the deed, Hamlet prays that he will not be corrupted by his act:

> . . . *Now could I drink hot blood,*
> *And do such bitter business as the day*
> *Would quake to look on. Soft, now to my mother.*
> *O heart lose not thy nature. Let not ever*
> *The soul of Nero [Claudius] enter this firm bosom;*
> *Let me be cruel, not unnatural.*[22]

Hamlet understands the laws of opposites and recognizes that good and evil are inextricably bound to each other. The human condition embraces all dualities, and freedom is found not in violent conquest or subduing, but in balancing, harmonizing, and unifying.

Yet in the end, as he fears all along, Hamlet becomes what he is fighting against. In a rash moment, during a highly emotional meeting with the Queen, he stabs the eavesdropper behind the arras, whom he takes to be Claudius, and finds instead that he has slain Polonius. In doing so, Hamlet kills another son's father and becomes the object of Laertes' revenge. To Horatio, Hamlet confesses:

> For by the image of my cause I see
> The portraiture of his [Laertes']. . . .[23]

Just as Claudius dies by the same poisoned cup that he has prepared for another, the prick to Hamlet's breast with the tainted rapier represents the seed of imbalance that exists within even the most noble heart.

THE BREATHING TIME OF DAY

Although Hamlet is initially in good physical and mental shape, the shock of the Ghost's revelation about his uncle and mother severely tries his balanced constitution and harmonious temperament. Like everyone else, Hamlet has physical strengths and weaknesses. In his case the heart is especially well developed, and he is able to endure enormous pressure and stress, avoiding extremes of both rashness of action and a paralyzed will. However, Hamlet's weakest organ is the lungs, and the play describes the progressive deterioration of its functions.

There are many references to Hamlet's worsening lung condition. His own coloring and thoughts are consistently described as pale, the hue associated with lung deficiencies in both traditional Western and Oriental medicine. For example, when the King and Queen ask what troubles him after he has seen the Ghost, he cites as one of the trappings of his woes the "windy suspiration of forc'd breath."[24] Later, he observes in himself:

> And thus the native hue of resolution [blood red]
> Is sicklied o'er with the pale cast of thought . . .[25]

Hamlet engages in special exercises to strengthen his lungs:

> *. . . If it please his*
> *Majesty, it is the breathing time of day with me.*[26]

During the climactic dual with Laertes, his mother describes him as "scant of breath."[27]

These and other references to Hamlet's pale countenance and breathing trouble are traditional symptoms of melancholy, the sickness associated with the lungs. In traditional Western philosophy and medicine, stretching back to Hippocrates and Galen, the four humors (see Figure 29) were conceived of as fluids or vital energies that circulated in the body. The humors were also influenced by environmental factors, such as wind, water, temperature, and direction. A person's physical and mental attributes were believed to depend upon the given balance of humors in the body. For example, Hamlet says,

> *I am but mad north-north-west. When the wind is*
> *southerly, I know a hawk from a handsaw.*[28]

This is a direct allusion to traditional humoral philosophy as expressed in Timothy Bright's *A Treatise of Melancholy*, published in 1586, in which therapeutic breathing is recommended for weakened lungs and the melancholy humor. "The air meet for melancholic folk ought to be . . . open and patent to all winds . . . especially to the south and south-east."[29] Each of the four winds rules a particular malady and can be counterbalanced by the complementary opposite force. Melancholy was believed to arise in the spleen from an excess of black bile, weakening the lungs and heart and producing chronic sadness and sorrow.

In addition to melancholy, there were three other humors. A choleric person was said to have yellow bile as the chief humor and to be governed by the liver. This humor produced an active, fiery personality and in excess led to the person's being bad-tempered and easily angered. Laertes is of this type. A phlegmatic person, demonstrating a more calm and self-possessed temperament, was ruled by the phlegm, or thick mucus in the body. Excessive phlegm rapidly led to sluggishness. Gertrude was essentially phlegmatic, as was Claudius, though he also exhibited strong choler. A sanguine individual, under the sovereignty of the heart

Figure 29. The Four Humors

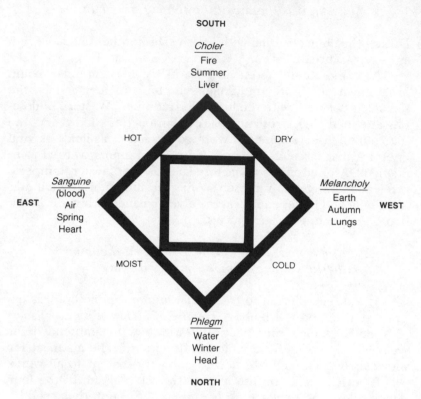

and the blood, presented a cheerful and optimistic countenance. Horatio is a good example of this type.

The doctrine of humors generally corresponds to the Far Eastern cycle of the five transformations (see Figure 30), which can be viewed as four cardinal energies encircling one central energy. From at least the sixth century B.C. until the seventeenth century A.D., when modern science arose and began to sever the connection between mind and body, this way of thinking prevailed in the West. The doctrine of humors formed the philosophical foundation of Elizabethan drama, and, like physiognomy, references to it permeate Shakespeare's plays.

For example, in *Hamlet,* just prior to the first visitation of his father's ghost, Hamlet philosophizes,

Figure 30. The Five Transformations

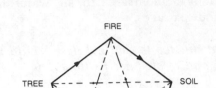

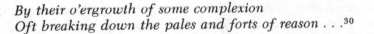

By their o'ergrowth of some complexion
Oft breaking down the pales and forts of reason . . .[30]

Complexion is a special term referring to the humors. It is defined by the *Oxford English Dictionary:* "In the physiology and natural philosophy of the Middle Ages: the combination of supposed qualities *(cold* or *hot,* and *moist* or *dry)* in a certain proportion, determining the nature of a body, plant, etc.; the combination of the four 'humours' of the body in a certain proportion, or the bodily habit attributed to such combination; 'temperament.' "

Following the play-within-a-play scene, in which he unmasks his uncle as his father's murderer, Hamlet and Guildenstern exchange observations following Claudius's angry departure,

GUILDENSTERN: *The King, sir—*
HAMLET: *Ay, sir, what of him?*
GUILDENSTERN: *Is in his retirement marvellous*
    distempered.
HAMLET: *With drink, sir?*
GUILDENSTERN: *No, my lord, with choler.*
HAMLET: *Your wisdom should show itself more richer to*
    signify this to the doctor, for for me to put him to
    his purgation would perhaps plunge him into
    more choler. [31]

There are many other references in the play to the four humors, and also to the four elements—earth, air, water, fire. One of the play's most famous passages,

> *O that this too too sullied flesh would melt,*
> *Thaw and resolve itself into a dew . . .*[32]

refers to the traditional remedy for melancholy. A cold, dry humor associated with congealing of the blood, melancholy was believed to result from an excess of the earth element to which it corresponded. To relieve this overabundance, earth was melted into water, which in turn resolved itself into a dew. Dew was also considered one of the secondary humors in medieval medicine.

These examples are meant to illustrate the traditional world view, which Shakespeare shared. The play as a whole, including the characters and complex motives of the protagonists, cannot really be understood without knowledge of the doctrine of the four humors. Similarly Ophelia's distribution of flowers to the King and Queen and her brother requires a familiarity with herbalism. When she gives Laertes rosemary, symbolic of remembrance, he is motivated to avenge the death of their father, Polonius, and thus Ophelia unwittingly serves the same function with respect to her brother as the Ghost does with respect to Hamlet. All these allusions, taken for granted by the Elizabethan mind, are usually lost on the modern reader.

Given a predisposition to weak lungs, it is not surprising that Hamlet chose to put on an "antic disposition" characteristic of certain forms of melancholy. Had he been choleric by nature, he might have chosen to conceal his method behind a mask of drunkenness. If phlegmatic, he might have withdrawn into a catatonic stupor or if overly sanguine, feigned epilepsy.

Much of Hamlet's paleness and breathing trouble can be laid to the shock of his father's murder and his mother's over-hasty remarriage. His heart is overburdened by the truth he has discovered and the demands expected of him. A strained heart, as we see in Oriental medicine and humoral doctrine, directly afflicts the lungs. However, dietary influences also played an important role. During the course of his madness, Hamlet forgoes meals and eats erratically. The action in the play spans four months, the exact time it takes for the quality of the red blood cells to change. While he was in excellent condition at the start of the play, neglect of diet over a period of 120 days would have completely transformed his blood quality, affecting the quality of his thoughts and feelings as well as his stamina and energy.

During this time, Hamlet's attitude toward life changes fundamentally and he becomes despondent and suicidal. The world that formerly held so much promise for him becomes stifling and unbearable.

> . . . *What piece of work is a man, how noble in reason, how infinite in faculties, in form and moving how express and admirable, in action how like an angel, in apprehension how like a god: the beauty of the world, the paragon of animals— and yet, to me, what is this quintessence of dust?* [33]

This pessimistic observation reflects underlying lung troubles, and Hamlet complains more and more about the poor quality of the air. In the same speech he declares:

> . . . *This brave o'erhanging firmament, this majestical roof fretted with golden fire, why, it appeareth nothing to be but a foul and pestilent congregation of vapours. . . .* [34]

He laments fate, which

> *Tweaks me by the nose, gives me the lie i'th' throat As deep as to the lungs . . .* [35]

The suffocation that he feels in his chest is projected onto the world, and he observes "Denmark's a prison." [36]

The humors were produced primarily by the type of food a person ate, and an imbalanced diet would lead to either an excess or deficiency and resultant physical, mental, or spiritual disorders. In an essay on *Melancholy* translated into English in 1594, about the time *Hamlet* was written, Peter de la Primaudaye, a member of the French Academy, defined humor as "a liquid and running body into which food is converted in the liver, to this end: that bodies might be nourished and preserved by them." [37]

Hamlet's worsening state of health, brought about by the shocking disclosures and an irregular way of eating, culminates in his cruelty to Ophelia. As his blood quality deteriorates, he becomes more suspicious, defensive, and withdrawn—true melancholic characteristics—and treats his friends as enemies. As his lungs decline, his kidneys—the seat of will—begin to suffer, and his resolve weakens.

At sea, on the voyage to England, Hamlet undergoes a major transformation. Irresolution and vacillation give way to resolve and new energy. Part of this change in behavior can be attributed to the change of environment and a more wholesome and regular diet. Aboard ship, spicy baked-meats, dairy food, Danish pastries, and other freshly prepared foods that were extremely imbalanced were probably not available. Instead, the shipboard regimen probably consisted primarily of dried salted fish, seafood, and whole grain biscuits and crackers. From his newly returned resolve, we also see that Hamlet's kidneys are functioning better, possibly as the result of some mineral-rich seaweed in his ocean-bound diet. As a result of this more yang fare, Hamlet returns to his senses, and his intuition begins to function again. Fortuitously, he discovers that the commission carried by Rosencrantz and Guildenstern from Claudius instructs the English court to put him to death.

From this point on, Hamlet acts every bit the true heir to the Danish throne. He jumps ship when the pirates attack in a display of nimble physical dexterity. Back in Denmark once again, he sends a bold letter to Claudius, defies Laertes, jumps in the open grave, declares his eternal love for Ophelia, and in the tragic finale makes up for his vacillation by making Claudius drink from the poisoned cup after stabbing him through the breast. As he lies dying from his own wounds, Hamlet turns to Horatio and implores,

> *If thou didst ever hold me in thy heart,*
> *Absent thee from felicity awhile,*
> *And in this harsh world draw thy breath in pain*
> *To tell my story.*[38]

Projected onto his only true friend in the world, Hamlet's last words, referring to the heart and lungs, echo the physical and psychological imbalance that has beset him. Horatio's response,

Now cracks a noble heart. Good night, sweet prince,
And flights of angels sing thee to thy rest.[39]

underscores the heart image that is the guiding metaphor of the play.

THE INCENSED POINTS OF MIGHTY OPPOSITES

At the social level, the contest between Hamlet and Claudius can be viewed as the conflict between traditional and modern society. According to two scholars in *Hamlet's Mill: An Essay Investigating the Origins of Human Knowledge and Its Transmission through Myth,* Shakespeare's play derives from an early Scandinavian myth portraying the precession of the equinoxes, or the change in world epochs. The original Ameleth is the custodian of a great mill (the stars revolving around the North Pole), which turns out peace and plenty until decay sets in and chaos takes over. According to one interpretation of this myth, *Ameleth,* Hamlet's original name, derives from the same root word of ambrosia and nourishment and means "the grain." His uncle is said to represent "the grinding" or maelstrom force.[40]

Whatever the exact mythological origins, Hamlet is the distillation of well-developed human culture. He has a deep sympathy for the natural world and in his life exhibits the qualities of moderation, balance, and harmony associated with health and vitality. Claudius is the embodiment of excess, novelty, overstimulation, and cleverness. In the King's person we find the seeds of the modern scientific mentality. Debating about how to rid himself of his nephew, Claudius reflects,

> *. . . Diseases desperate grown*
> *By desperate appliance are reliev'd,*
> *Or not at all.*[41]

Deciding to send Hamlet to his death, the King soliloquizes, extending the medical metaphor,

> ... *Do it, England;*
> *For like the hectic in my blood he rages,*
> *And thou must cure me.* ... [42]

Again, when his plans are thwarted and Hamlet returns, Claudius convinces Laertes to challenge him to a duel with an image of sickness and disease:

> ... *But to the quick of th'ulcer:*
> *Hamlet comes back* ... [43]

Modern society, rather than reflecting on the internal origin of its private and public ills, seeks an external cause to be rooted out and destroyed. The two methods that Claudius uses—poisonous drugs and the knife blade—are the methods of modern warfare and the operating room.

In contrast, Hamlet, the very incarnation of the self-reflective soul, is always looking within himself for the source of his troubles and is ever mindful of becoming what he is fighting against. "Taint not thy mind," his father's Ghost—the voice of ancestral tradition —warns him.[44] While Hamlet also adopts some of the imagery of disease to refer to his uncle, he tries not to adopt his methods. These two ways of viewing the world are the real combatants on the stage. In describing to Horatio the fates of Rosencrantz and Guildenstern, Hamlet remarks,

> *'Tis dangerous when the baser nature comes*
> *Between the pass and fell incensed points*
> *Of mighty opposites.*[45]

It is this inner battle raging between reason and appetite, forgiveness and revenge, moderation and intemperance, and order and chaos that the outer struggle mirrors. Just before taking up swords with Laertes at the end, Hamlet confesses to Horatio,

> ... *in my heart there was a kind of fighting*
> *That would not let me sleep.* ... [46]

LET BE

The Elizabethan society for which this play was performed stood on the threshold of the modern age. Shakespeare saw clearly the approaching philosophy that would separate mind and body and reduce life to mechanistic functioning. Claudius embodies this mechanistic spirit: the impulse to uproot nature without considering the consequences and to use others as instruments to our own ends. This way of thinking is what is rotten in Denmark—and the entire modern world.

Hamlet represents traditional society that dies to make way for the new and whose spirit will live on when technique, novelty, and excess have run their course. Such is the order of things. Yin follows yang, yang succeeds yin. A period of artistic culture, spiritual development, and peace gives way to an era of technological progress, material development, and conflict. Meat and sugar (symbolized by the final triumph of Fortinbras, another choleric type) replace grains and vegetables. And so the spiral unfolds, each turn resulting in a slightly different expression of the cycle and leading eventually to a higher synthesis. This is the order of the universe—the alternation of yin and yang, of tragedy and comedy.

In *Hamlet*, Shakespeare, the poet laureate of traditional society, poses the basic dilemma of the modern age: How to live in and transform a world that appears "weary, stale, flat, and unprofitable." All about Hamlet is death and disorder, corruption and degeneration. It is interesting that Shakespeare chose an ancient Danish legend as the vehicle for this purpose. However remote and medieval the setting, the Scandinavian environment is surprisingly modern regarding nutrition. The Viking diet—heavy animal food, dairy products, sweetmeats, and alcohol—has pretty much conquered the modern world. Today the world's highest consumption of fat and cholesterol—and the highest rate of heart disease—are still found in regions of Scandinavia.

Hamlet's aversion to the atmosphere of meat and alcohol is a recurrent theme. He abhors the effects of Claudius's drinking parties on the common wealth and health:

This heavy-headed revel east and west
Makes us traduc'd and tax'd of other nations—

> *They clepe us drunkards, and with swinish phrase*
> *Soil our addition . . .*[47]

He upbraids his mother's faithless conduct,

> *Nay, but to live*
> *In the rank sweat of an enseamed bed,*
> *Stew'd in corruption . . .*[48]

The image is drawn from seam, a type of saturated animal fat used in cooking and making stews. The metaphor is carried further when he tells her in a subsequent passage,

> *. . . Forgive me this my virtue;*
> *For in the fatness of these pursy times*
> *Virtue itself of vice must pardon beg . . .*[49]

The word *pursy*, meaning flabby or puffed up, reinforces the image.

Despite this violent, oppressive environment, Hamlet learns to come to terms with existence. At the close, he no longer curses that "the world is out of joint" but accepts his obligation to set it right and restore harmony. He no longer views the world in the dualist terms of "to be or not to be" but, embracing the evil along with the good, says "the readiness is all. . . . Let be."[50] He no longer rejects death and disorder as chaotic and random but finds "a special providence in the fall of a sparrow."[51] As his own physical strength and vitality return, Hamlet's faith in the meaning of life is renewed, and he accepts his own tragic part in the universal drama,

> *There's a divinity that shapes our ends,*
> *Rough-hew them how we will—*[52]

Hamlet's heart is at peace at last.

Such, in brief, is the philosophical foundation to Shakespeare's play. The many levels to *Hamlet* spring from a deep understanding of nature and the order of the universe, including the art of physiognomy and the doctrine of the four elements. In the same way that

Figure 31. Correspondences in *Hamlet*

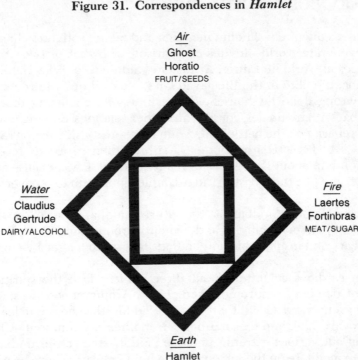

Air
Ghost
Horatio
FRUIT/SEEDS

Water
Claudius
Gertrude
DAIRY/ALCOHOL

Fire
Laertes
Fortinbras
MEAT/SUGAR

Earth
Hamlet
Ophelia
GRAINS/VEGETABLES

> . . . *Heaven's face does glow*
> *O'er this solidity and compound mass [the Earth's four*
> *elements]* . . . [53]

so Shakespeare looks upon human nature as conditioned by the four humors. Each of his characters, as we have seen, embodies traditional qualities, eats specific foods, and suffers from specific illnesses associated with one of these vital energies (see Figure 31). Although this harmonious and orderly way of looking at life has disappeared and the modern world draws its breath in pain, *Hamlet* remains to tell the story under the starlit sky until whole grains (the staff of life), native common sense, and felicity return.

GOOD NIGHT, SWEET PRINCE

Hamlet's dilemma—finding meaning and taking action to change a degenerate world—invites comparison with that of two other princes in world literature, Arjuna and Siddhartha. Like Hamlet, Arjuna, the hero of the Bhagavad Gita, is called upon to revenge the wrong done his household and finds himself facing mortal combat with his uncles, cousins, and other relations. Sinking down in his chariot on the battlefield, Arjuna casts away his weapons and refuses to fight. His charioteer, Krishna, then proceeds to enlighten him about the nature of reality and the laws of cause and effect, and like the Ghost of Elder Hamlet spurs him to recover his resolve.

Like Hamlet, Siddhartha, the future Buddha, is put off by the suffering, sorrow, ugliness, and brutality around him. The palace is dreary and insufferable and he finds he can no longer live in its midst.

In cardiovascular terms, all three princes face the spiritual "flight or fight" syndrome. Hamlet and Arjuna choose to stand their ground and accept their destiny. Siddhartha chooses to leave the royal estates and seek harmony in another environment. After trying out various extreme practices, Siddhartha settles under a tree to meditate on the sorrows of the human heart. There he eats brown rice and seeks to unify his mind with the infinite. After a long period of self-reflection, Siddhartha attains enlightenment. As the Buddha, he goes on to devote his life to teaching a middle way between extremes of yin and yang and a philosophy grounded in serving others, forgiveness, endless gratitude, and a simple way of eating. As the New York Times art critic observed in a recent review of a Buddhist art exhibit, "In all these sculptures and paintings we see the Asian equivalent of a Prince Hamlet who took the right turning."[54]

Hamlet was relatively enlightened, and in the end he and Laertes forgave each other. However, through most of the performance, Hamlet was not able to reconcile all the opposites within himself. Had he been able to see all phenomena as complementary and antagonistic, he would have initially pacified the spirit of his father's Ghost, pointing out that the seeds of his murder lay in his own past misdeeds, and prayed for the smooth journey of his soul to the next world. He would have forgiven

Claudius and Gertrude and shown them a better way. He would not have turned against Ophelia but married her and, if the King and Queen couldn't be changed, set off with her for Vinland and a new life together. If the court at Elsinore had observed a more natural way of life, including a more centrally balanced diet, the "carnal, bloodly, and unnatural acts" might have been averted and "purposes mistook" might not have "fall'n on th'inventors' heads."[55]

For modern society today, poised between "the pass and fell incensed points of mighty opposites"—such as heart disease and cancer, capitalism and communism, and nuclear war and biological degeneration—there is still time to transmute tragedy into comedy and create a happy ending.

PART III
Recipes and Exercises

30

Kitchen Utensils

Bamboo Mats

Small bamboo mats may be used in covering food. They are designed to allow heat to escape and air to enter so that food does not spoil quickly if unrefrigerated.

Cutting Board

It is important to cut vegetables on a clean, flat surface. Wooden cutting boards are ideal for this purpose. They should be wiped clean after each use. A separate board should be used for the preparation of dishes containing animal foods.

Electrical Applicances

Avoid all electrical appliances as far as possible when preparing foods or cooking. Electricity produces a chaotic vibration that is transmitted to the energy of the food. Instead of toasting bread, steam or bake it. Instead of using an electric blender, use a suribachi to puree sauces and dressings. Occasionally, however, an automatic blender may be used to grind the soybeans for making tofu or when cooking for a party or large numbers of people. Use common sense.

Flat Grater

A small enamel or steel hand-style grater that will grate finely is recommended.

Foley Hand Food Mill

This utensil is useful for pureeing, especially when preparing baby foods or dishes requiring a creamy texture.

Glass Jars

Large glass jars are useful for storing grains, seeds, nuts, beans, or dried foods. Wood or ceramic containers, which allow air to circulate, are better but may be difficult to locate.

Metal Heat Deflectors

These are especially helpful when cooking rice and other grains as they help distribute heat more evenly and prevent burning. Avoid asbestos pads.

Oil Brush

A small brush used to brush oil on a skillet, especially when oil needs to be carefully regulated for medical purposes, is useful. A new, clean paintbrush may be kept for this purpose.

Pickle Press

Several pickle presses or heavy crocks with a plate and weight should be available for regular use in the preparation of pickles and pressed salads.

Pressure-Cooker

A pressure-cooker is an essential item in preparing the Diet for a Strong Heart, especially in preparing brown rice and other whole grains. Stainless steel is recommended.

Saucepans

A variety of saucepans with covers is essential for everyday cooking. A 2-quart saucepan made of stainless steel is good for boiling small quantities of vegetables and heating up leftovers, and also serves as the top of a double boiler when set inside a 4-quart saucepan. A 4-quart saucepan made of stainless steel, glass, or ceramic is useful for making soups, boiling vegetables, and preparing sauces. A 6-quart saucepan made of enamelized cast iron is ideal for the long, slow cooking of grains, beans, and vegetable casseroles or for quick soups and vegetables.

Skillets

Several frying pans are essential in the natural foods kitchen. A 9-inch, heavy cast-iron or enamel cast-iron skillet is ideal for long slow sautéing of vegetables, for kinpura- and nishime-style dishes, and for making fried rice and noodles. Cast-iron heats up slowly, holds the heat, and cooks evenly, especially over a medium-low flame. A light 6- or 9-inch stainless steel skillet is ideal for quick sautéing, for tempura, for crêpes, and for dry-roasting grains, seeds, nuts, and flour. Stainless steel does not hold heat or cook as evenly as cast-iron but heats up quickly and gives good results at medium to high temperatures.

Soup Pot

A heavy kettle of cast iron, enameled cast iron, or stainless steel with a tight-fitting lid used for boiling noodles or pasta, steaming (with a rack set inside), preparing stock and large volumes of soup. Heavy cookware allows for more careful cooking. An 8-quart kettle is a good size for family use.

Steamer Basket

The small stainless steamers are suitable. Bamboo steamers are also fine for regular use.

Stove

A high-quality source of heat is one of the most important elements in cooking. Wood is the ideal fuel, and food cooked on a woodstove is more delicious and peaceful than food cooked by other methods. Charcoal and coal are also superior sources of fuel. For the modern urban home, natural gas is the most practical. Gas gives clean, even, easily controllable heat. It respects the natural vibration of the food. Electric heat is very hard to adjust and produces irregular energy in the food. Microwave methods, which step up the vibration of the food even more than do electric methods, create the most chaotic cooking. Until a regular gas stove can be obtained, a small propane gas cooking stove may be set up in the kitchen or apartment equipped with an electric or microwave range. Small portable gas burners are also ideal for traveling and for use in offices instead of electric hot plates.

Suribachi (Grinding Bowl)

A suribachi is a ceramic bowl with grooves set into its surface. It is used with a wooden pestle and is needed in preparing condiments, pureed foods, salad dressings, and other items. A 6-inch size is generally fine for regular use.

Tamari Dispenser

This small glass bottle with a spout is very helpful in controlling the quantity of tamari soy sauce used in cooking.

Tea Strainer

Small, inexpensive bamboo strainers are ideal, but small mesh strainers may also be used.

Utensils

Wooden utensils such as spoons, rice paddles, and cooking chopsticks are recommended since they will not scratch pots and pans or leave a metallic taste in your foods.

Vegetable Brush

A natural-bristle vegetable brush is recommended for cleaning vegetables.

Vegetable Knife

A sharp, high-quality Oriental knife with a wide rectangular blade allows for the more even, attractive, and quick cutting of vegetables. Stainless steel and carbon steel varieties are recommended.

Wire Mesh Strainer

A large strainer is useful for washing grains, beans, sea vegetables, some vegetables, and draining noodles. A small, fine mesh strainer is good for washing smaller items such as millet or sesame seeds.

31

Menus

The following weekly menus are typical of the kinds of meals that might be prepared by a macrobiotic household during each of the four seasons in a temperate climate. As an example of the Standard Macrobiotic Diet, they include fresh salad, fresh fruit, desserts, and other supplemental foods that may be eaten for variety and enjoyment several times a week by those in generally good health.

For those with existing heart or circulatory problems or other serious diseases, a more limited form of the diet may need to be prepared for an initial period of several months or more, depending on the individual case. After the condition has stabilized, a broader form of the diet, including most of the dishes listed here, may be implemented. Please refer to the appropriate chapter for your condition in Part II and to Table 24 on pages 255–257 for appropriate modifications and important information on the use of salt, oil, and length and style of cooking.

Most of the dishes listed below can be made from the recipes in this book. However, for a more comprehensive and thorough explanation of proper cooking methods, please see *Aveline Kushi's Complete Guide to Macrobiotic Cooking for Health, Harmony, and Peace,* from which these menus are adapted.

SPRING MENU

	Breakfast	Lunch	Dinner

S
U
N
D
A
Y
	Soft rice
	Miso soup with
	  celery
	Bancha
		Udon and broth
		Pressed salad
		Grain coffee
			Pressure-cooked
			  brown rice
			Tamari broth
			Tofu with arame
			Boiled carrots and
			  onions
			Steamed kale
			Quick lemon-miso
			  pickles
			Oatmeal cookies
			Bancha

M
O
N
D
A
Y
	Whole oats
	Rice kayu bread
	Bancha
		Miso soup with
		  wakame and daikon
		Brown rice and
		  seitan
		Bancha
			Pressure-cooked
			  brown rice and
			  wheat berries
			Red lentil soup
			Broccoli with tofu
			  cream dressing
			Boiled kombu
			Tamari onion
			  pickles
			Dandelion tea

T
U
E
S
D
A
Y
	Miso soft rice with
	  chives
	Bancha
		Tofu sandwich
		Tamari broth
		Boiled salad with
		  dandelions
		Bancha
			Pressure-cooked
			  brown rice
			Steamed tempeh
			  and sauerkraut
			Boiled mustard
			  greens with
			  tamari-ginger sauce
			Boiled wakame and
			  onion
			Amasake pudding
			Bancha

	Breakfast	Lunch	Dinner

W
E
D
N
E
S
.
	Miso soup with
	  onion and wakame
	Toasted mochi
	Grated daikon with
	  nori strips
	Grain coffee
		Rice balls
		Chinese cabbage
		  with tamari-lemon
		  sauce
		Bancha
			Pressure-cooked rice
			  and barley
			Clear soup
			Chick-peas
			Nishime vegetables
			Broccoli and
			  cauliflower pickles
			Bancha

T
H
U
R
S
D
A
Y
	Miso soup with
	  wakame
	Soft millet
	Sprouted wheat
	  bread
	Bancha
		Fried soba
		Natto
		Dulse, carrots,
		  celery
		Grain coffee
			Brown rice with
			  wild vegetables
			Carrot soup
			Hiziki
			Carrot tops with
			  sesame seeds
			Kanten
			Bancha

F
R
I
D
A
Y
	Brown rice cream
	Miso soup with
	  scallions
	Bancha
		Seitan and
		  sauerkraut
		Sourdough bread
		Small garden salad
		  with sprouts
		Bancha
			Pressure-cooked
			  brown rice
			Azuki beans and
			  wheat berries
			Clear broth
			Wakame with
			  umeboshi dressing
			Chinese-style
			  sautéed vegetables
			  with kuzu sauce
			Bancha

S
A
T
U
R
D
A
Y
	Miso soup
	Soft buckwheat
	Mustard green
	  pickles
	Grain coffee
		Boiled millet
		Tamari broth
		Tempeh with
		  watercress
		Bancha
			Pressure-cooked rice
			  and rye
			Fu and broccoli in
			  broth
			Kombu, carrots, and
			  burdock
			Nori condiment
			Fruit compote
			Bancha

SUMMER MENU

	Breakfast	Lunch	Dinner
S U N D A Y	Miso soup with wakame and daikon Boiled tofu with ginger-parsley sauce Bancha	Boiled millet Fresh corn soup Boiled string beans and almonds Watermelon Corn silk tea	Brown rice salad Black beans Wakame with scallions Tamari rutabaga pickles Bancha
M O N D A Y	Soft rice with nori flakes Red radish pickles Bancha	Cold somen noodles Steamed cabbage, celery, and carrots Grain coffee	Brown rice with fresh corn Cool chick-pea soup Sautéed snowpeas and chinese cabbage Hiziki salad with tofu Bancha
T U E S D A Y	Scrambled tofu and corn Sourdough bread Bancha	Miso soup with sesame seeds and broccoli Corn on the cob with umeboshi Boiled onions Green coffee	Rice salad Clear broth Kombu, carrots and burdock Baked zucchini with miso-lemon sauce Strawberry shortcake Barley tea
W E D N E S D A Y	Soft barley with scallions and nori strips Chinese cabbage pickles Bancha	Barley stew Arepa Bancha	Buckwheat salad Lentils Celery soup Boiled cabbage with sesame and umeboshi sauce Bancha

	Breakfast	Lunch	Dinner
T	Creamy onion miso	Udon and broth	Pressure-cooked
H	soup	Wakame cucumber	brown rice
U	Whole oats	salad with	Corn on the cob
R	Rice kayu bread	tamari-vinegar	Cauliflower soup
S	Bancha	sauce	Arame with tempeh
D		Grain coffee	and onions
A			Quick lemon-miso
Y			pickles
			Steamed kale
			Fruit salad
			Bancha
F	Soft rice with	Bulghur	Brown rice and
R	scallions	Sautéed tofu and	lotus seeds
I	Corn on the cob	vegetables	Boiled carrots,
D	Bancha	Parsley with ginger	onions, and chinese
A		sauce	cabbage
Y		Brown rice tea	Red radishes and
			kuzu sauce
			Shio kombu
			Barley tea
S	Soft millet with	Rice balls	Brown rice with
A	sweet corn	Fried tempeh	whole dried corn
T	Tamari onion pickles	Sliced cucumber	Barley soup
U	Bancha	Bancha	Hiziki with soybeans
R			Boiled turnip greens
D			with sesame-tamari
A			sauce
Y			Fresh cantaloupe
			Bancha

AUTUMN MENU

	Breakfast	Lunch	Dinner

S
U
N
D
A
Y
	Whole oats
	Miso bread
	Bancha
		Wild rice
		Miso soup with
		  daikon and
		  wakame
		Broiled tofu
		Bancha
			Brown rice
			Clear broth
			Nishime daikon and
			  vegetables
			Chinese cabbage with
			  tamari-lemon sauce
			Hiziki
			Tamari turnip pickles
			Applesauce
			Bancha

M
O
N
D
A
Y
	Soft rice with
	  corn and
	  umeboshi
	Tamari daikon
	  pickles
	Bancha
		Roasted rice
		Creamy onion
		  miso soup
		Bancha
			Millet with squash
			Barley soup
			Boiled cauliflower and
			  broccoli
			Bran pickles
			Bancha

T
U
E
S
D
A
Y
	Soft barley with
	  scallions
	Miso soup with
	  squash and
	  millet
	Bancha
		Fried noodles and
		  tempeh
		Pressed mixed
		  salad
		Grain coffee
			Pressure-cooked brown rice
			Azuki beans and chestnuts
			Baked butternut squash
			  and onions
			Boiled cabbage with
			  sesame seeds and
			  umeboshi sauce
			Shio kombu
			Daikon green pickles
			Bancha

W
E
D
N
E
S
D
A
Y
	Soft rice with
	  squash
	Bancha
		Seitan stew
		Steamed mustard
		  greens
		Bancha
			Brown rice and walnuts
			Clear soup
			Lotus root stuffed with
			  miso
			Boiled collard greens with
			  tamari-vinegar sauce
			Arame with onions
			Chinese cabbage pickles
			Squash pie
			Grain coffee

	Breakfast	Lunch	Dinner
T	Soft barley	Rice ball	Pressure-cooked brown rice
H	Rice kayu bread	Onion wakame	Squash soup
U	Grain coffee	soup	Burdock kinpura with
R		Sautéed tofu and	seitan
S		vegetables	Parsley with ginger sauce
D		Bancha	Dulse, carrots, and celery
A			Bancha
Y			
F	Soft buckwheat	Whole wheat	Sweet brown rice and
R	with scallions	sourdough bread	azuki beans
I	Sauerkraut	Broccoli with tofu	Clear soup
D	Bancha	dressing	Endive with kuzu sauce
A		Lotus root salad	Steamed kale with
Y		Roasted brown	tamari-ginger sauce
		rice tea	Kombu and dried daikon
			Bancha
S	Soft millet with	Rye and	Fried rice
A	squash	vegetables	Corn soup
T	Tamari onion	Chick-pea soup	Boiled watercress
U	pickles	Boiled salad	Baked carrots
R	Bancha	Grain coffee	Wakame with scallions
D			Rutabaga tamari pickles
A			Azuki beans, chestnuts, and
Y			raisins
			Bancha

WINTER MENU

	Breakfast	Lunch	Dinner

S
U
N
D
A
Y
	Miso soup with
	  wakame and
	  cauliflower
	Soft rice with
	  parsley
	Chinese cabbage
	  pickles
	Bancha
		Fried soba
		Boiled carrots and
		  onions
		Grain coffee
			Brown rice and
			  sesame seeds
			Azuki bean soup
			Sautéed cabbage,
			  celery, and carrots
			Boiled kombu
			Bran pickles
			Cooked pears
			Bancha

M
O
N
D
A
Y
	Whole oats with
	  dulse
	Rice kayu bread
	Bancha
		Tofu sandwich
		Tamari broth
		Bancha
			Pressure-cooked
			  brown rice
			Oden
			Colorful soybean
			  casserole
			Turnip greens with
			  sesame-tamari
			  dressing
			Arame with dried
			  tofu and carrots
			Bancha

T
U
E
S
D
A
Y
	Soft millet with
	  squash
	Miso soup with
	  jinenjo
	Bancha
		Boiled udon with
		  seitan
		Tamari turnip
		  pickles
		Bancha
			Brown rice and
			  azuki beans
			Clear daikon soup
			Burdock kinpura
			Boiled watercress
			  salad
			Wakame with
			  scallions and
			  miso-vinegar sauce
			Turnip green
			  pickles
			Baked apple with
			  kuzu-raisin sauce
			Bancha

	Breakfast	Lunch	Dinner
W	Miso soft rice	Buckwheat soup	Pressure-cooked
E	Pickled daikon	Cabbage roll	brown rice
D	greens	Tempeh	Seitan stew
N	Bancha	Grain coffee	Steamed kale and
E			carrots
S			Hiziki
D			Broccoli and
A			cauliflower pickles
Y			Bancha
T	Buckwheat pancakes	Brown rice	Fried rice
H	with apple-kuzu	Tofu and vegetables	Black soybeans
U	sauce	Roasted brown rice	Baked buttercup
R	Grain coffee	tea	squash
S			Boiled collard
D			greens with a
A			tamari-ginger sauce
Y			Wakame and onions
			Daikon pickles
			Amasake pudding
			Bancha
F	Miso soup with	Rice ball	Sweet brown rice
R	wakame and onion	Azuki beans with	and chestnuts
I	Toasted mochi	lotus seeds	Cauliflower soup
D	Grated daikon and	Tamari onion pickles	Burdock kinpura
A	nori strips	Bancha	Daikon greens and
Y	Bancha		kombu
			Ginger pickles
			Grain coffee
S	Genuine brown rice	Pressure-cooked	Boiled brown rice
A	cream	brown rice	Vegetable tempura
T	Creamy onion miso	Boiled broccoli with	Grated daikon and
U	soup	tofu cream dressing	ginger
R	Bancha	Bancha	Kidney beans
D			Steamed kale
A			Amasake
Y			Bancha

32

Recipes

This chapter includes some of the basic recipes for the Standard Macrobiotic Diet. For those with existing cardiovascular conditions, please read carefully the nutritional guidelines in the chapters on specific heart and circulatory conditions in Part II and consult Table 24 on pages 255–257 for important information on seasoning, use of oil, length of cooking, and other considerations. After these basic recipes are learned, you may wish to consult a cookbook with a wider selection of recipes, such as *Aveline Kushi's Complete Guide to Macrobiotic Cooking for Health, Harmony, and Peace,* from which some of these recipes have been adapted. Other macrobiotic cookbooks are listed in the bibliography.

GRAINS

PRESSURE-COOKED BROWN RICE

2 cups organic brown rice
1 1/4–1 1/2 cups spring water
per cup of rice

pinch of sea salt per cup of
rice

Gently wash rice (short- or medium-grain) and quickly place it in a pressure-cooker. Smooth out the surface of the rice so that it is level. Slowly add spring water, pouring it down the side of the pressure-cooker so that the surface of the rice remains calm and even. If time permits, soak rice for 2 to 3 hours. This makes it much more digestible. After water has boiled in uncovered pressure-cooker or with lid on but unfastened, add salt, place cover on pressure-cooker, and slowly bring up to pressure on a gas or wood-stove. Reaching pressure takes 10 to 15 minutes and is signified by the hissing, jiggling, or spinning of the gauge, depending on the model pressure-cooker used. When pressure is up, place underneath it a metal heat deflector and turn to low. Cook for 50 minutes. When rice is done, remove pressure-cooker from burner and allow to stand for at least 5 minutes before reducing pressure and opening. If you wait 10 to 15 minutes for pressure to come down naturally before opening, the rice will be even better. This wait allows any scorched grain on the bottom to loosen. With a bamboo rice paddle or wooden spoon, lift rice from the pressure-cooker one spoonful at a time and smooth into a large wooden bowl. Distribute evenly, with the heavier rice at the bottom and the lighter rice at the top. Alternating scoops in this way makes for a more balanced bowl of rice. Rice pressure-cooked in this way will have a delicious, nutty, naturally sweet taste and impart a very peaceful, strong feeling.

To rewarm leftover rice, place rice in a small ceramic bowl or container and set inside a large pot. Add about ½ inch of water, pouring down the side of the pot, cover, and bring to a boil. Be careful not to get water in the bowl with the rice. The method is similar to using a double boiler. After the rice has steamed for a few minutes, remove bowl and serve. This method allows the rice to retain its sweetness and strength without becoming moist or soggy. Leftover rice may also be added directly to soups, sautéed with vegetables to make fried rice, or cooked in other styles.

Note: Each cup of uncooked rice makes about 3 cups of cooked rice. Allow about 1 cup per person. In general, you will want to start with 3 or more cups of uncooked rice and store the remainder. Leftover rice will keep for several days. After rice cools off, place in a closed container in the refrigerator.

Variation: One-third of an umeboshi plum may be added instead of salt for each cup of uncooked rice. Long-grain rice may occasionally be used in summer.

BOILED RICE

1 cup brown rice   *pinch of sea salt*
2 cups spring water

Wash rice and place in heavy pot or saucepan. Add water and salt. Cover with a lid. Bring to a boil, lower flame, and simmer for about 1 hour or until all water has been absorbed. Remove and serve.

SOFT BROWN RICE (RICE KAYU)

1 cup brown rice   *pinch of sea salt*
5 cups spring water

Wash rice and pressure-cook or boil as in either of the above recipes. However, not all of the water will be absorbed. Rice should be creamy and some of the grains should be visible after cooking. In case water boils over while pressure-cooking, turn off flame and allow to cool off. Then turn on flame again and continue to cook until done.

Note: Makes a nourishing and appetizing breakfast cereal. Especially recommended for those who are sick and who have difficulty swallowing or holding food down.

Variation: Vegetables such as daikon or Chinese cabbage or an umeboshi plum may be added while cooking. A 1-inch square of dried kombu is also highly recommended.

GENUINE BROWN RICE CREAM

1 cup brown rice   *½ umeboshi plum or a pinch*
10 cups spring water   *of sea salt per cup of rice*

Dry roast rice in a cast-iron or stainless-steel skillet until golden brown. Place in pot, add water and plum or salt, and bring to a boil. Cover, lower heat, and place heat deflector beneath pot. Cook until water is one-half of original volume. Let cool and place in cheesecloth or unbleached muslin, tie and squeeze out the pulp. Heat the cream again, then serve. Add salt if needed. The pulp is also very good to eat and can be made into a small ball and steamed with grated lotus root or carrot.

Note: Makes a delicious breakfast cereal and is also good for those who have difficulty eating. The lives of many people who otherwise could not eat have been saved with rice cream. The love, care, and energy of the cook can be imparted to the food with his or her hands.

Variation: Garnish with scallions, chopped parsley, nori, gomashio, or roasted sunflower seeds.

FRIED RICE

1 tablespoon dark sesame oil	*4 cups cooked brown rice*
1 medium onion, sliced	*1-2 tablespoons tamari soy*
diagonally or diced	*sauce*

Brush skillet with sesame oil. Heat for a minute or less but do not let oil start to smoke. Add onion; place rice on top. If rice is dry, moisten with a few drops of water. Cover skillet and cook on low heat for 10 to 15 minutes. Add tamari soy sauce and cook for another 5 minutes. There is no need to stir. Just mix before serving.

Note: Those in good health may have fried rice several times a week, though the amount of oil may need to be reduced depending on the individual's condition. Those who need to restrict their oil may use 2 to 3 tablespoons of water to replace the oil. Check dietary recommendations carefully.

Variation: Use scallions, parsley, or a combination of vegetables such as carrots and onion, cabbage and mushroom, and daikon and daikon leaves.

RICE WITH BEANS

1 cup brown rice	*1¼-1½ cups spring water*
¹/₁₀ to ⅛ cup of beans per	*pinch of sea salt*
cup of rice	

Wash rice and beans. Cook beans ½ hour beforehand following basic recipes in bean section below. Allow beans to cool; add with salt and cooking water to rice. Bean water counts as part of the total water in the recipe. Pressure-cook for 45 to 50 minutes and serve as with plain rice.

Note: Heart patients should generally use only azuki, chickpeas, or lentils. Those in good health may use a variety of other beans as well. Cooking grains and beans together make for a substantial meal and save the time and fuel needed for cooking each dish separately.

RICE AND VEGETABLES

1 cup brown rice
¼ cup dried daikon
½ cup carrots (finely diced or small matchsticks)
⅛ cup burdock (finely diced or small matchsticks)

1¼–1½ cups spring water per cup of rice
pinch of sea salt per cup of rice

Place washed rice in pressure-cooker and mix with vegetables. Add water and salt, cover, and cook as for plain rice.

Variation: A small amount of tamari soy sauce may be added with salt before cooking. Other vegetables that go well with rice are sweet rice, green beans, green peas, carrots, etc. Soft vegetables such as onion and green leafy vegetables tend to become mushy and should be avoided for this dish. Rice and vegetables may also be cooked with sesame seeds, walnuts, or lotus seeds, as well as with azuki beans or black soy beans.

RICE BALLS WITH NORI SEA VEGETABLE

1 sheet toasted nori
pinch of sea salt

1 cup cooked brown rice
½–1 umeboshi plum

Roast a thin sheet of nori by holding the shiny side over a burner about 10 to 12 inches from the heat. Rotate for 3 to 5 seconds until color changes from black to green. Fold nori in half and tear into two pieces. Fold and tear again. You should now have four pieces that are about 3 inches to a side. Add a pinch of sea salt to a dish of water and wet your hands. Form a handful of rice into a solid ball. Press a hole in the center with your thumb and place a small piece of umeboshi inside. Then close hole and compact ball again until solid. Cover rice ball with nori, one piece at a time, until it sticks. Wet hands occasionally to prevent rice and nori from sticking to them, but do not use too much water.

Note: Rice balls make a tasty, convenient lunch or snack because they can be eaten without utensils. They are great to take along when traveling and keep fresh for a few days. Use less or no umeboshi when making rice balls for children.

Variation: Rice can be made into triangles instead of balls by cupping your hands into a V-shape. Balls or triangles can be rolled in toasted sesame seeds and eaten without nori. Small pieces of salt or bran pickles, vegetables, pickled fish, or other condiments can be inserted inside instead of umeboshi. Instead of nori sheets, use roasted crushed sesame seeds, shiso leaves, pickled rice leaves, dried wakame sheets, or green leafy vegetable leaves.

BROWN RICE WITH FRESH CORN

1 cup fresh uncooked corn kernels, removed from the cob
2 cups brown rice

pinch of sea salt per cup of grain
1 1/4–1 1/2 cups spring water per cup of rice

Remove corn from the cob. Wash rice and place in pressure-cooker. Add corn and water. Mix corn in with rice. Pressure-cook as for plain brown rice.

MILLET

1 cup millet
2 1/2 cups boiling water

pinch of sea salt per cup of millet

Wash millet. Lightly roast millet in dry skillet for about 5 minutes or until slightly golden. Stir gently during this time to prevent burning. Add boiling water and salt. Bring to boil, cover, lower heat, and simmer 30 to 35 minutes.

Note: Millet has a delicious nutty flavor and light, fluffy consistency.

Variation: Roast millet with a little sesame oil, or sauté onions 3 to 5 minutes on low heat, add millet and sauté another 3 to 5 minutes, add boiling water and cook as above. The sautéing methods are not recommended for those who need to avoid oil. Millet can also be topped with a sauce to reduce its somewhat dry taste. A nourishing breakfast cereal of soft millet can be made by adding 4 cups of boiling water to the basic recipe instead of 2½ cups.

BARLEY

1 cup barley
1¼–1½ cups spring water
per cup of barley

pinch of sea salt per cup of
barley

Follow same method as basic pressure-cooked brown rice.

Note: Barley is very strengthening and recommended for regular use by heart patients.

Variation: Barley may also be boiled, fried, and cooked with a variety of other grains, beans, and vegetables, and used in soups. For soft barley cereal, combine 1 cup barley, 4 to 5 cups water, and a pinch of sea salt and boil for 1¼–1½ hours. Serve hot and garnish with scallions, chopped parsley, nori, or gomashio.

WHOLE OATS

1 cup whole oats
5–6 cups spring water

pinch of sea salt per cup of
oats

Wash oats and place in pot. Add water and salt. Cover and bring to a boil. Reduce heat and simmer on low for several hours or overnight until water is absorbed. Use a heat deflector to prevent burning. Makes an excellent cereal.

Note: Whole oats are very strengthening for heart patients and are to be preferred to steel-cut oats or rolled oats.

Variation: Cooking time can be reduced by pressure-cooking following the basic brown rice recipe. For a very nourishing and peaceful dish, combine 1½ cups barley, 1 cup whole oats, and ½ cup partially cooked beans. Add 3 pinches of sea salt, about 4 cups of water, and pressure-cook as usual.

BUCKWHEAT (KASHA)

1 cup buckwheat   *pinch of sea salt*
2 cups boiling spring water

Roast buckwheat in dry skillet for 4 to 5 minutes. Put grain in pot and add boiling water and salt. Bring to boil, reduce heat, and simmer for 30 minutes or until water has been absorbed.

Note: Buckwheat is a strong, warm grain. Patients with more yin heart disease may eat buckwheat frequently in this form or in noodle form as soba. Patients with more yang heart disease should avoid it. See specific dietary recommendations.

Variation: Cook buckwheat with sautéed cabbage and carrots or with onion and chopped parsley. For a hearty cereal, use 4 to 5 cups of boiling water and cook as above.

SWEET RICE

1 cup sweet rice   *pinch of sea salt*
1 cup spring water

Wash rice, add water and salt, and cook in pressure-cooker following basic rice recipe.

Note: Sweet rice is more glutinous than regular rice and should be used only occasionally. It may also be added in small volume to regular rice for a sweeter taste.

MOCHI

Mochi is sweet rice served in cakes or squares made by pounding cooked sweet rice with a heavy wooden pestle in a wooden bowl. Pound until grains are crushed and become very sticky. Wet pestle occasionally to prevent rice from sticking to it. Form rice into small balls or cakes, or spread on a baking sheet that has been oiled and dusted with flour and allow to dry. Cut into pieces and roast in a dry skillet, bake, or deep-fry. For occasional use and special celebrations.

RYE

1 cup rye   *pinch of sea salt*
1¼–1½ cups spring water

Cook the same as basic pressure-cooked brown rice, or boil, in which case 2 cups of water are used.

Note: Since rye is hard and requires a lot of chewing, it is usually mixed with other grains or consumed in flour form as rye bread. For a delicious, chewy dish, add 1 part rye to 3 parts brown rice. Rye may be dry-roasted in a skillet for a few minutes prior to cooking to make it more digestible.

WHOLE DRIED CORN

2 cups whole dried corn,   *4 cups spring water*
  especially dent corn   *pinch of sea salt*
1 cup sifted wood ash

Soak corn overnight. Place corn kernels in pressure-cooker. Add wood ash and water. Cover, turn up heat to high, and bring to pressure. When pressure is up, reduce heat to medium low, place a heat deflector under the pot, and pressure-cook for 1 hour. Remove from heat and allow pressure to come down naturally. When pressure is completely down, remove cover and place corn in a strainer or collander. Rinse all wood ashes thoroughly from the corn. Place corn back into a cleaned pressure-cooker and pressure-cook again for 1 hour with sea salt and water. When cooked, remove from burner, place in a serving bowl, and use in soups, vegetable dishes, or salads.

BAKED CORN ON THE COB

This traditional method of baking the corn in its husk makes for a sweeter and more delicious corn on the cob than either boiling or steaming.

4–8 ears of fresh corn

With husks still on, place corn on a baking sheet in oven and cook at 350° for 30 minutes. The silk and husks will retain the corn's natural juices during baking. When done, simply remove husks and silk and serve hot.

Seasoning: Instead of butter, margarine, salt, or pepper, umeboshi plums may be used to season corn. Simply puree 1 or 2 pickled salt plums in a suribachi with a little water or a little corn oil if desired, or use ready-made umeboshi paste, and apply lightly to corn. The umeboshi gives a salty taste. It is strong, so don't use too much.

BASIC CORN DOUGH

Dough made from dry whole corn taken from corn on the cob is the basis for tortillas, arepas, empanadas, and other traditional Indian corn dishes. In Spanish, corn dough is called *masa.* Flour, flint, or cracked corn available from Latin American markets is recommended for this preparation. Leftover dough will keep for about a week in the refrigerator. With aging it begins to sour and can be used in making corn doughnuts and other naturally sweetened items. Pink or red spots indicate that the dough has spoiled.

4 cups whole dry corn　　　　*8–10 cups spring water*
1 cup sifted wood ash in a　　*pinch of sea salt*
tied muslin bag

Place corn, ash, and water in a pot and pressure-cook for 20 minutes. Drain water after cooking and wash corn thoroughly to remove residue from wood ash. Use at least four changes of water. The loosened skins of the corn should float off in the rinse water.

If they don't, add more ash and cook 10 to 15 minutes longer. After rinsing off wood ash, return to cooker. Add fresh water to cover and pressure-cook for 50 to 60 minutes further. Remove grain from cooker and let cool completely. Grind in a hand grinder (do not use a blender) and knead for 10 to 15 minutes by hand. Add water for consistency and sea salt to taste. Use in one of the following recipes.

AREPAS

These delicious corn dough balls are the traditional staple in many parts of Latin America and are eaten instead of wheat bread. They can be made plain or stuffed with a variety of ingredients.

1 ½ pounds corn dough (see recipe, page 379)

¼ teaspoon sea salt water to moisten

Crumble dough, add salt, and knead with a small amount of water until soft and the consistency of an ear lobe. If you use too much liquid, add more dough or let dry for a few minutes in the open air. Form dough into 6 to 8 fist-sized balls. Brush cast-iron skillet with sesame oil. Flatten the arepas into ovals several inches across and a half-inch thick, or make into biscuits or muffins. Cook 2 to 3 minutes on each side until crust forms and then bake on a cookie sheet for 20 minutes at 350° or until arepas begin to puff up. They are done when they make a hollow, popping sound when tapped.

Variation: Arepas can also be made without baking by pan-frying for 5 minutes on each side in a covered skillet over low heat. Then uncover, turn up heat, and cook for an additional 7 to 8 minutes on each side. For variety, try adding 2 cups of sesame seeds or chopped sautéed vegetables and knead thoroughly into the dough. Fancier arepas can also be made by serving with a tofu, tempeh, or miso-tahini spread.

BOLLOS POLONES

These stuffed corn balls are boiled and especially good for those whose oil intake is restricted.

2 pounds corn dough (see
recipe, page 379)

8 cups spring water
pinch of sea salt

Moisten hands, knead dough for a few minutes, adding salt and water to moisten. Form into 10 to 12 fist-sized balls. Make a hole in the middle of each ball and insert filling (such as cooked beans, seitan, vegetables, or fish). Close hole, using more dough if needed, turning ball clockwise with thumb on the middle. Bring water to boil in a large pot. Put balls in, reduce heat, and cook for 20 minutes, turning the stuffed balls from time to time to ensure even cooking. Garnish with parsley or chopped scallion. Serve with a miso sauce, a carrot sauce, or other topping.

WHOLE WHEAT

1 cup wheat berries
1 1/4–1 1/2 cups spring water

pinch of sea salt

Cook following basic pressure-cooked brown rice recipe or boiled-rice recipe. Boiled wheat will usually cook longer than rice.
Note: Wheat is difficult to digest in whole form and must be thoroughly chewed. It also requires longer cooking time. Soaking wheat berries 3 to 5 hours beforehand reduces cooking time and makes a softer, more digestible dish. For a tasty combination, combine 1 part wheat berries and 3 parts rice or other grain.

NOODLES AND BROTH

8 cups spring water
1 package soba or udon
noodles
1 piece of kombu, 2–3 inches
long

2 dried shiitake mushrooms
2–3 tablespoons tamari soy
sauce

Boil water. Oriental noodles already contain salt so no salt needs to be added to the water. Add noodles to 4 cups water and boil. After about 10 minutes, check to see if they are done by breaking the end of one noodle. Buckwheat cooks faster than whole wheat, and thinner noodles cook faster than thicker ones. If the inside and outside are the same color, noodles are ready. Remove noodles from pot, strain, and rinse with cold water to stop them from cooking and prevent clumping. To make the broth, place kombu in pot, add remaining 4 cups water and mushrooms that have been soaked, their stems cut off, and sliced. Bring to boil. Reduce heat and simmer for 3 to 5 minutes. Remove kombu and mushrooms. Add tamari soy sauce to taste for 3 to 5 minutes. Place cooked noodles into the broth to warm up. Do not boil. When hot, remove and serve immediately. Garnish with scallions, chives, or toasted nori.

Note: Soba buckwheat noodles are very strengthening. In summer they can be cooked and enjoyed cold. Udon wheat noodles are much lighter. Western-style whole grain noodles and pasta may also be used regularly. These include whole wheat spaghetti, shells, spirals, elbows, flat noodles, lasagna, etc. Use pinch of salt in water when cooking.

FRIED NOODLES

1 package soba or udon
1 tablespoon sesame oil
2 cups cabbage

1–2 tablespoons tamari soy
sauce
½ cup sliced scallions

Cook noodles as in previous recipe, rinse under cold water, and drain. Oil skillet and put in cabbage; place noodles on top. Cover and cook on low heat for several minutes or until noodles become warm. Add tamari soy sauce and mix noodles and vegetables well. At the very end of cooking, add scallions. Serve hot or cold.

Note: If you cannot take oil, use 2 tablespoons of water for sautéing.

Variation: Many combinations of vegetables may be used, including carrots and onions, scallions and mushrooms, cabbage and tofu.

WHOLE WHEAT BREAD

8 cups whole wheat flour
¼–½ teaspoon sea salt

2 tablespoons sesame oil
(optional)
spring water

Mix flour and salt, add oil, and sift thoroughly together by hand. Form a ball of dough by adding just enough water and knead 300 to 350 times. Oil two bread pans with sesame oil and place dough in pans. Place damp cloth over pans and let sit for 8 to 12 hours in a warm place. After dough has risen, bake at 300° for 15 minutes and then 1¼ hours longer at 350°.

Note: Flour products, including bread, are not recommended for regular use by those who are seriously ill.

Variation: A delicious sourdough starter for bread can be made by combining 1 cup of flour and enough water to make a thick batter. Cover with damp cloth and allow to ferment for 3 to 4 days in a warm place. After starter has soured, add 1 to 1½ cups of starter to bread dough, knead, and proceed as above. For rye bread, use 3 cups rye flour to 5 cups whole wheat flour.

RICE KAYU BREAD

2 cups brown rice   *8 cups spring water*

Pressure-cook rice in water for 1 hour or more. Take out rice and allow to cool in large bowl. While still slightly warm, add to rice:

2 teaspoons sesame oil   *enough whole-wheat flour to*
(optional)   *form into a ball of dough*
½ teaspoon sea salt

Add oil and salt to rice and mix well. Add enough flour to make soft ball of dough. Knead 300 to 350 times, adding flour to ball from time to time to keep from getting too sticky. Place dough in two oiled bread pans, shape into loaves, cover with damp cloth, set in warm place, and let rise 8 to 12 hours. Bake at 300° for 30 minutes and 350° for another hour, or until golden brown.

Note: This bread is better for heart patients than whole wheat bread, but should still be used sparingly.

SEITAN (WHEAT GLUTEN)

3½ pounds whole wheat flour   *8–9 cups spring water*

Place flour in large bowl and add 8 to 9 cups of warm water. Consistency should be like oatmeal or cookie batter. Knead for 3 to 5 minutes or until flour is mixed thoroughly with water. Cover with warm water and allow to sit a minimum of 5 to 10 minutes. Knead again in soaking water for 1 minute. Pour off cloudy water into jar. Place remaining gluten (the part of the wheat high in protein) into a large strainer and put strainer in a large bowl or pot. Pour cold water over gluten to cover and knead in the strainer. Repeat until the bran and starch (reddish outer coating) of the wheat are completely separated. It is customary to save the first rinse water containing bran and starch (see below). Repeat the rinsing and kneading process in the strainer and pot until all the starch and bran are washed off. Alternate between cold and hot water when rinsing and kneading gluten. Always start and finish with cold water to contract the gluten. Gluten should form a sticky mass. Separate into 5 to 6 pieces and form balls. Drop balls into 6 cups boiling water and boil for 5 minutes, or until balls rise to surface. Put balls on top of a piece of kombu, add 3 to 5 tablespoons of tamari soy sauce and 1 teaspoon grated ginger, bring to a boil, lower heat, and cook for 45 to 60 minutes. Leftover seitan may be stored in a closed container with a little liquid from the pot. Save the rest of the kombu tamari broth for soup or noodles. The water containing the washed off starch and bran can be saved as a thickening agent for soups, stews, and sauces. This recipe makes about 1 and a half pounds of seitan and will serve from 6 to 8 people.

Note: Seitan is very versatile, tasty, and full bodied in texture. It is especially appealing for people making a transition to natural foods. Spring-wheat flour has a softer texture than winter wheat and is often preferred.

Variation: Seitan can be cut into cubes for soups and salads; used in a stew with carrots, burdock, brussels sprouts, onion, radish, or other vegetables; combined with bread crumbs, onions, mushrooms, and celery to stuff a squash; fried in larger slices for sandwiches and grainburgers.

FU

Fu is a wheat gluten product similar to seitan but toasted, steamed, and dried. Light in consistency, fu absorbs liquid and expands several times in volume when cooked. Like seitan, it is easy to digest and gives energy. Fu can be enjoyed plain; garnished with grated ginger and toasted black sesame seeds; added to miso soup, tamari soy sauce broth, stews, and salads; or cooked together with vegetables.

At home, fu can be made using the basic method for preparing seitan. Then gently toast in oven that is moderately hot. After cooling, lightly steam to allow fu to puff up, then cut into rounds, and let dry in a cool place. Store in an airtight container. Fu is also available prepackaged in many natural foods stores.

SOUPS

BASIC VEGETABLE MISO SOUP

1 3-inch strip dry wakame sea vegetable
1 cup thinly sliced onions

1 quart spring water
1 ¼–1 ½ tablespoons miso

Rinse wakame quickly in cold water and soak for 3 to 5 minutes and slice into ½-inch pieces. Place wakame and onions in pot and add water. Bring to a boil, cover pot, and simmer for 10 to 20 minutes or until tender. Reduce heat to very low but not boiling or bubbling. Place miso in a bowl or suribachi. Add ¼ cup of broth and puree until miso is completely dissolved in liquid. Add pureed miso to soup. Simmer for 3 to 5 minutes and serve. Garnish with scallions, parsley, ginger, or watercress.

Note: Be careful to reduce the heat while the miso is cooking to preserve the beneficial enzymes in miso. As a general rule, use about 1 teaspoon of miso for each cup of water in the broth. Soup shouldn't taste too salty or too bland.

Variation: Barley miso is highly recommended, especially for heart patients and for people with other sicknesses. Hatcho (100 percent soybean) miso is strong, but not salty, and also may be used to help restore health. Other misos, such as brown rice miso, may be used occasionally. In terms of aging, select miso that has fermented one-and-a-half years or more. All types of miso may be eaten year round and slightly modified in proportion according to the season or condition of health. Vegetables may be varied often.

Other basic combinations include wakame, onions, and tofu; onions and squash; cabbage and carrots; daikon and daikon greens. If your health allows for oil, you may brush pot with 1 teaspoon or less of unrefined vegetable oil, especially dark sesame oil, sauté the vegetables first, and then add to the wakame in the pot.

MISO SOUP WITH DAIKON AND WAKAME

1½ cups daikon
1 quart spring water

½ cup wakame
3 teaspoons miso

Wash and slice daikon into ½-inch slices and add to water. Cook for 5 minutes. Meanwhile, soak wakame for 3 to 5 minutes and chop into small pieces. Add wakame to pot and cook over low heat until vegetables are soft. Dilute and add miso to stock. Simmer for 3 minutes. Garnish with chopped scallion.

Note: Daikon is particularly helpful to eliminate excess mucus, fat, protein, and water from the body. Cooking time of wakame depends on how soft or hard it is.

MISO SOUP WITH MILLET

½ cup millet
½ cup celery
1 cup sliced onions
1 cup butternut squash

1 quart spring water
¼ cup miso
1 sheet toasted nori

Wash millet and dry-roast in an unoiled skillet by stirring gently for 5 to 10 minutes at low to medium heat until light brown or golden in color and a nutty aroma is released. In a pot, layer vegetables, starting with celery, then onions, and squash on top. Spread millet evenly on top of layered vegetables. Carefully add water to just below the level of the squash. Cook over a medium heat. Add water gradually as the millet expands to keep the water level at a constant below the squash. To preserve the layers, do not stir. After millet becomes very soft, add the rest of the soup stock or water. Bring to a boil. Reduce heat. Mix miso with small amount of soup water and puree. Add pureed miso to the soup a couple of minutes before serving. Garnish with nori and parsley.

Variation: Other grains may be substituted for millet, including barley, rice, buckwheat, oats, or cracked wheat. Alternate vegetables as well.

TAMARI OR CLEAR BROTH

2 shiitake mushrooms
1 3-inch piece kombu sea
vegetable
4 cups spring water

2 tofu cakes, cubed
2–3 tablespoons tamari soy
sauce
¼ cup sliced scallions

Soak shiitake 10 to 20 minutes. Place kombu and shiitake in spring water (including soaking water) and boil for 3 to 4 minutes. Take kombu and shiitake out and save for another recipe. Add tofu and boil until tofu comes to the surface. Do not boil tofu too long or it will become too hard. Tofu in soup is best enjoyed soft. Add tamari soy sauce and simmer for 2 to 3 minutes. Garnish with scallions and nori.

Variation: This clear broth soup can be made with chopped watercress and other vegetables instead of tofu. The shiitake too is optional but very good for heart patients with overly yang conditions.

LENTIL SOUP

1 cup lentils
2 onions, diced
1 carrot, diced
1 small burdock root, diced

1 quart spring water
¼–½ teaspoon sea salt
1 tablespoon chopped parsley

Wash lentils. Layer vegetables in soup pot, starting with onions, then carrot, burdock, and place lentils on top. Add water and pinch of salt. Bring to a boil. Reduce heat to low, cover, and simmer for 45 minutes. Add chopped parsley and remaining salt. Simmer 20 more minutes and serve. Tamari soy sauce may be added for flavor.

Variation: For those who can use oil, vegetables may first be sautéed and then cooked with lentils as above.

AZUKI BEAN SOUP

1-inch square dried kombu
1 cup azuki beans
1 quart spring water
1 medium onion, sliced

½ cup sliced carrots
¼–½ teaspoon sea salt
tamari soy sauce to taste
(optional)

Soak kombu 5 minutes and slice. Wash beans, place in pot, and add water. Bring to a boil. Reduce heat and simmer until beans are 80 percent done, about 1¼ hours. Take out cooked beans or use other pot. Put onion on bottom of pot, then carrots, then azuki beans, and place kombu on top. Add salt. Cook for 20 to 25 minutes more or until vegetables are soft. At very end, add tamari soy sauce to taste. Garnish with scallions or parsley and serve.

Variation: Instead of carrots and onion, winter squash may be used. This is particularly recommended for kidney, spleen, pancreas, and liver troubles.

CHICK-PEA SOUP

1 3-inch piece kombu
1 cup chick-peas soaked
overnight
4–5 cups spring water

1 onion, diced
1 carrot, diced
1 burdock stalk quartered
¼–½ teaspoon sea salt

Place kombu, chick-peas, and water in pressure-cooker and cook for 1 to 1½ hours. Bring pressure down. Place beans in another pot. Add vegetables and salt. Cook for 20 to 25 minutes on medium-low heat. Garnish with scallions, parsley, or bread crumbs.

BARLEY SOUP

½ cup barley
¼ cup lentils
1 celery stalk
3 onions, diced

1 carrot
5–6 cups spring water
¼–½ teaspoon sea salt

Wash barley and lentils. Layer vegetables in pot starting with celery on bottom, then onions, carrot, lentils, and barley on top. Add water just enough to cover and bring to a boil. Add sea salt just before boiling. Lower flame and simmer until barley becomes soft and milky. Check taste. You may add a drop of tamari soy sauce for flavor and garnish with nori or parsley.

Note: Barley broth is very nourishing for heart patients. The amount of barley may be increased and other variations of vegetables may be used.

Variation: You may cook barley before using for soup, adding ½ cup of barley to 1½ cups of water. Cook 20 to 30 minutes, then follow recipe.

BROWN RICE SOUP

3 shiitake mushrooms
1 3-inch piece kombu
1 quart of spring water
2 cups cooked brown rice

¼ cup dried celery
1–2 tablespoons tamari soy
  sauce

Boil mushrooms and kombu in water for 2 to 3 minutes. Remove and slice into thin strips or pieces. Place them back in water, add rice, and bring to a boil. Lower flame and cook for 30 to 40 minutes. Add celery and simmer for 5 minutes. Add tamari soy sauce to taste and simmer for final 5 minutes, garnish with scallion and serve.

Variation: You may also add miso for a wonderful, warming soup.

BUCKWHEAT SOUP

1 teaspoon sesame oil
1 onion, diced
½ cup roasted buckwheat
5–6 cups spring water

pinch of sea salt
tamari soy sauce to taste
½ cup minced parsley

Brush a small amount of sesame oil in pot. Sauté onion until translucent. Add buckwheat and water and salt. Bring to boil, cover, reduce heat, and simmer 25 to 30 minutes. Season with tamari soy sauce and simmer 10 more minutes. Garnish with minced parsley.

Note: Not recommended for those heart patients who need to restrict oil or buckwheat intake.

Variation: Without oil, you can make a light-tasting soup. For a rich, dynamic soup, add carrots, cabbage or a variety of other vegetables.

CORN SOUP

4 ears fresh uncooked corn　　*5–6 cups spring water or*
1 celery salk, diced　　　　　　*kombu stock*
2 onions, diced　　　　　　　　*¼ teaspoon sea salt*
　　　　　　　　　　　　　　　tamari soy sauce to taste

Strip kernels from corn with knife. Place celery, onions, and corn in pot. Add water and pinch of salt. Bring to a boil, lower heat, cover and simmer until celery and corn are soft. Add rest of salt and tamari soy sauce to taste if desired. Serve with chopped parsley, watercress, or scallions and nori.

SQUASH SOUP

1 large buttercup squash　　*4–5 cups spring water*
1 onion, diced　　　　　　　*½ teaspoon sea salt*

Remove skin from squash. Place diced onion in pot and add cubed squash, along with water. Add pinch of sea salt. Bring to boil, cover, and lower heat. Simmer 20 to 30 minutes or until squash is soft. Remove squash and puree in a Foley food mill. Place pureed squash in a pot; add rest of salt. Bring to a boil, lower heat, and cook for 20 minutes. Garnish with scallions or parsley.

Variation: This thick, creamy, and delicious soup may also be made with other autumn and winter squashes or pumpkins. You may add a little powdered kuzu (kudzu) after pureeing squash to make a creamy soup with a nice smooth texture.

CARP AND BURDOCK SOUP (KOI-KOKU)

*1 fresh carp
burdock in weight at least
  equal to fish
½–1 cup used bancha tea
leaves and twigs wrapped in
cheesecloth sack*

*1 tablespoon grated ginger
miso to taste
spring water and bancha
  (kukicha) tea*

Select a live carp and express your gratitude for taking its life. Ask fishseller to carefully remove gallbladder and yellow bitter bone (thyroid) and leave the rest of the fish intact. This includes all scales, bones, head, and fins. At home, chop entire fish into 1- to 2-inch slices. Remove eyes if you wish. Meanwhile, chop at least an equal amount of burdock (ideally 2 to 3 times the weight of fish) into thinly shaved slices or matchsticks. This quantity of burdock may take a while to prepare. When everything is chopped up, place burdock and fish in pressure-cooker. Tie old bancha (kukicha) twig leaves and stems from your teapot in cheesecloth. It should be the size of a small ball. Place this ball in pressure-cooker on top or nestled inside fish. The tea twigs will help soften the bones while cooking. Add enough liquid to cover fish and burdock, approximately ⅓ bancha tea and ⅔ spring water. Pressure-cook 1 hour. Bring down pressure, take off lid, add miso to taste (½ to 1 teaspoon per cup of soup), and grated ginger. Simmer for 5 minutes. Garnish with chopped scallions and serve hot.

Note: This delicious, invigorating soup is excellent for restoring strength and vitality and opening the electromagnetic channel of energy in the body. It may be eaten occasionally by all heart and circulatory disease patients, even those who otherwise shouldn't eat animal products. It is also good for mothers who have just given birth or who are breastfeeding. In cold weather it is particularly warming. Be careful, however, to eat only a small volume (1 cup or less) at a time. Otherwise you will become too yang and be attracted to liquids, fruits, sweets, and other strong yin. Soup will keep for a week in the refrigerator or several months in the freezer where it can be taken out from time to time as needed.

Variation: For those whose oil isn't restricted, the burdock may be sautéed for a few minutes in sesame oil at the start, prior to cooking with the fish. Soup may also be made by boiling in lidded pot for 4 to 6 hours or until all bones are soft and dissolved. As liquid evaporates, more water or bancha tea should be added. If carp is unavailable, substitute another more yin fish such as perch, red snapper, or trout. If burdock is scarce, use carrots instead, or use half burdock and half carrots.

KOMBU SEA VEGETABLE STOCK

Quickly wipe kombu with a dried brush to remove dust. Minerals are lost by wiping so, if not dusty, place immediately in pot containing cold spring water. Boil 3 to 5 minutes. Remove kombu and use in other dishes or dry out and use as a condiment or side dish. Use stock for miso, grain, bean, or vegetable soups.

SHIITAKE MUSHROOM STOCK

Soak 5 to 6 shiitakes in water for 30 minutes. Add shiitake and its soaking water to 1 to 2 quarts of spring water and bring to a boil. Boil 5 to 10 minutes. Remove shiitake and save for the soup (in which case be sure to remove stems) or use in another recipe. Kombu may also be combined with shiitake to make a stock.

FRESH VEGETABLE STOCK

Save vegetable roots, stems, tops, and leaves for a nutritious soup stock. Boil in 1 to 2 quarts of spring water for 5 to 10 minutes. Remove vegetable pieces and compost or discard.

FISH STOCK

Boil fish heads or bones for a few minutes. You may tie the fish parts in a cheesecloth sack and place in water or remove fish parts from stock by straining after boiling through a cheesecloth. Use fish stock for vegetable or grain soups, or thicken with pastry flour to make a fish sauce and season with tamari soy sauce.

Note: Not recommended for heart patients whose fish intake is limited. Commercially available bonito flakes are not recommended. However, home-prepared, freshly shaved, smoked and dried, traditional bonito is suitable.

VEGETABLES

Waterless Cooking (Nishime Style)

Use a pot with a heavy lid or one made for waterless cooking. Soak 1 or 2 long strips of kombu about 10 minutes, or until they are soft, and cut into 1-inch pieces. Place kombu in bottom of pot. Add vegetables such as carrots, daikon, turnips, burdock, lotus root, onions, dried shiitake mushrooms, and cabbage. These should be cut into 2-inch chunks and layered on top of the kombu. Add enough water to come just below the top layer of vegetables. Sprinkle several pinches of sea salt or drops of tamari soy sauce over the vegetables. Cover and set flame to high until a high steam is generated. Lower heat and cook peacefully for 15 to 30 minutes or longer depending on the kind of vegetables used. If water evaporates during cooking, add more water to the bottom of the pot. At end of cooking, turn off heat and allow vegetables to sit for about 2 minutes. The cooked juice may be served along with the vegetables and is very delicious.

Note: This way of cooking vegetables without oil is highly recommended for heart patients. It helps restore general strength and vitality.

Sautéing

There are two basic ways of sautéing: with oil and with water. In the first, cut the vegetables into small pieces such as matchsticks, thin slices, or shaved slices. Lightly brush skillet with dark or light sesame oil. Heat oil, but before oil begins to smoke add vegetables and a pinch of sea salt to bring out their natural sweetness. Occasionally turn over or move vegetables with chopsticks or wooden spoon to ensure even cooking. However, do not stir. Sauté for 5 minutes on medium heat, followed by 10 minutes on low flame.

Gently mix from time to time to avoid burning. Season to taste with sea salt or tamari soy sauce and cook 2 to 3 minutes longer.

The second method combines water and oil. Vegetables may be prepared either in small pieces or in large, thick pieces. Sauté as above in lightly oiled skillet for about 5 minutes. Then add enough cold water to cover the vegetables half way or just enough to cover the surface of the skillet. Add a pinch of sea salt, cover, and cook until almost tender. When 80 percent done, season with sea salt or tamari soy sauce and cook 3 to 4 minutes more. Remove cover and simmer until water evaporates.

Note: Sautéing with oil is not recommended for many heart patients or others who need to avoid or reduce oil. However, for those in good health, sautéed vegetables may be prepared daily. For those who cannot use oil, use 1 to 2 tablespoons of water instead.

Variation: Delicious combinations include burdock and carrots; onion and carrots; cabbage, onion, and carrots; parsnips and onions; mushrooms and celery; broccoli and cauliflower; Chinese cabbage, mushrooms, and tofu; kale and seitan. Soft vegetables take only 1 to 2 minutes to sauté, while cooking time is longer for root vegetables. Other unrefined vegetable oils may be used in this way. However, only sesame and corn oil are recommended for regular use.

Boiling

Place about ½ to 1 inch of cold spring water in pot and add a pinch of sea salt. Bring to a boil and add vegetables. Vegetables should be tender but crisp.

Note: To keep a green color, cook watercress, parsley, scallions, and other green leafy vegetables at a high flame for only 1 to 2 minutes. To preserve the taste, it is also better not to add salt after boiling. Tamari soy sauce may be added at end of cooking for flavor.

Variation: For an especially sweet taste, place a 3-inch piece of kombu on bottom of pot when cooking round vegetables such as carrots or daikon. Vegetables may be seasoned with tamari soy sauce or miso instead of salt. Tasty combinations of boiled vegetables include broccoli and cauliflower; cabbage, corn, and tofu; carrots, onions, and green peas.

Steaming

Place ½ inch of spring water in pot. Insert a vegetable steamer inside pot or a wooden Japanese steamer on top of pot. Place sliced vegetables in steamer and sprinkle with a pinch of sea salt. Cover and bring water to boil. Steam until tender but slightly crisp. Greens will take only 1 to 2 minutes, other vegetables 5 to 7 minutes depending on type, size, and thickness.

Note: Lightly steamed greens can be eaten every day. These include leafy tops of turnip, daikon, and carrot; watercress; kale; mustard greens; Chinese cabbage; parsley.

Variation: If you don't have a steamer, place ½ inch of water in bottom of pot. Add vegetables and pinch of sea salt. Bring to a boil, lower heat to medium, and steam until tender. Save vegetable water for soup stock or sauces.

Other Cooking Styles

Vegetables may be prepared in a variety of other styles including baking, broiling, and tempuraing (deep-frying). However, these are not generally recommended for most heart and circulatory patients. For those in good health who wish to try these methods, seek proper instruction and guidance or consult another macrobiotic cookbook.

BOILED CARROTS AND ONIONS

2 1-inch pieces dried kombu   *spring water*
2–3 onions, sliced   *½ teaspoon sea salt*
4–5 carrots, cut into large
  chunks

Place kombu squares in a saucepan. Add sliced onions and put carrots on top. Add water to cover the onions and sprinkle ½ teaspoon of sea salt on vegetables. Cover and cook over medium heat about 10 minutes. If carrots are soft, dish is done. At end, mix so that onion juice covers carrots. Take out kombu and save for another recipe. If the kombu is soft, it may be sliced thinly and served alongside the carrots.

Variation: To thicken the remaining juice, add about ½ teaspoon of kuzu, stir for a few minutes, and pour over carrots and onions.

KINPURA-STYLE BURDOCK

2 pieces of dried tofu, soaked and sliced into rectangular shapes
1 teaspoon dark sesame oil
1 cup burdock, shaved or cut into matchsticks

2 cups carrots, cut into matchsticks
spring water
tamari soy sauce

Place the dried tofu in warm or hot water and soak for 3 to 4 minutes. Rinse in cold water. Remove and squeeze out water. Slice the tofu into rectangular shapes. Place a small amount of oil in a skillet and heat. Place the burdock in the skillet and sauté for 2 to 3 minutes. Add carrots and dried tofu and sauté 2 to 3 minutes. Place a small amount of the spring water to about half-cover the vegetables. Add a small amount of of tamari soy sauce. Bring to a boil, reduce heat to low, cover, and simmer about 30 minutes or until all liquid is gone.

Variation: Fresh sliced lotus root may be substituted for burdock to create a different taste. Other good kinpura combinations are turnip and carrots; carrots and cabbage; parsnips and onion; onion, carrots, and turnip; and celery and parsley stems. The dried tofu may be omitted or fresh tofu or tempeh used instead. For those who wish to avoid oil, sauté with 1 to 2 tablespoons of water instead and boil at a high temperature to keep the vegetables crispy. A light kuzu sauce seasoned with tamari soy sauce goes well over this dish.

BOILED DAIKON

As a side dish, daikon may be boiled in large slices and served with a sauce, with miso, or with toasted black sesame seeds. This is a typical recipe.

2 8-inch strips kombu, soaked
and sliced into ¼–½-inch
rectangles

1 medium daikon, cut into
½-inch rounds (3–4 cups)
1–2 teaspoons miso

Place kombu on bottom of the pot. Layer daikon on top of kombu. Add water to half-cover and bring to a boil. Cover, reduce heat to low, and simmer until daikon is translucent and soft, about 30 to 40 minutes. Season with miso diluted in a little juice and cook 5 to 10 minutes longer. The dish should be sweet, not salty, to the taste. If overcooked, it may become bitter.

DRIED DAIKON WITH KOMBU AND TAMARI

2 6-inch strips kombu
½ cup dried daikon

tamari soy sauce to taste

Soak kombu and slice lengthwise into ¼-inch strips and place in bottom of heavy pot with a heavy lid. Soak daikon until soft. If daikon is very dark in color, wash first. Place dried daikon on top of kombu in pot. Add enough kombu and daikon soaking water and spring water if needed to just cover top of daikon. Cover pot, bring to boil, lower heat, add tamari soy sauce, and simmer 30 to 40 minutes until kombu is tender. Cook away excess liquid.

Note: This dish helps to dissolve fat deposits around the heart, in the arteries, and elsewhere throughout the body.

Variation: Fresh daikon has more power than dried daikon. Slice fresh daikon and cook as above until very tender. If daikon is unavailable, red radish may be used, though the effect is not so strong.

BOILED CABBAGE WITH SESAME AND UMEBOSHI SAUCE

4 cups very finely sliced
cabbage
2 cups spring water

2 teaspoons kuzu
1–2 umeboshi plums
1 tablespoon sesame seeds

Slice cabbage very fine and boil just until the cabbage is a bright, colorful green, about 2 to 3 minutes. Drain cabbage. Make a sauce with the cabbage-boiling water, kuzu, and umeboshi plums. Pour the sauce over the cabbage. Wash sesame seeds and roast until golden brown. Place seeds on a cutting board and chop. Sprinkle the chopped seeds on top of the cabbage.

Variation: A little grated ginger may also be added to the sauce. Another good topping is ½ teaspoon of pureed miso, 1 tablespoon of brown rice vinegar, and some sesame seeds mixed together.

STEAMED CHINESE VEGETABLES

spring water
sea salt
2 cups finely sliced cabbage
1 cup thinly sliced onions
½ cup thinly sliced celery

2–4 teaspoons chopped
parsley
1 sheet toasted nori, cut into
squares

Place a little water in a skillet. Add vegetables and steam. When water starts to evaporate, add just a little more water and a small amount of sea salt, a pinch or two. Salt will draw water out of the vegetables. With chopsticks or a wooden utensil, gently move the vegetables around to help them cook. Use high heat to help keep the vegetables crisp. Finish cooking and add a little chopped parsley. The vegetables should cook altogether only about 2 to 3 minutes and be almost raw and crispy. Place in a bowl and serve with garnish of toasted nori.

AZUKI, KOMBU, AND SQUASH

1 cup azuki beans
2 3-inch strips kombu

1 hard winter squash
sea salt

Wash and soak azuki beans with kombu. Remove kombu after soaking and chop into 1-inch-square pieces. Place kombu at bottom of pot and add chopped hard winter squash such as acorn, butternut, or hokkaido. Add azukis on top of squash. Cover with water and cook over a low heat until beans and squash are soft. Sprinkle lightly with sea salt. Cover and let cook for 10 to 15 minutes. Turn off heat and let sit for several minutes before serving.

Note: This dish is helpful in regulating blood sugar levels, especially in those who are hypoglycemic, diabetic, or have pancreatic or liver disorders. It is naturally sweet and delicious and will reduce the craving for sweets. May be prepared 1 to 2 times per week.

Variation: You may cook azuki beans 50 to 70 percent, then add on top of squash, and proceed as above.

BROCCOLI AND TOFU CREAM DRESSING

1 head broccoli, cut into   *16 ounces tofu*
flowerets   *2–3 umeboshi plums*

Boil broccoli until done, about 2 to 3 minutes, in a little water. Vegetable should be slightly crisp and bright green in color. Place tofu between two cutting boards for about 15 to 30 minutes and press out liquid or squeeze by placing the tofu in a cotton cloth. Place pitted umeboshi in a suribachi and puree. Add tofu and grind until smooth and creamy. Mix thoroughly. Mix tofu cream and broccoli together.

STEAMED KALE AND CARROTS

spring water   *1 cup sliced (in rounds)*
4 cups washed and thinly   *carrots*
sliced kale

Place a small amount of liquid in a pot. Place a steamer in the pot and put carrots in the steamer. Bring to a boil, cover, and steam until the carrots are done. They should be slightly crisp. Remove carrots and place in a bowl. Place kale in the steamer and steam a few minutes until done. Kale should be bright green and slightly crisp when done. Remove the kale and mix with the steamed carrots.

STEAMED COLLARD GREENS WITH
TAMARI-VINEGAR SAUCE

spring water
3 cups finely sliced collard
greens

tamari soy sauce
brown rice vinegar

Place a small amount of water in a pot and bring to a boil. Place a steamer in the pot. Set the collards in the steamer and steam several minutes or until done. The greens should be bright green and slightly crisp. Remove and place in a serving dish. Mix a small amount of tamari soy sauce, brown rice vinegar, and water together to make a sauce. Place 1 teaspoon of sauce over each serving of collard greens.

CHINESE CABBAGE WITH
TAMARI-LEMON SAUCE

spring water
4 cups finely sliced Chinese
cabbage
2–3 teaspoons fresh lemon
juice

½ cup spring water
2–3 tablespoons tamari soy
sauce

Place about ½ inch of water in a pot and bring to a boil. Add the Chinese cabbage, cover, and simmer 1 to 2 minutes. Stir occasionally to cook the cabbage evenly. Remove the vegetable when tender and drain. It should be brightly colored and slightly crisp. To make the sauce, combine lemon juice, ½ cup spring water, and tamari soy sauce and mix. Serve the sauce and Chinese cabbage separately and pour a teaspoon on each serving before eating.

BOILED MUSTARD GREENS WITH
TAMARI-GINGER SAUCE

4 cups finely sliced mustard
greens
spring water

tamari soy sauce
grated ginger

Place ¼ inch of water in a pot and bring to a boil. Drop in the mustard greens and cook several minutes or until done. Mix often to cook the greens evenly, making sure to bring the greens from the bottom of the pot up to the top. When done the greens should be bright green and slightly crisp. For the sauce, mix ¼ cup of water and ¼ cup of tamari soy sauce with ½ teaspoon fresh grated ginger. Serve greens with a spoonful of sauce over each serving.

BOILED WATERCRESS

2 bunches watercress   *spring water*

Wash the watercress very well. Place ¼ to ½ inch of water in a pan and bring to a boil. Place about a quarter of the watercress in the water and cook about 30 to 40 seconds, moving it around with chopsticks to make sure it cooks evenly. Remove, drain, and allow to cool. Repeat with the remaining watercress, cooking about a quarter of it at a time. After cooking, draining, and cooling all the watercress, slice and place on a plate or in a serving bowl.

SALADS

RAW SALAD

1 head lettuce   *1 box alfalfa sprouts*
5–6 red radishes, sliced thin   *1 ear corn, kernels removed*
1 cucumber, sliced into thin   *1 carrot, shredded*
rounds

Arrange lettuce attractively on a serving plate. A nice, soft variety, like Boston lettuce, opens up easily and the leaves can be torn by hand. Distribute sliced radishes and cucumbers evenly in a circle on the lettuce leaves. Place the sprouts in small groupings in the center of the circle on top of the lettuce or around the outside edge or both. Boil the corn kernels in about ¼ inch of water in a saucepan for 2 to 3 minutes. Let cool and sprinkle over the salad. Finally, add shredded carrot on the very top. Serve with a separate sauce, such as umeboshi plum dressing with a little onion and sesame seeds; tofu dressing with a little umeboshi; a miso-brown rice vinegar dressing with a little mirin; or a tamari-ginger dressing with a little mirin.

BOILED SALAD

spring water
sea salt
1 cup sliced Chinese cabbage
½ cup sliced onion

½ cup thinly sliced carrots
½ cup sliced celery
1 bunch watercress

When making a boiled salad, boil each vegetable separately. All vegetables, however, may be boiled in the same water. Cook the mildest tasting vegetables first, so that each will retain its distinctive flavor. Place 1 inch of water and a pinch of sea salt in a pot and bring to a boil. Drop Chinese cabbage slices into water and boil 1 to 2 minutes. All vegetables should be slightly crisp, but not raw. To remove vegetables from water, pour into a strainer that has been placed inside a bowl so as to retain the cooking water. Put the drained-off water back into the pot and reboil. Next boil the sliced onion. Drain as above, retaining water and returning to boil. Next boil sliced carrots followed by sliced celery. Last, drop watercress into boiling water for just a few seconds. For vegetables to keep their bright color, each vegetable should be allowed to cool off. Sometimes you can run under cold water while in the strainer, but it is not ideal. Mix vegetables together after boiling. A dressing of 1 umeboshi plum or 1 teaspoon of umeboshi paste may be added to ½ cup of water (vegetable stock from boiling may be used) and pureed in a bowl or suribachi for seasoning.

Note: A refreshing way to prepare vegetables in place of raw salad. Especially recommended for heart patients who cannot have uncooked foods. This method just takes out the raw taste and preserves the crispy freshness.

PRESSED SALAD

Wash and slice desired vegetables into very thin pieces, such as ½ cabbage (may be shredded), 1 cucumber, 1 stalk celery, 2 red radishes, 1 onion. Place vegetables in a pickle press or large bowl and sprinkle with ½ teaspoon sea salt and mix. Apply pressure to the press. If you use a bowl in place of the press, place a small plate on top of the vegetables and place a stone or weight on top of the plate. Leave it for at least 30 to 45 minutes. You may leave it up to 3 to 4 days but the longer you press the vegetables the more they resemble light pickles.

Note: This is a method to remove excess liquid from raw vegetables. For many heart patients, a boiled salad is preferable.

Variation: A press is not necessary when using soft vegetables. Just mix with salt and serve after 30 minutes.

BROWN RICE SALAD

2 cups brown rice
1¼–1½ cups spring water
  per cup of rice
1 cup diced carrots
1 cup fresh green peas

½ cup quartered and sliced
  cucumbers
½ cup diced celery
¼ cup very finely chopped
  shiso leaves
pinch of sea salt

Wash and pressure-cook rice. When rice is done, remove and place it in a bowl to cool. Fluff up the rice to remove steam and lighten it. Boil the carrots and peas separately in a saucepan containing a little water until tender. Remove and allow to cool off. Add the carrots and peas to the rice, along with the cucumber and celery, and mix together well. Mix in the chopped shiso leaves, which come pickled with umeboshi plums and may sometimes be obtained whole by themselves. Garnish with sliced scallions or parsley and serve.

Variation: Instead of shiso leaves, salad may be served with a dressing made of brown rice vinegar, salt, and mirin or lemon and salt. Roasted sesame seeds make a nice garnish.

SAUCES AND DRESSINGS

KUZU SAUCE

1 tablespoon kuzu
1½ cups vegetable stock or
water

tamari soy sauce

Dilute kuzu (a white starch, also known as kudzu) in small volume of cold water and add to pot containing stock or water. Bring to a boil, lower heat, and simmer 10 to 15 minutes. Stir constantly. Add tamari soy sauce to taste. Serve over vegetables, tofu, noodles, grains, or beans.

Variation: Arrowroot powder may be used instead of kuzu. Avoid thickeners such as cornstarch.

TAMARI-VINEGAR DRESSING

¼–½ teaspoon sesame oil (optional)
1 tablespoon tamari soy sauce

4 tablespoons brown rice vinegar
1 tablespoon grated onion
½ cup spring water

If using oil, heat for about 1 minute over low heat. Puree all the ingredients together in a suribachi and serve.

TAMARI-LEMON DRESSING

2–3 tablespoons tamari soy sauce
½ cup spring water

2–3 teaspoons freshly squeezed lemon juice

Combine the ingredients and mix. For variety, a little minced onion and ½ teaspoon of heated sesame oil may be added.

TAMARI-GINGER DRESSING

2 tablespoons tamari soy sauce
2–3 tablespoons spring water

¼ teaspoon fresh grated ginger
2 tablespoons roasted sesame seeds, 70% crushed

Combine ingredients and mix.

MISO-GINGER SAUCE

1 teaspoon barley miso   *spring water*
½ teaspoon freshly grated
ginger

Place 1 teaspoon of miso and a little freshly grated ginger in a suribachi. Puree with a small amount of water to make a smooth, creamy sauce.

TOFU DRESSING

½ teaspoon pureed umeboshi   *2 teaspoons spring water*
plum   *8 ounces of tofu*
¼ onion, grated or diced   *chopped scallions or parsley*

Puree umeboshi, onion, and water in suribachi. Add tofu and puree until creamy. Add water to increase creaminess if desired. Garnish with scallions or parsley. Serve with salad.

UMEBOSHI DRESSING

2 umeboshi plums   *½ teaspoon sesame oil*
¼–½ teaspoon grated onion   *½ cup spring water*

Puree umeboshi and onion in suribachi. Add slightly heated oil and mix. Add water and mix to smooth consistency. Serve on salad.

Note: This dressing can also be made without oil by adding a little bit more water.

Variation: Umeboshi paste may be used instead of plums. Use 1 teaspoon of paste per plum. Also, chives and scallions may be substituted for onions and the mixture used as a dip for crackers or chips.

PICKLES

PRESSED SALT PICKLES

2 large daikon and their
leaves
¼–½ cup sea salt

heavy ceramic or wooden
crock or keg

Wash daikon and their leaves with enough cold water 2 to 3 times, making sure all dirt is removed, especially from the leaves. Set aside and let dry for about 24 hours. Slice the daikon into small rounds. Sprinkle sea salt in the bottom of the crock. Next layer some of the daikon leaves, followed by a layer of daikon rounds. Then sprinkle with sea salt again. Repeat this until the daikon is used or the crock is filled. Place a lid or plate that will fit inside the crock on top of the daikon, daikon leaves, and salt. Place a heavy rock or brick on top of the lid or plate. Cover with a thin layer of cheesecloth to keep out dust. Soon water will begin to be squeezed out and rise to the surface of the plate. When this happens, replace heavy weight with a lighter one. Store in a dark, cool place for 1 to 2 weeks or longer. If water is not entirely squeezed out, add more salt. And make sure water is always covered or it will spoil. When ready, remove a portion, wash under cold water, slice and serve.

Note: Pickles are a naturally fermented food and aid in digestion. A small volume may be eaten daily. However, commercial pickles such as dill pickles that have been made with vinegar and spices should be strictly avoided.

Variation: Pickles may also be made from Chinese cabbage, carrots, cauliflower, and other vegetables in this manner.

TAMARI SOY SAUCE PICKLES

Mix equal parts spring water and tamari soy sauce in a bowl or glass jar. Slice vegetables such as turnips or rutabaga and place in this liquid. Soak for 4 hours to 2 weeks, depending on the strength desired.

RICE BRAN PICKLES (NUKA)

Long Time *(Ready in 3 to 5 months)*
10–12 cups of nuka *(rice bran)* or wheat bran
1½–2 cups sea salt
3–5 cups spring water

Short Time *(Ready in 1 to 2 weeks)*
10–12 cups nuka
⅛–¼ cup sea salt
3–5 cups spring water

Roast nuka or wheat bran in a dry skillet until it gives off a nutty aroma. Allow to cool. Combine roasted nuka or wheat bran with salt and mix well. Place a layer of bran mixture in the bottom of a wooden keg or ceramic crock. A single vegetable such as daikon, turnips, rutabaga, onion, or Chinese cabbage may be used. Slice vegetables into 2- to 3-inch pieces and layer on top of the nuka. If more than one type of vegetable is used, layer one on top of another. Then sprinkle a layer of nuka on top of the vegetables. Repeat this layering until the nuka mixture is used up or until the crock is filled. Always make sure that the nuka mixture is the top layer. Place a wooden disk or plate to fit inside the crock, on top of the vegetables and nuka. Place a heavy weight, such as a rock or brick, on top of the plate. Soon water will begin to be squeezed out and rise to the surface of the plate. When this happens, replace heavy weight with a lighter one. Cover with a thin layer of cheesecloth and store in a cool room. To serve, take out pickled vegetables as needed and rinse under cold water to remove excess bran and salt. The same nuka paste may be used for several years. Just keep adding vegetables and a little more bran and salt.

SCALLION-MISO PICKLES

1 bunch scallions   miso

Wash scallions and place in a jar so they are completely covered with miso. Leave for 1 to 2 days. Remove, wash off miso, and save it for cooking. Slice scallions and serve.

BEANS AND BEAN PRODUCTS

AZUKI BEANS

1 cup azuki beans
2½ cups spring water per cup
of beans

¼ teaspoon sea salt per cup
of beans

Wash beans and place in pressure-cooker. Add water, cover, and bring to pressure. Reduce flame to medium low and cook 45 minutes. Remove pressure-cooker from burner and rinse cold water over it to bring pressure down quickly. Open, add salt, cook uncovered until liquid evaporates.

Note: Most other types of beans can be pressure-cooked in this way. Chick-peas and yellow soybeans should first be soaked. Black soybeans should not be pressure-cooked because they clog up the gauge.

Variation: Beans may also be boiled by putting in a pot, adding 3½ to 4 cups of water per cup of beans, and cooking for about 1 hour and 45 minutes. When 80 percent cooked, add salt and cook for another 15 to 20 minutes until liquid is evaporated. To reduce cooking time, add flavor, and make beans more digestible, lay a 3-inch piece of kombu under beans at the beginning. A small volume of vegetables may also be cooked along with beans, such as chopped squash, onions, or carrots.

LENTILS

1 cup lentils
2½ cups spring water

¼ teaspoon sea salt

Wash lentils and place in pot. Add water, cover, and bring to a boil. Reduce flame to medium-low. After 30 minutes, add salt and cook another 15 to 20 minutes. Remove cover and allow liquid to cook off.

Variation: Chopped onions and celery go well with lentils and may be cooked together.

CHICK-PEAS

1 cup chick-peas   *½ teaspoon sea salt*
3 cups spring water

Wash beans and soak overnight. Place beans and soaking water in pressure-cooker. Add more water if necessary. Bring to pressure, turn down heat to medium low, and cook 1 to 1½ hours. Take off burner and allow pressure to come down. Remove lid, add salt, and return to burner. Cook uncovered for another 45 to 60 minutes.

Variation: Diced onion and carrots may be added to beans during last hour of cooking.

COLORFUL SOYBEAN CASSEROLE

soaking water   *1 burdock, sliced*
2 cups yellow soybeans   *1 stalk celery, sliced*
2 3-inch pieces kombu   *1 dried daikon, shredded*
1 shiitake mushroom   *1½ tablespoons tamari soy*
5 large pieces dried lotus root   *sauce*
6 dried tofu   *1 teaspoon kuzu*
1 carrot, sliced

Soak soybeans in cold water overnight in 2½ cups of water per cup of soybeans. Next day, place beans and soaking water in pressure-cooker and bring to pressure. Soak kombu, shiitake, lotus root, and dried tofu for 10 minutes. After beans have cooked 70 to 80 percent (approximately 15 minutes) reduce pressure, open, and layer kombu, shiitake, lotus root, and dried tofu on top. Bring back to pressure and cook 10 more minutes. Reduce pressure, open, skim off hulls from beans and take out vegetables and put on separate plates. Meanwhile, cut up carrot, burdock, celery, and dried daikon. Slice up cooked kombu and put in bottom of a large saucepan in a little water. On top of kombu add soft vegetables such as celery, shiitake, daikon, and tofu; then root vegetables including carrots, burdock, and lotus root; and finally soybeans and any origi nal water remaining in pressure-cooker. Add 1½ tablespoons of tamari soy sauce, cover, cook 30 minutes. Add 1 teaspoon of kuzu to make creamy and a little grated ginger for flavoring. Soybeans should be very tender and sweet.

Note: This dish is extremely nourishing and highly recommended for heart patients. However, those with a yin condition should be careful not to use more than one shiitake mushroom. Those with a yang condition or healthy persons may use 5 to 6 shiitake.

Variation: Depending on availability, some vegetables may be omitted or added. Also, seitan makes this dish especially delicious.

BLACK SOYBEANS

2 cups black soybeans   *1 teaspoon sea salt*
spring water   *tamari soy sauce*

Wash beans quickly and soak overnight in cold water, adding ¼ to ½ teaspoon of sea salt per cup of beans. The salt will prevent the skins from peeling. In the morning, place beans and soaking water in pot. If necessary, add additional water to cover surface of beans. Bring to a boil, reduce heat, and simmer uncovered. When a dark foam rises to the surface, skim and discard. Continue in this way until no more foam rises. Cover beans and cook for 2½ to 3 hours. Add water to cover surface of beans if necessary. Toward end of cooking, uncover and add a little tamari soy sauce to give the skins a shiny, black color. Cook away excess liquid. Shake pot up and down to coat beans with remaining juice, and serve.

Note: This dish is particularly beneficial for the sexual organs and to relieve an overly yang condition caused by excess meat or fish. Avoid pressure-cooking black beans since they may clog the gauge.

MISO

Miso (fermented soybean paste) is highly recommended for daily use. Heart patients and others with illness, weakness, or fatigue should use barley miso that has aged for 3 years. Hatcho miso (100% soybean) and brown rice miso may be used occasionally. Avoid misos that have aged less than 1½ years. Store-bought miso should be made with organic or all-natural ingredients. Miso sold in bulk is usually preferable to miso sold in sealed plastic, which has been pasteurized, thereby reducing the beneficial enzymes and bacteria that aid digestion. Instant miso mixes are not recommended for daily use if regular miso is available. Instant miso is all right for traveling, and if circumstances permit should be cooked for a few minutes in water rather than steeped like a tea bag. Miso can be made at home with a grain called *koji*, which contains a special bacteria that enables the soybeans to ferment. Koji is available in some natural foods stores or can be made at home with a koji starter available from American Type Culture Collection, 12301 Park Lawn Drive, Rockville, Maryland 20852. (Request koji culture, aspergilus oryzae, Ahlburg Cohn, Code No. 14805.) Miso is used primarily in making miso soup (see recipe in soup section). However, it can also be used in cooking with vegetables, as a seasoning in place of salt, and in spreads, dips, dressings, pickles, relishes, and condiments. For complete miso recipes, see *How to Cook with Miso* by Aveline Kushi (Japan Publications, 1978).

HOMEMADE TOFU

3 cups organic yellow
soybeans

6 quarts spring water
4½ teaspoons natural nigari

Soak beans overnight, strain, and grind in an electric blender. Place ground beans in pot with 6 quarts of water and bring to a boil. Reduce flame to low and simmer for 5 minutes, stirring constantly to avoid burning. Sprinkle cold water on beans to stop bubbling. Gently boil again and sprinkle with cold water. Repeat a third time. Place a cotton cloth or several layers of cheesecloth in a strainer and pour this liquid into a bowl. This is soy milk. Fold corners of the cloth to form a sack or place cloth in a strainer and squeeze out remaining liquid. Pulp in sack is called *okara* and may be saved for other recipes. In a suribachi or blender, grind the nigari, which is a special salt made from sea water and available in many natural foods stores. Sprinkle powdered nigari over soy milk in a bowl. With a wooden spoon carefully make a large,

X-shaped cut with two deep strokes in this mixture and allow to sit 10 to 15 minutes. During this time it will begin to curdle. The next step calls for a wooden or stainless-steel tofu box (available in many natural foods stores) or a bamboo steamer. Line box or steamer with cheesecloth and gently spoon in soy milk. Cover top with layer of cheesecloth and place lid on top of box or steamer so it rests on cheesecloth and curdling tofu. Place small stone or weight on lid and let stand for about 1 hour or until tofu cake is formed. Then gently place tofu in a dish of cold water for 30 minutes to solidify. Keep tofu covered in water and refrigerate until used. Tofu will stay fresh for several days in the refrigerator. However, it is best to change water daily.

Note: Raw tofu is somewhat difficult to digest, so it is preferably eaten cooked. Tofu bought at the store should be made from organically grown soybeans and natural nigari. Refined solidifiers are sometimes used instead of natural nigari and should be avoided when possible. Those on an oil-restricted diet should avoid tofu mayonnaise, tofu dips, and other tofu products that contain oil, vinegar, or spices.

Variation: Tofu is very versatile, picks up the taste of the foods it is combined with, and has a variety of textures depending upon how it is cooked. It may be sliced, cubed, diced, pressed, or mashed and boiled in soups, sautéed with vegetables or grains, or baked in casseroles. It may also be used in dips, sauces, dressings, and desserts. The okara or pulp can be added to soups or cooked with vegetables.

BOILED TOFU WITH GINGER-PARSLEY SAUCE

spring water
16 ounces tofu, sliced into 5
 pieces about ½-inch thick

tamari soy sauce
fresh grated ginger
chopped parsley or scallions

Place about ¼-inch of water in a pot and bring to a boil. Place tofu slices in the water and cover pot. Reduce heat to low and simmer 1 to 2 minutes. Keep the heat low, or the tofu will become hard. Remove tofu, drain, and place slices on individual serving plates. Prepare a sauce by mixing a small amount of water, tamari soy sauce, and grated ginger. Place a teaspoon of sauce over each slice of boiled tofu and garnish with chopped parsley or scallions.

SCRAMBLED TOFU AND CORN

3 tablespoons dark sesame or corn oil
16 ounces firm tofu

3 cups fresh sweet corn, removed from cob
½–1 teaspoon sea salt
sliced scallions

Place the oil in a pot and heat. Crumble the tofu and add to the pot. Place the sweet corn on top of the tofu. Cover and cook over low heat for 3 to 4 minutes or until the tofu becomes hot and the corn is done. Sprinkle a small amount of sea salt on top of the corn. Mix and serve hot. Just before serving, add scallions as a garnish but to retain their bright green color don't cook them.

Variation: The tofu, corn, and scallions may also be sautéed with 2 to 3 tablespoons of water for those who need to limit their oil. Other vegetables may be added or substituted, including cabbage, onions, carrots (cut in matchsticks), and mushrooms. The colors of the vegetables should be bright and the texture slightly crispy.

TEMPEH (SOY MEAT)

Tempeh is a traditional fermented soyfood originating in Indonesia. In the last decade it has become increasingly popular in the Far East and West and is now available in many natural foods stores. Tempeh is crisp, delicious, and nourishing and may be steamed, boiled, baked, or sautéed. It is enjoyed with a wide variety of grains, vegetables, and noodles and may be used in soups, salads, or sandwiches. Tempeh should always be cooked before eating. Tempeh may also be made at home. A special culture is available in many natural foods stores or may be ordered from The Farm, 156 Drakes Lane, Summertown, Tennessee 38483. For recipes and further information on tempeh making, see *The Book of Tempeh* by William Shurtleff and Akiko Aoyagi (Harper & Row, 1980).

CABBAGE-ROLL TEMPEH

2 strips kombu
Several outer layers of
  cabbage leaves

8 ounces tempeh
2 onions

Soak kombu 1 hour or more. Steam cabbage until soft. Cut the tempeh into 2-inch rectangles and steam or boil. Place on cabbage leaves and roll up. Slice soaked kombu and onions thinly. Layer kombu and onions in bottom of pot. Add water and cabbage rolls. Add sea salt to taste if desired. Cook until very soft.

Note: Avoid cooking with salt or tamari soy sauce when serving tempeh to children. Tempeh is very energizing and salt could make them overactive.

NATTO

Natto is a fermented soy product that aids digestion and strengthens the intestines. It looks like baked beans connected by long slippery strands and has a unique odor. Natto is available in macrobiotic specialty stores or can be made at home (see recipe in *Aveline Kushi's Complete Guide to Macrobiotic Cooking,* Warner Books, 1985. Natto is usually eaten with a little tamari soy sauce, mixed with rice, or served on top of buckwheat noodles.

SEA VEGETABLES

HIZIKI OR ARAME

2 cups soaked hiziki or arame
1 medium onion, sliced
1 carrot sliced in matchsticks

spring water
3–4 tablespoons tamari soy
  sauce

Wash hiziki quickly under cold water. Place in bowl, cover with water, and rinse quickly 3 times with cold water. Drain and save the last rinse water. Slice hiziki in 1- to 2-inch pieces. Place hiziki on top of other vegetables in pot. Add enough soaking water to cover top of hiziki. Bring to a boil, cover, reduce heat to low. Add

1 tablespoon of tamari soy sauce. Cook on low heat for 45 to 60 minutes. Season with additional tamari soy sauce to taste and simmer for 20 more minutes until liquid evaporates. Mix vegetables only at end and serve.

Note: Hiziki is thicker and coarser in texture than arame. Arame is milder, softer, has less of a briny taste, takes less time to cook, and is usually the sea vegetable preferred by those new to macrobiotic cooking. One ounce of dried arame or hiziki cooks up to about 2 cups.

Variation: Both hiziki and arame can be cooked with lotus root, daikon, and other vegetables; combined with grains or tofu; added to a salad; or put into a pie crust and baked as a roll. For those who can use oil, a strong, rich dish can be created by adding a little oil at the beginning of cooking.

WAKAME

2 cups soaked wakame   *1 medium onion, sliced*
soaking water   *2 teaspoons tamari soy sauce*

Rinse wakame quickly under cold water and soak 3 to 5 minutes. Slice into 1-inch pieces. Put onion in pot and wakame on top. Add soaking water to cover vegetables. Bring to boil, lower heat, and simmer for 30 minutes or until wakame is soft. Add tamari soy sauce to taste and simmer 10 to 15 more minutes.

Note: Wakame is the chief vegetable added to miso soup. It also makes a tasty side dish or can be used as an alternative in most recipes calling for kombu.

KOMBU

1 12-inch strip kombu   *1 carrot cut in triangular*
spring water   *pieces*
1 onion, quartered   *1 tablespoon tamari soy sauce*

Soak kombu 3 to 5 minutes, slice in half, and then slice diagonally into 1-inch pieces. Place in pot and add vegetables and enough soaking water to cover vegetables halfway. Add 1 tablespoon of tamari soy sauce. Bring to a boil. Reduce the heat to low and simmer for 30 minutes. Add additional tamari soy sauce to taste if desired, and cook for 5 to 10 more minutes.

Note: Kombu is delicious as a side dish or can be used as a stock for soups. Adding a 3-inch piece of kombu beneath beans will speed up cooking, add flavor, and make beans more digestible. When cooking with kombu, oil is usually not used.

NORI

Nori comes in thin sheets and can be used for wrapping rice balls (see recipe in grain section). It is also used to make sushi and makes an attractive garnish for soups, noodles, and salads. Toast lightly by holding nori, shiny side up, 10 to 12 inches from flame and rotate about 3 to 5 seconds until the nori changes from black to green.

DULSE

Dulse may be eaten dry as a snack or dry-roasted and ground into a powder in a suribachi to make a condiment. Dulse can also be used to season soups at the very end of cooking, salad, and main dishes.

AGAR-AGAR

This whitish sea vegetable forms into a gelatin when cooked and is used to make vegetable aspics and delicious fruit desserts. See recipe for kanten in dessert section.

CONDIMENTS

GOMASHIO (SESAME SALT)

For ordinary adults, we recommend about 1 part salt to 10 to 12 parts sesame seeds. For extremely active adults, such as those engaged in manual labor, 1 part salt to 8 to 10 parts sesame seeds may be used for a stronger condiment. For small children, 1 part salt to 16 to 20 parts sesame seeds makes a lighter, less salty side dish. Separate batches of gomashio should be made and clearly labeled for adults and children, since too much salt will make children overactive. A half teaspoon to 1 teaspoon of gomashio on a bowl of rice is plenty for both adults and children.

Adult Gomashio
2½–3 tablespoons sea salt
1 cup sesame seeds

Very Active Adult Gomashio
3½–4 tablespoons sea salt
1 cup sesame seeds

Childrens' Gomashio
1½–2 tablespoons sea salt
1 cup sesame seeds

Wash seeds in a very fine mesh strainer, as in preparing rice, and let drain. Seeds that float to the top while washing should be discarded. Roast the sea salt in a skillet a short time. For both sea salt and sesame seeds, stainless steel is lighter, easier to handle, and heats up and cools off more quickly than cast iron. However, cast iron cooks more evenly and may be used instead if desired. Roasting the sea salt releases moisture in the salt and helps to make fluffy gomashio. Roasting also releases a strong chlorine from the salt. The salt is done when it becomes shiny.

The sesame seeds are roasted after the salt has been roasted, ground, and set aside. Always roast sesame seeds when they are wet; they will cook more evenly. Dry seeds will burn easily. Roast seeds over medium heat. Do not roast too many seeds at once or some will burn, while others will not be roasted enough. Add only enough seeds to cover the bottom of the skillet. While roasting, push the seeds back and forth in the skillet with a rice paddle or wooden spoon. Shaking the pan occasionally will also help to roast seeds evenly and avoid burning. The seeds are done when they crush easily between the thumb and index finger, about 5 to 10 minutes. Do not overroast the seeds as they tend to become a little darker after removal from the skillet on account of the heat held inside. The seeds will also begin to pop and give off a nutty fragrance when done.

Place the roasted sea salt in a suribachi and grind until it becomes a fine powder and all small lumps are dissolved. Add hot roasted sesame seeds to the roasted, ground sea salt. Hot seeds grind more easily and should always be added after first grinding the salt. If seeds are ground first, they will turn darker when salt is added. Slowly grind the salt in an even, circular motion with a wooden pestle, making sure to grind against the grooved sides of the suribachi instead of the bottom of the bowl. Grind until each seed is half-crushed and thoroughly coated with salt. Do not grind into a powder. If you grind gently, the gomashio will taste sweeter. More powerful or quicker grinding crushes the seeds and makes them saltier to the taste. Allow gomashio to cool off when done grinding, and then place in an airtight glass or ceramic container to store. Do not place warm gomashio in the container, but let it cool. Otherwise, moisture will collect on the top and sides of the jar, causing the gomashio to spoil quickly. Gomashio will keep fresh for several weeks and may be reroasted if it begins to dry out. Avoid making too much at a time, preparing it fresh at least once a week.

Variation: For variety, sesame seeds may be prepared with miso, tamari soy sauce, roasted umeboshi plums, roasted powdered kombu or wakame, or shiso leaves. Roasted sesame seeds may also be used as a condiment or garnish without salt or other seasoning.

TAMARI SOY SAUCE

Tamari soy sauce is the name given by George Ohsawa to traditional, naturally made soy sauce to distinguish it from the commercial, chemically processed soy sauce found in many Oriental restaurants and supermarkets. Tamari soy sauce is also called *natural shoyu.* In natural foods stores there is now also available a wheatless soy sauce, known as genuine or real tamari. It is stronger in flavor. Tamari soy sauce, however, is recommended for regular use and should be used primarily in cooking and not added to rice or vegetables at the table.

ROASTED SEA VEGETABLE POWDER

Use either wakame, kombu, dulse, or kelp. Roast sea vegetable in oven until nearly charred (approximately 10 to 15 minutes at 350°) and crush in a suribachi.

Note: For more yin heart conditions, this powder can be used more frequently in larger amounts (up to 1 teaspoon per day). For more yang conditions, slightly less volume is advisable (about ½ teaspoon per day). For conditions caused by a combination of both, an in-between volume is recommended.

UMEBOSHI PLUMS

Umeboshi are special plums (imported from Japan and now also grown in this country) that have been dried and pickled with sea salt and aged from one to three years. They usually come with shiso (beefsteak) leaves, which contribute to their distinctive red color. Umeboshi may be eaten by themselves or used to enhance grains and vegetables. They may also be pureed for making a tart and tangy dressing, sauce, or tea. The umeboshi contains a harmonious balance of more yin factors, such as the natural sourness of the plum, and more yang factors created by the salt, pressure, and aging used in their preparation. Umeboshi are excellent for strengthening the intestines and may be used regularly by persons with all types of heart disease. Some natural foods stores also sell umeboshi paste without the pits. The paste is not as strong or balanced, and heart patients are advised to use the whole plums.

TEKKA (ROOT VEGETABLE CONDIMENT)

⅓ cup finely minced burdock　*½ teaspoon grated ginger*
⅓ cup finely minced carrot　*¼ cup sesame oil*
⅓ cup finely minced lotus　*⅔ cup hatcho miso*
root

Prepare vegetables, mincing as finely as possible. Heat oil in a skillet and sauté vegetables. Add miso. Reduce heat to low and cook 3 to 4 hours. Stir frequently until liquid evaporates and a dry, black mixture is left.

Note: Tekka is very strengthening for the blood but should be used sparingly because of its strong contractive nature. For more yin heart conditions, it can be used daily (about ½ teaspoon). For more yang conditions or those caused by a combination of yin and yang, use small volume only on occasion.

TAMARI-NORI CONDIMENT

Place dried nori or several sheets of fresh nori in ½ to 1 cup of spring water and simmer until most of the water cooks down to a thick paste. Add tamari soy sauce several minutes before end of cooking for a light to moderate taste.

Note: This special condiment helps the body recover its ability to discharge toxins. It may be eaten by persons with all types of heart disease. For more yang conditions, use a slightly smaller volume (approximately ½ teaspoon per day). For more yin conditions, use up to 1 teaspoon daily. For conditions caused by a combination of both, an in-between volume may be eaten.

SHIO-KOMBU CONDIMENT

1 cup sliced kombu   *½ cup tamari soy sauce*
½ cup spring water

Soak kombu until soft and chop into 1-inch-square pieces. Add sliced kombu to water and tamari soy sauce. Bring to a boil and simmer until the liquid evaporates. Cool off and place in a covered jar to keep for several days.

Note: This condiment is very high in minerals and aids in the discharge of toxins. Heart patients may eat several pieces daily. If it is too salty, reduce the tamari.

SAUERKRAUT

A small amount of sauerkraut made from organic cabbage and sea salt may be used as a condiment occasionally.

VINEGAR

Brown rice vinegar, sweet brown rice vinegar, and umeboshi vinegar may be used moderately. Avoid red wine or apple cider vinegars.

GINGER

Fresh grated or squeezed gingerroot may be used occasionally in a small volume as a garnish or flavoring in vegetable dishes, soups, pickled vegetables, and especially with fish or seafoods. Usually about ¼ teaspoon of grated ginger or a few drops of ginger juice squeezed from grated gingerroot is sufficient to garnish a dish for 4 to 5 people.

GRATED DAIKON

A small volume of grated daikon is traditionally served with fish or seafood. It helps to neutralize the effects of animal food.

1 cup grated daikon   *sliced scallions*
tamari soy sauce

Grate the daikon and place in a serving bowl. In the center of the daikon pour several drops of tamari soy sauce. Garnish with a few scallion slices. When served, each person can take a tablespoon of daikon and put 1 or 2 more drops of tamari soy sauce on it when eating. A tiny bit of grated ginger may also be added.

HORSERADISH

May be used occasionally by those in good health to aid digestion, especially for fish and seafood.

DESSERTS AND SNACKS

COOKED APPLES

Wash apples and peel unless organically grown, in which case skins may be eaten. Slice and place in a pot with a small amount of water to keep from burning (about ¼ to ½ cup). Add pinch of sea salt and simmer for 10 minutes, or until soft.

Note: Those with yin forms of heart disease should avoid desserts completely. Those with yang heart conditions may have a small volume of cooked fruit on occasion if craved.

Variation: Puree in a Foley food mill to make applesauce. Other fruits may be cooked in this way.

KANTEN (GELATIN)

3 apples, sliced
2 cups spring water
2 cups apple juice

pinch of sea salt
agar-agar flakes

Wash and slice fruit and place in pot with liquid and salt. Add agar-agar flakes in amount according to directions on package (varies from several teaspoons to several tablespoons). Stir well and bring to boil. Reduce heat to low and simmer 2 to 3 minutes. Place in shallow dish or mold and put in refrigerator to harden.

Note: This delicious natural gelatin is not recommended for some heart patients because of the high fruit and fruit juice content.

Variation: Kanten may also be made with other temperate-climate fruits, including strawberries, blueberries, peaches, or melons. Nuts and raisins may be added to the fruit. Vegetable aspics may be made in this same way with vegetable soup stock instead of fruit juice and vegetable pieces instead of fruit. Azuki beans and raisins are a delicious combination.

AZUKI BEANS, CHESTNUTS, AND RAISINS

This nice dish needs no additional sweetener other than the beans and fruit. It is traditionally served over hot baked or dry pan-fried mochi.

1 cup azuki beans
1 cup dried chestnuts
5 cups spring water

1 strip kombu, about 6 inches
 long
½–¾ cup raisins
½–1 teaspoon sea salt

Soak beans and chestnuts together 5 hours in 5 cups of water. When finished soaking, place kombu in bottom of a pot. Add azuki beans, chestnuts, and raisins. Add soaking water to cover mixture and bring to a boil. Cover, reduce heat to low, and simmer about 3 hours. Add extra cold water if necessary from time to time. Season with a little sea salt and simmer several more minutes before serving.

Variation: To prepare more quickly, mixture may be pressure-cooked about 40 to 45 minutes instead of boiled. Add salt at the end of cooking.

RICE PUDDING

½ cup almonds
3–4 tablespoons tahini
¾ cup spring water
3½ cups cooked brown rice

1½ cups apple juice
¼ teaspoon sea salt
⅓–½ cup spring water

Boil almonds and tahini in ¾ cup water and puree in a blender. Place mixture and other ingredients in pressure-cooker for 45 minutes. After pressure has come down, take out and place mixture in a baking dish or covered casserole, and bake at 350° for 45 to 60 minutes.

Note: A tasty dessert for those in good health but not recommended for some forms of heart disease.

COUSCOUS CAKE

2 cups couscous
2 cups apple juice

1½–2 cups spring water
pinch of sea salt

Wash the couscous and place it in a fine mesh steamer or line the bottom of a steamer with cheesecloth to keep it from falling through. Steam about 5 minutes. Remove and place in a bowl. Fluff up couscous to cool off. Bring apple juice, water, and salt to a boil. Boil 1 to 2 minutes. Pour hot liquid over the couscous and mix in. Place the couscous in a glass cake pan or baking dish and press it down so that it occupies about half the pan and is a little dense. Cover and let sit a few minutes.

Topping
1 cup spring water
2 cups apple juice
pinch of sea salt

4–5 tablespoons agar-agar
flakes or 1 bar (read
directions first)
2 cups fresh strawberries,
sliced

Place water, juice, sea salt, and agar-agar in a saucepan and bring to a boil. Reduce heat to low and simmer 2 to 3 minutes. Add the strawberries and remove from the heat. Let liquid cool off a little and then pour it over the couscous. Place the cake in a cool place or refrigerate and let sit until the topping jells. When done the cake should be firm and cover the bottom half of the pan. The strawberry topping should be firm and cover the top half of the pan. Slice in squares and serve.

Note: This is a wonderful cake, traditionally served at macrobiotic parties and other special occasions. Instead of the strawberry topping, apricots, apples, cherries, and other fresh fruits may be used. Until their condition improves, heart patients may need to avoid this dessert because of the high juice and fruit content.

SQUASH PIE

1 medium buttercup squash
1 cup spring water
pinch of sea salt

¼–½ cup barley malt
1 tablespoon kuzu
1 cup chopped walnuts

Wash squash and remove skin and seeds (which may be saved for roasting). Cut squash into chunks and place in a pot with 1 cup of water. Add a pinch of salt, bring to a boil, reduce heat to medium low, and cover. Simmer until the squash is soft, about 20 minutes or until tender. Place the squash in a hand food mill and puree until smooth. Place the pureed squash in a pot and add the barley malt. Simmer about 5 minutes. Dilute the kuzu in a little water and add it to the pureed squash, stirring constantly to avoid lumping. Simmer 2 to 3 minutes. Remove from heat and allow to cool. Roll out pastry dough (using a basic pie crust recipe). Bake the bottom crust at 350° for about 10 minutes. Add the squash filling to the empty shell, smooth out the top of the filling, and sprinkle the chopped walnuts on top. Bake 30 to 35 minutes or until the crust is golden brown.

Note: Not recommended for certain forms of heart disease. Check dietary recommendations.

RICE CAKES

Made from puffed brown rice and sea salt, rice cakes are a tasty crunchy snack. They are available ready-made in most natural foods stores and may be eaten plain or enjoyed with sesame or peanut butter, natural fruit jellies and jams, or spreads made with miso, tofu, or other ingredients. In addition to regular brown rice cakes, there are varieties made with sesame seeds, buckwheat, millet, oats, or other grains. Rice cakes store well but dry out with age. To restore their crispness, place for a few minutes in a low oven.

MISO-TAHINI SPREAD

6 tablespoons tahini   *1 tablespoon barley or rice miso*

Dry-roast tahini in a skillet over medium-low heat until golden brown. Stir constantly to prevent burning. In suribachi stir tahini with miso. Add chopped scallions for variation. Delicious with bread or crackers.

Note: This spread is high in oil and may need to be avoided by most heart patients until their condition stabilizes.

ROASTED SEEDS

Dry-roast sesame, sunflower, pumpkin, or squash seeds by placing several cups of seeds in a skillet. Turn on heat to medium low and gently stir with wooden roasting paddle or spoon for 10 to 15 minutes. When done, seeds should be darker in color, crisp, and give off a fragrant aroma. Seeds may be lightly seasoned with tamari soy sauce while roasting.

Note: Heart patients may occasionally have roasted seeds in small volume.

BEVERAGES

BANCHA TWIG TEA

Add 2 tablespoons of roasted twigs to 1½ quarts of spring water and bring to a boil. Lower heat and simmer for several minutes. Place bamboo tea strainer in cup and pour out tea. Twigs in strainer may be returned to teapot.

Note: This tea, also known as kukicha tea, is the main beverage in macrobiotic cooking. It may be eaten at the end of every meal and in between meals. However, everyone should watch his or her liquid consumption and drink only when thirsty.

BROWN RICE OR MILLET TEA

Dry-roast uncooked brown rice or millet over medium heat for 10 minutes or until a fragrant aroma develops. Stir and shake pan occasionally to prevent burning. Add 2 to 3 tablespoons of roasted grain to 1½ quarts of spring water. Bring to a boil, reduce heat, and simmer 10 to 15 minutes.

Note: Millet is strengthening to the heart.

ROASTED BARLEY TEA

Prepare same way as roasted brown rice or millet tea above. This tea is especially good for melting animal fat from the body.

Roasted barley tea also makes a very nice summer drink and may also aid in the reduction of fever.

CORN SILK TEA

Native peoples in North America traditionally enjoyed a beverage made from the golden silk strands of fresh corn. To prepare, place ½ cup fresh corn silk in a quart of spring water and bring to a boil. Reduce heat and simmer several minutes. Corn silk tea is good in hot weather and beneficial to the kidneys and heart.

GRAIN COFFEE

Roast separately each of the following: 3 cups of uncooked brown rice, 2½ cups of wheat, 1½ cups of azuki beans, 2 cups of chick-peas, 1 cup chicory root. Roast ingredients until dark brown, then mix together and grind into a fine powder in a grain mill. This mixture is known as yannoh. For a coffeelike drink, use 1 tablespoon per cup of water. Bring to a boil, lower heat, and simmer for 5 to 10 minutes.

Note: There are also a variety of grain coffees available in natural foods stores. Avoid any that contain dates, figs, molasses, or honey. Others may be used occasionally as an alternative to bancha tea at the meal.

MU TEA

Mu tea is a medicinal tea made with a variety of herbs, including ginseng. Mu #9 is excellent for strengthening the female sex organs and for stomach troubles and may also be used therapeutically by men. Mu tea is sold prepackaged in most natural foods stores. Stir package in 1 quart of water and simmer for 10 minutes. Except for medicinal purposes, macrobiotic cooking does not recommend ginseng, which is extremely yang, and fragrant and aromatic herbs, which are too yin, for ordinary daily consumption.

UMEBOSHI TEA

Umeboshi tea has a nice sour taste. It helps cool the body in summer and prevent loss of minerals through perspiration. It can be made by boiling 2 to 3 pitted umeboshi plums in a quart of spring water, reducing the heat, and simmering for about 20 to 30 minutes. It may also be made by cooking 3 to 4 umeboshi pits leftover from other cooking. A few shiso leaves may be added to enhance flavor. Umeboshi tea is usually served cool in the summertime, though it also may be prepared hot. The taste should not be overly salty or will contribute to thirst rather than quench it.

AMASAKE (SWEET RICE BEVERAGE)

4 cups sweet brown rice   *½ cup koji*
8 cups spring water

Wash rice, drain, and soak in 8 cups of water overnight. Place rice in pressure-cooker and bring to pressure. Reduce heat and cook for 45 minutes. Turn off heat and allow to sit in pressure-cooker for 45 minutes. When cool enough, mix koji into rice by hand and allow to ferment 4 to 8 hours. During fermentation, place mixture in a glass bowl, cover with wet cloth or towel, and place near oven, radiator, or other warm place. During fermentation period, stir the mixture occasionally to melt the koji. After fermenting, place ingredients in a pot and bring to boil. When bubbles appear, turn off heat. Allow to cool. Refrigerate in a glass bowl or jar.

Note: Amasake may be served hot or cold as a nourishing beverage or used as a natural sweetener for making cookies, cakes, pies, or other desserts. As a beverage, first blend the amasake and place in a saucepan with a pinch of sea salt and spring water in volume to desired consistency. Bring to a boil and serve hot or allow to cool off.

Note: Heart patients may have amasake occasionally as a beverage, especially to satisfy craving for a sweet taste.

33

Cooking
Self-Reflection

When people first come to macrobiotics, a strong commitment to the new way of living is more important than anything else. Whether they are in good health or very sick, whether they are intelligent or not so smart, whether they are beautiful or not so beautiful, do not matter. Perseverance is the key to lasting happiness, and even a strong will can be blunted by occasionally taking sugar, too many sweets, or too much fish or other animal food. We must constantly evaluate our own condition and awareness. From time to time we can reflect on the ten factors below to help judge whether we are preparing balanced meals and strengthening our hearts.

1. Are we using the highest-quality ingredients available? Organic foods are not always affordable, but within our family's shopping budget, are we allocating enough funds for the best-quality brown rice, other whole grains, sea salt, unrefined vegetable oil, and spring water? Are we cutting corners on the basics by purchasing processed foods and convenience foods and by eating out too much? Are we using wood, gas, or other healthful source of energy to cook our food? Are our pots and pans of good quality or are they made of inferior materials? Have we weighed the social costs of lower-quality foods and materials on the soil, the air, and the water as well as the personal costs of increased medical and insurance payments for our family in the future?

2. Are we carefully cleaning and washing grains and vegetables before cooking? Do we take time to sift through dry ingredients for pebbles and other debris? Do we separate individual leaves of leafy green vegetables when washing? Do we budget enough time for proper soaking? Is our cutting technique careful and calm rather than hurried and sloppy? Are we envisioning how the dishes will look prior to cooking them? Often, cooking will turn out better if we let the foods cook themselves rather than following preconceived ideas and combinations. But an overall design for the meal and a sense of the mood we want to create can guide us as we cook, allowing us to complement our intuitive decisions.

3. Are we preparing whole foods? Foods cooked in whole form, such as brown rice and whole wheat berries, help center us and provide more complete energy than foods that are processed. Are we regularly consuming whole oats instead of rolled oats? Are we using too many flour or baked products and serving noodles too often? Are we always slicing vegetables or do we sometimes cook them whole?

4. Are we using a variety of foods in our daily cooking? Are we preparing just brown rice or also making other grains? Are we cooking just short-grain rice or also including other varieties from time to time? Are we serving root, round, and leafy green vegetables each day? Are we preparing some of our vegetables raw as well as cooked? Are we preparing sea vegetables in different ways? Are we changing our meals to reflect the passage of the seasons? Serving the same type of food day after day is one of the main causes of binging, sickness, failure to recover from sickness, or even going off the diet altogether.

5. Are we using a variety of cooking methods? Are we utilizing the different types of boiling, steaming, and sautéing in preparing vegetables? Do we occasionally cook grains and beans together? Do we combine sea vegetables with other foods from time to time? Are we making pickles in various styles and changing the ingredients? Are we making a variety of salads served fresh, marinated, pressed, and boiled? Do we make tempura or deep-fried foods, if our health permits, now and then? Changing our style of cooking will provide variety and satisfaction.

6. Do we frequently vary our cooking time? Do we make both short- and long-time pickles, quick and well-aged condiments, slow-cooked dishes and rapidly prepared ones?

7. Do we use a variety of seasonings such as sea salt, tamari soy sauce, and miso? Do we occasionally season dishes with umeboshi plums, rice vinegar, and grated ginger? Do we always use the same kind of miso or do we use different types? Do we occasionally use other good-quality unrefined oils as well as dark sesame oil? Do our meals offer a full range of tastes? Whole grains and vegetables constitute the principal part of the meal and pro vide a naturally sweet taste. Are other tastes—sour, bitter, pungent, and salty—available at every meal in side dishes, garnishes, or condiments? Are family members craving certain foods, binging, or eating out frequently? These desires can arise not only from improperly cooked food but also from an imbalance in tastes.

8. Is our food prepared fresh and are we using leftovers wisely? Are we making miso soup fresh each day or storing it for several days at a time so that it loses much of its energy? Some foods, such as leftover rice and noodles, make wonderful fried dishes and are even better the next day. Inedible ends, skins, and tips of vegetables may be saved and reused in soup stocks. Tempura oil may be recycled. By changing the style and appearance of leftovers, we can create food that is fresh and interesting. However, sometimes there is a tendency to cook too much at once to save time or stretch out cooking for the week. Preparing foods as freshly as possible for each meal retains their natural energy and provides optimal nourishment.

9. Are our meals served beautifully and do we vary the presentation of our foods? A variety of colors in the meal, different serving bowls and dishes, and changing garnishes will stimulate the appetite, add flavor, and enhance the enjoyment of the meal. Sometimes just the touch of color (whether green, yellow, orange, red, white, or black) will create a completely different mood.

10. Are our meals peaceful? It is important to be in a calm, peaceful frame of mind when preparing food, to concentrate on our cooking, and express our gratitude to all who have contributed to producing or helping with the meal. Cooking and meals should be a time of harmony and fellowship. Are we bringing our troubles

and anxieties to the kitchen, allowing this energy to affect our meals? Are we trying to cook and do something else at the same time? At the table, do we take a moment to express inwardly or outwardly our appreciation for the miracle of life and our daily bread or rice? Are we chewing our food well and dedicating our life to creating a more peaceful world?

34

Home Cares

The following home remedies arc based on traditional macrobiotic Oriental medicine and folk medicine, modified and adjusted for more practical use in modern society. Similar remedies have been used for thousands of years to help alleviate various imbalances caused by a faulty diet or unhealthy life-style. They should be followed only after complete understanding of their uses. If there is any doubt as to whether these remedies should be used, please seek out an experienced macrobiotic counselor or medical professional for proper guidance.

Bancha Stem Tea

Used for strengthening the metabolism in all sicknesses. Use 1 tablespoon tea to 1 quart water, bring to a boil, reduce heat, and simmer 4 to 5 minutes.

Brown Rice Cream

Used in cases when a person in a weakened condition needs to be nourished and energized or when the digestive system is impaired. Dry-roast brown rice evenly until all the grains turn yellow. To 1 part rice, add a tiny amount of sea salt and 3 to 6 parts water and pressure-cook for at least 2 hours. Squeeze out the creamy part of the cooked rice cereal through a cheesecloth sanitized in boiling water. Eat with a small volume of condiment, such as umeboshi plum, gomashio, tekka, kelp or other sea vegetable.

Brown Rice Plaster

Used to help reduce the fever around the infected area when the swelling of a boil or infection is not opened by the taro plaster. Hand grind 70 percent cooked brown rice, 30 percent raw leafy vegetables, and a few crushed sheets of raw nori in a suribachi—the more grinding the better. (If the mixture is very sticky, add water.) Apply the paste to the affected area. If the plaster begins to burn, remove it, since it is no longer effective. To remove, rinse with warm water.

Buckwheat Plaster

This plaster draws retained water and excess fluid from swollen areas of the body. Mix buckwheat flour with enough hot water to form a hard, stiff dough, and then combine thoroughly with 5 to 10 percent fresh grated ginger. Apply in a 1-half-inch layer to the affected area; tie in place with a bandage or piece of cotton linen. This plaster can be applied anywhere on the body. Replace about every 4 hours. After removing the plaster, you may notice that fluid is coming out through the skin or that the swelling is starting to go down. A buckwheat plaster will usually eliminate the swelling after only several applications or at most after 2 to 3 days.

Burdock Tea

Used for strengthening vitality. To 1 portion fresh burdock shavings, add 10 times the amount of water. Bring to a boil, reduce heat, and simmer for 10 minutes.

Carrot-Daikon Drink

To help eliminate excessive fats and dissolve hardening accumulations in the intestines. Grate 1 tablespoon each raw daikon and carrot. Cook in 2 cups spring water for 5 to 8 minutes with a pinch of sea salt or 7 to 10 drops tamari soy sauce.

Daikon Radish Drink

Drink No. 1: Serves to reduce a fever by inducing sweating. Mix a half cup grated, fresh daikon with 1 tablespoon tamari soy sauce and ¼ teaspoon grated ginger. Pour hot bancha tea or hot water over this mixture, stir, and drink while hot.

Drink No. 2: Induces urination. Use a piece of cheesecloth to squeeze the juice from the grated daikon. Mix 2 tablespoons of this juice with 6 tablespoons of hot water to which a pinch sea salt or 1 teaspoon tamari soy sauce has been added. Boil this mixture and drink only once a day. Do not use this preparation more than 3 consecutive days without proper supervision and never use it without first boiling.

Drink No. 3: Helps dissolve fat and mucus. In a teacup place 1 tablespoon fresh grated daikon and 1 teaspoon tamari soy sauce. Pour hot bancha tea over mixture and drink. It is most effective when taken just before sleeping. Do not use this drink longer than 5 days unless guided by an experienced macrobiotic counselor.

Dandelion Root Tea

Used to strengthen the heart and small intestine function and increase vitality. Use 1 teaspoon of root to 1 cup water. Bring to a boil, reduce heat, and simmer 10 minutes.

Dentie

Helps to prevent tooth problems, promotes a healthy condition in the mouth, and stops bleeding anywhere in the body by contracting expanded blood capillaries. Bake an eggplant, particularly the calix or cuplike top part, until black. Crush into a powder and mix with 30 to 50 percent roasted sea salt. Use daily as a tooth powder or apply to any bleeding area—can even be used inside the nostrils in case of nosebleed by inserting squeezed, wet tissue dipped in dentie into the nostril.

Dried Daikon Leaves

Used to warm the body and to treat various disorders of the skin and female sex organs. Also helpful in drawing odors and excessive oils from the body. Dry fresh daikon leaves in the shade, away from direct sunlight, until they turn brown and brittle. (If daikon leaves are unavailable, turnip greens may be substituted.) Boil 4 to 5 bunches of the leaves in 4 to 5 quarts water until the water turns brown. Stir in a handful of sea salt and use in one of the following ways: (1) Dip cotton linen into the hot liquid and wring lightly. Apply to the affected area repeatedly, until the skin becomes completely red. (2) Women experiencing problems in their sexual organs should sit in a hot bath to which the daikon-leaves liquid described above has been added along with a handful of sea salt. The water should come to waist level with the upper portion of the body covered with a towel. Remain in the water until the whole body becomes warm and sweating begins. This generally takes about 10 minutes. Repeat as needed, up to 10 days. Following this bath, douche with warm bancha tea, ½ teaspoon sea salt, and juice of half a lemon or similar volume of brown rice vinegar.

Ginger Compress

Stimulates blood and body fluid circulation; helps loosen and dissolve stagnated toxic matter, cysts, and tumors. Place a handful of grated ginger in a cheesecloth and squeeze out the ginger juice into a pot containing 1 gallon very hot water. Do not boil the water or you will lose the power of the ginger. Dip a cotton hand towel into the ginger water, wring it out tightly and apply to the area of the body to be treated. It should be very hot but not uncomfortably hot. A second, dry towel can be placed on top to reduce heat loss. Apply a fresh hot towel every several minutes until the skin becomes red. For more yin conditions, the ginger compress should be applied for only a short time (about 5 minutes maximum) to activate circulation in the affected area. For such a condition, repeated applications over an extended time may accelerate the expansive condition. Please seek more specific recommendations from a qualified macrobiotic adviser.

Ginger Sesame Oil

Activates the function of the blood capillaries, circulation, and nerve reactions. Also relieves aches and pains. Mix the juice of grated, fresh ginger with an equal amount of sesame oil. Dip cotton linen into this mixture and rub briskly into the skin of the affected area. This is also helpful for headache, dandruff, and hair growth.

Grated Daikon

A digestive aid, especially for fatty, oily, heavy foods and for animal food. Grate fresh daikon (red radish or turnip may be used if daikon is not available). Sprinkle with tamari soy sauce and eat about 1 tablespoon. You may also add a pinch of grated ginger.

Green Magma Tea

Good for reducing and melting fats, cysts, and tumors arising from animal foods. Young barley grass powder is available in many natural foods stores. Pour hot water over 1 to 2 teaspoons and drink. Consult an experienced macrobiotic counselor for length of time to use.

Kombu Tea

Good for strengthening the blood. Use 1 3-inch strip of kombu to 1 quart of water. Bring to a boil, reduce heat, and simmer for 10 minutes. Another method is to dry kombu in a 350° oven for 10 to 15 minutes, or until crisp. Grate ½ to 1 teaspoon of kombu into a cup and add hot water.

Kuzu Drink

Strengthens digestion, increases vitality, and relieves general fatigue. Dissolve a heaping teaspoon kuzu powder in 2 teaspoons of water, then add to 1 cup cold water. Bring the mixture to a boil, reduce the heat to the simmering point, and stir constantly until the liquid becomes a transparent gelatin. Stir in 1 teaspoon tamari soy sauce and drink while hot. Kuzu is also known as kudzu.

Lotus Root Plaster

Draws stagnated mucus from the sinuses, nose, throat, and bronchi. Mix grated, fresh lotus root with 10 to 15 percent pastry flour and 5 to 10 percent grated, fresh ginger. Spread a ½-inch layer onto cotton linen and apply the lotus root directly to the skin. Keep on for several hours or overnight and repeat daily for several days. A ginger compress can be applied before this application to stimulate circulation and to loosen mucus in the area being treated.

Lotus Root Tea

Helps relieve coughing and dissolves excess mucus in the body. Grate ½ cup fresh lotus root, squeeze the juice into a pot, and add a small amount of water. Cook for 5 to 8 minutes, add a pinch of sea salt or tamari soy sauce, and drink hot.

Mustard Plaster

Stimulates blood and body fluid circulation and loosens stagnation. Add hot water to dry mustard powder and stir well. Spread this mixture onto a paper towel and sandwich it between two thick cotton towels. Apply this "sandwich" to the skin area and leave on until the skin becomes red and hot, and then remove. After removing, wipe off remaining mustard plaster from the skin with towels.

Nachi Green Tea

Helps dissolve and discharge animal fats and reduce high cholesterol levels. Place ½ teaspoon tea into the serving kettle. Pour 1 cup hot water over the tea and steep for 3 to 5 minutes. Strain and drink 1 cup per day.

Ranshio

Used to strengthen the heart and to stimulate heartbeat and blood circulation. Crush a raw egg and mix with 1 tablespoon tamari soy sauce. Drink slowly. Use only once a day and for no more than 3 days. Do not use for easing overly yang conditions.

Salt Bancha Tea

Used to loosen stagnation in the nasal cavity or to cleanse the vaginal region. Add enough salt to warm bancha tea (about body temperature) to make it just a little less salty than sea water. Use the liquid to wash deep inside the nasal cavity through the nostrils or as a douche. Salt bancha tea can also be used as a wash for problems with the eyes, sore throat, and fatigue.

Salt Pack

Used to warm any part of the body. For the relief of diarrhea, for example, apply the pack to the abdominal region. Roast salt in a dry pan until hot and then wrap in thick cotton linen pillowcase or towel and tie with string or cord like a package to prevent spilling. Apply to the troubled area and change when the pack begins to cool.

Salt Water

Cold salt water will contract the skin in the case of burns while warm salt water can be used to clean the rectum, colon, and vagina. When the skin is damaged by fire, immediately soak the burned area in cold salt water until irritation disappears. Then apply vegetable oil to seal the wound from the air. For constipation or mucus or fat accumulation in the rectum, colon, and vaginal regions, use warm water (body temperature) as an enema or douche.

Sesame Oil

Used to relieve stagnated bowels or to eliminate retained water. Take 1 to 2 tablespoons of raw sesame oil with ¼ teaspoon each ginger and tamari soy sauce on an empty stomach to induce the discharge of stagnated bowels. To eliminate water retention in the eyes, put a drop or two of pure sesame oil (preferably dark sesame oil) in the eyes with an eyedropper, ideally before sleeping. Continue up to a week, until the eyes improve. Before using the sesame oil for this purpose, boil and then strain it through a sanitized cheesecloth to remove impurities, and let cool before use.

Shiitake Mushroom Tea

Used to relax an overly tense, stressful condition and to help dissolve excess animal fats. Soak a dried black shiitake mushroom cut in quarters. Cook in 2 cups of water for 20 minutes with a pinch of sea salt or 1 teaspoon of tamari soy sauce. Drink only ½ cup at a time.

Tamari Bancha Tea

Neutralizes an acidic blood condition, promotes blood circulation, and relieves fatigue. Pour 1 cup of hot bancha twig tea over 1 to 2 teaspoons tamari soy sauce. Stir and drink hot.

Taro Potato (Albi) Plaster

Often used after a ginger compress to collect stagnated toxic matter and draw it out of the body. Taro potato can usually be obtained in most major cities from Chinese, Puerto Rican, or Armenian grocery shops or natural foods stores. The skin of this vegetable is brown and covered with "hair." Smaller potatoes are the most effective for use in this plaster. Peel off taro potato skin and grate the white interior. Mix with 5 to 10 percent grated fresh ginger. Spread this mixture in a ⅔- to 1-inch-thick layer onto a fresh cotton linen and apply the taro side directly to the skin. Change every 4 hours. If taro is not available, a preparation using regular white potato can be substituted. While not as effective as taro, it will still produce a beneficial result. Mix in a suribachi 50 to 60 percent grated white potato with 40 to 50 percent grated or mashed green leafy vegetables. Add enough wheat flour to make a paste and add 5 to 10 percent grated ginger. Apply as before. If, when the plaster is removed, the light-colored mixture has become dark or brown, or if the skin where the plaster was applied also takes on a dark color, this indicates that excessive carbon and other elements are being discharged through the skin. Repeat once or twice daily. If the person feels chilly from the coolness of the plaster, a hot ginger compress applied for 5 minutes while changing plasters will help relieve this. If chill persists, roast sea salt in a skillet, wrap it in a towel, and place it on top of the plaster. Be careful not to let the patient become too hot from this salt application.

Tofu Plaster

This method draws out a fever more effectively than an ice pack. Squeeze the water from the tofu, mash it, and then add 10 to 20 percent pastry flour and 5 percent grated ginger. Mix the ingredients together and apply directly to the skin and fasten with a light cloth or towel. Change every 2 or 3 hours or sooner if plaster becomes very hot.

Ume Extract

A concentrated form of umeboshi plums, available in some natural foods stores. Good for neutralizing an acid or nauseous condition and diarrhea. Pour hot water or bancha tea over ¼ to ⅓ teaspoon of ume extract.

Umeboshi Plum

Baked umeboshi plum or powdered baked whole umeboshi plum neutralizes an acidic condition and relieves intestinal problems, including those caused by microorganisms. Take ½ to 1 umeboshi plum (baked is stronger than unbaked) with 1 cup bancha tea. If you bake and crush into a powder, add a teaspoon to 1 cup of hot water.

Ume-Sho-Bancha

Strengthens the blood and the circulation through the regulation of digestion. Pour 1 cup of bancha tea over the meat of ½ to 1 umeboshi plum and 1 teaspoon of tamari soy sauce. Stir and drink hot. Also helps relieve headaches in the front part of the head.

Ume-Sho-Bancha with Ginger

Helps to increase blood circulation. Prepare as above, but add ¼ teaspoon ginger juice squeezed from fresh grated gingerroot and pour 1 cup of hot bancha tea over. Stir and drink.

Ume-Sho-Kuzu Drink

Strengthens digestion, revitalizes energy, and regulates the intestinal condition. Prepare the kuzu drink according to the instructions for Kuzu Drink and add the meat of ½ to 1 umeboshi plum. One-eighth teaspoon of fresh grated ginger may also be added.

35

Breathing and
Chanting Exercises

The exercises in the next four chapters will help to stabilize the physical, mental, and spiritual condition. They may be performed individually or together as a sequence. Wherever applicable, they have been directed to strengthening the heart and other circulatory organs and vessels. For further information on physical and spiritual exercises, please see my book, *The Book of Dō-In* (Tokyo: Japan Publications, 1979).

RIGHT SITTING POSTURE

Select any of the following sitting postures, allowing the force of Heaven to pass straight through the body vertically so that you can align yourself with the center of the Earth. These sitting postures are basic to most of the exercises that follow.

Seiza Posture: Sit on either the ground or the floor with natural straight posture, the muscles relaxed, the shoulders and elbows also relaxed, and the legs bent and the feet tucked up under the buttocks (see Figure 32). Leave a distance the size of one fist between the knees and the hands, which are at the sides resting lightly on the thighs, palms down.

Right Sitting on a Chair: Sit deeply in the chair with natural straight posture, the knees bent at a 90-degree angle (see Figure 33). There should be a distance the size of one fist between the knees, as in the Seiza posture.

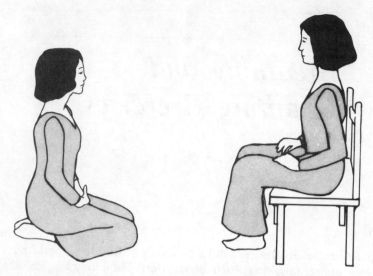

Figure 32.   Figure 33.

Right Sitting Postures

Lotus Flower Posture: Sit on either the ground or the floor, the legs crossed with each foot on the opposite thigh. Hold the spine naturally straight by putting a cushion about 4 inches in height under the buttocks.

Half-Lotus Flower Posture: Sit on the ground or floor, the legs crossed, with one foot resting on the opposite thigh and the other on the floor. To keep naturally straight posture, a cushion approximately 4 inches in height may be placed under the buttocks.

Rounded Sitting: Sit with normally straight posture, the legs open more than 90 degrees, the soles of the feet flat against each other. To keep the spine naturally straight, a cushion may be placed under the buttocks.

After selecting one of the above postures, rest the left hand on the right, palms up, thumbs touching each other so that the spirals at the tips of the thumbs meet. Keep the eyes either half-open or lightly closed. Relax the eyes, looking forward to the ground approximately 10 to 15 feet away, without focusing upon any particular object.

Begin low, deep breathing through the nose. Breathe in deeply, breathing downward toward the lower abdomen, the region of the *hara*. Hold the breath for several seconds, allowing the abdomen to remain expanded toward the front. Then exhale with a slow, long breath. Repeat this breathing for about three to five minutes. During this period, visualize that you are stabilizing yourself firmly upon the Earth, as if you were immovable under all circumstances.

The purpose of this exercise, traditionally called *Heavenly Foundation*, is to unify the physical, mental, and spiritual constitution as a part of the natural environment and to establish an unshakable inner confidence in the order of the universe. It also actively harmonizes the entire metabolism of the body, including the heart and circulatory system.

PRINCIPLES OF BREATHING

In addition to the breathing exercise above, further breathing exercises may be performed to stabilize the cardiovascular condition and one's health in general. Basically, breathing is the interchange of energy between ourselves and the atmospheric environment—the air. Just as the proper way of eating and drinking is essential to our physical, mental, and spiritual development, the proper way of breathing is essential for us to adapt, with the utmost effectiveness, to the atmospheric environment. Proper breathing is essential for the development of universal understanding and consciousness as well as for personal health and happiness.

Breathing is the manifestation of the yin centrifugal expanding function and the yang centripetal contracting function, alternately exercised in harmonious movement, mainly through our respiratory organs. However, not only the respiratory organs such as the nasal and bronchial cavities and the lungs but also the heart and blood vessels and their functions are closely coordinated with breathing. The nervous system, including autonomic nervous reactions and brain functions, is also closely related to the function of breathing.

Generally, the active functioning of these systems and organs accelerates active breathing, and active breathing in turn accelerates the active functioning of these systems and organs. On the other hand, their slow and inactive functions bring forth slow and inactive breathing; and slow and inactive breathing results, in time, in their slow and inactive functions. Accordingly, the volume of air during inhalation and exhalation, the duration of the inhalation and exhalation relative to each other, and the speed of breathing all have different effects upon all the body's systems and functions. They also directly and indirectly influence our psychological and spiritual conditions, changing the kinds, volume, direction, and dimensions of image and thought.

Slower breathing slows down the heartbeat, blood circulation, and other body fluid circulation. Body temperature tends to become slightly lower. Mentally, slower breathing produces a more tranquil and peaceful state, clearer thinking, and more objective understanding, as well as a more sensitive response to the environment. Spiritually, it contributes to greater perception and deeper insight, and leads toward more universal consciousness. In contrast, faster breathing results in increased metabolism of various body functions. The heartbeat, as well as the circulation of blood and other body fluids, is accelerated. Body temperature tends to rise. Mentally, faster breathing produces a more unstable and excitable condition, paralleling emotional changes. Spiritually, it contributes to a more subjective and egocentric observation and evaluation of surrounding conditions, with greater attachment to fragmented and partial affairs, rather than broad and universal awareness.

Deeper breathing results in more profound and active metabolism and harmony among the systems and organs of the body. Body temperature tends to be stable. Mentally, deeper breathing produces deeper satisfaction, emotional stability, and stronger confidence, and helps maintain a steady and even expression. Spiritually, it makes one more thoughtful and steadfast and reinforces the tendency to become all-embracing, ultimately producing a more loving personality. In contrast, shallow breathing results in a more inactive metabolism as well as a lack of coordination and disharmony among various physical functions. Body temperature tends to change irregularly. Mentally, shallow breathing produces a tendency to be more anxious, unstable, frustrated, and discontented, often leading to fear. Spiritually, it can lead to shallow perception, frequent changes in evaluation, loss of confidence, lack of courage, and loss of memory and vision of the future.

Longer breathing results in better coordination among the metabolism of various functions. Body temperature tends to be stable and, in general, the activities of all organs and glands tend to slow down. Mentally, it produces a more peaceful and satisfied feeling. Greater endurance, patience, and quietness also result, along with reduced emotional excitement and irritability. Spiritually, longer breathing contributes to more objective and wider perception, as well as deeper understanding. Past memories and visions of the future tend to become more extended. In contrast, shorter breathing creates a tendency toward faster and more irregular metabolism. Body temperature tends to increase slightly. Mentally, there are more frequent changes of image and thought, as well as more frequent changes of mind. Impatience, lack of endurance, and shortness of temper are evident. Spiritually, shorter breathing creates disharmony with the environment. Conflicting and antagonistic feelings are enhanced, together with an increase in shortsightedness and a more subjective viewpoint.

It is advisable to maintain a breathing pattern that is slower, deeper, and longer, rather than faster, shallower, and shorter. One's physical, mental, and spiritual development reflects the nature of one's breathing and the adjustment of these variables. However, any conscious adjustment of the speed, depth, and length of breathing should be aimed at developing more natural breathing, which works without any artificial intention or special effort. Slow, deep, and long breathing can, in fact, be developed automatically by practicing the macrobiotic way of eating—a diet that is centered around whole cereal grains and supplemented by vegetables grown on the land and in the sea, locally and seasonally, with a minimum consumption of animal food. Drinking a larger volume of liquid as well as eating sugar, sweets, fruit, raw food, and too much oil also tends to make breathing faster, shallower, and shorter. Eating and drinking a larger volume of food in general also tends to increase the speed of breathing, making it shallower and shorter. Proper chewing, as well as a more moderate intake, contributes to more steady, even breathing and stabilizing of the overall condition.

There are many traditional exercises to develop the breath. Three of the most basic, which are good for the heart and circulation in general, are as follows:

Breathing with the Center of the Abdomen

This breathing exercise is done deeply and slowly with the natural movement of the *hara* region, the central region of the abdomen and vital electromagnetic energy center of the body. At the time of slow but deep inhalation, the hara is filled with energy and the lower abdomen naturally expands toward the front. At the time of slower, longer exhalation, the same region naturally contracts.

Between inhaling and exhaling, the breath should be held for several seconds. The exhalation should be generally two or more times longer than the inhalation. The effectiveness of this breathing is to generate physical energy, mental stability, and spiritual confidence. It results in the firm establishment of the self upon this Earth, and the ability to avoid being influenced by changing surroundings. It produces an increase in body temperature. This breathing also accelerates active digestive and circulatory functions throughout the body, which results in total health and longevity.

With practice, the duration of exhalation can be extended, from two to three times the length of the inhalation to five to seven times the length. This increases the effects of the exercise.

Breathing with the Heart Region

In this breathing exercise, both the inhalation and the exhalation are slow and long, concentrating in the heart region or the central region of the chest. The duration of inhaling is almost equal to the duration of exhaling, and the breath is not held between inhaling and exhaling—both naturally and smoothly continue in slow, long movements.

The effect of this breathing is to harmonize the beating of the heart and to generate smooth circulation of the blood and other body fluids. Mentally, it generates a feeling of harmony and love with all aspects of the environment as well as with the surrounding people. It also develops sensitivity, sympathy, understanding, and compassion.

Breathing with the Region of the Midbrain

This breathing exercise is done at the region of the midbrain, the inner center of the head. The inhalation is made slowly but sharply, as if breathing up toward the zenith of the head, giving the feeling of lifting the body upward. This inhalation should be made smoothly and continuously, as long as possible, and at its extreme point, the breath is suddenly but gently released. The exhalation should be made downward toward the mouth. This exercise may be beneficial to circulatory disorders in the head, including stroke.

CHANTING AND SOUND

In our daily conversation, we use various words and pronunciations to express ourselves. The sounds of these words are vibrations that are formed in the mouth, nasal, and throat cavities in coordination with the vibrating uvula, the walls of the cavities, the teeth, the motions of the throat muscles, and the vocal cords, as well as with respiratory movement. The forces that create these vibrations, however, descend originally from Heaven through the hair spiral in the center of the head and ascend from the Earth through the lower region of the body. Accordingly, when our physical and mental conditions are in harmony with the environment through the daily practice of proper diet, thought, activity, and breathing, the sound of our words is able to represent the powerful forces of Heaven and Earth, and our verbal expressions are able to carry the true vision of nature and the universe. Words or verbal sounds pronounced in such a healthy state, in harmony with the environment, represent the universal spirit and give a powerful influence both to ourselves and to all beings surrounding us.

Each sound that is pronounced when we are in a healthy condition carries its own meaning and power, and also has a special effect on our physical, mental, and spiritual condition. Among these sounds, some are pronounced with the mouth open—yin sounds—and others are pronounced with the mouth closed—yang sounds. There are many varieties in between. When our physical and mental conditions are more peacefully adapted to nature through a dietary practice of eating grains and vegetables, these sounds become clearer in pronunciation. If our conditions become disharmonious with the environment through eating other varieties of food, including heavy animal food, our sounds become more rough.

In India and in the Far East generally, traditional peoples classified sounds by their vibratory effects on certain parts of the body —for example, "I" for the stomach and middle region of the body, "O" for the kidneys and back side of the middle region, "Ha" for the lungs and respiratory function. Properly used, selected sounds can physicalize and spiritualize our daily activity. Historically, these sounds have often been sung or chanted to produce various effects.

The following two common sounds may be sung or chanted to strengthen the entire physical, mental, and spiritual constitution, including the heart and circulatory system. This may be done individually or together with other people, which increases their effects.

The Prolonged Sound of SU: This sound brings us in harmony with all surrounding people and all forms of life in the world. In breathing out, sound *SU* as long as comfortably possible. Vocalization may be deep and strong at first and diminish naturally toward the end as the breath is released. Then breathe in and chant *SU* again during the next exhalation. Repeat several times. Note: Chanting may also be performed silently if desired and will still have a beneficial effect.

The Prolonged Sound AUM: The sound *A*, which is pronounced with the mouth open, represents the infinite universe, and physically it vibrates the lower part of our body. The sound *U* represents harmony and physically vibrates the upper region of the body, including the heart, and the lower region of the head. The sound *M*, which is pronounced with the mouth closed, represents the infinitesimal world and physically vibrates the most compacted area, the brain.

Thus *AUM* is an expression of the whole universe and vibrates our body and spiritual channel from the lowest part to the highest part, resulting in the active charge of vibrations and electromagnetic currents in our physical, mental, and spiritual functions. This sound, the Sanskrit *OM,* has been used in Asia for centuries to generate life activity as well as to establish human existence as a part of the universe. In the West, *AMEN* and *SHALOM* traditionally served similar functions and may also be sung or chanted for health and harmony at all levels.

36

Meditation Exercises

MEDITATION TO OPEN THE HEART

The purpose of this exercise is to develop love and feelings of harmony toward a certain person, toward many people, or toward a certain idea or thought. It also helps to dissolve emotional conflicts and obstacles that may exist in our relation with some other person or unfamiliar thought.

Although there may be no particular person to whom we wish to dedicate our love and no particular thought with which we wish to realize our harmony, if we practice this exercise every so often, dedicated to all people and beings, we will be able to achieve a spirit of universal love and harmony.

This exercise can be practiced alone or with another person. Especially for two persons between whom mutual love and harmony are to be achieved, the practice of this exercise, performed by looking gently into each other's eyes, can heighten the inspiration of love and harmony and contribute to realization of oneness (see Figure 34).

This exercise generates the active flow of the electromagnetic force running through our spiritual channel and especially illuminates the region of the heart, accelerating the circulation of the blood. It produces active vibrations that are spirally radiated from the center of the chest area, resulting in the rapid elevation of loving and harmonious feelings.

To begin, make the back naturally straight in the Right Sitting

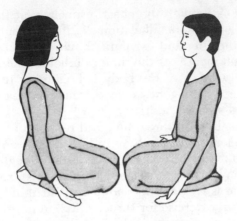

Figure 34. Heart Meditation

Posture described in Chapter 35 while sitting on a chair, the ground, or the floor so that the spiritual channel may smoothly carry the forces of Heaven and Earth. Keeping the eyes half-open, look toward the infinite distance without focusing on any particular point. Opening both arms wide, as if ready to accept and embrace all things, let the hands naturally open toward the front (see Figure 35). The outstretched palms should be a few inches from the ground, and there should be no tension.

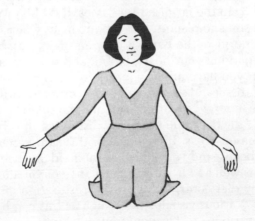

Figure 35. Heart Meditation

Start to breathe with the chest, especially at the area of the heart, with a long, gentle inhalation slightly longer than the exhalation. Both inhaling and exhaling should be done through the slightly opened mouth. At the time of inhaling, slightly move the chest area forward, as if the body is beginning to glide toward flying in space. As you gently exhale, your body naturally returns to the original straight position.

While repeating this breathing and motion of the body, keep an intensive clear image in the mind of the person or persons to whom your love is to be dedicated, or of the thought or idea with which harmony is to be realized. During this exercise, silently repeat the words *love* and *harmony* in your mind.

Continue this exercise for three to five minutes. Then return to the normal meditating posture and gradually diminish the image and words.

HEART VISUALIZATION

Persons with heart or circulatory disease may wish to use this exercise to visualize the strengthening of their cardiovascular system. To do this, they may concentrate on a mental image of their heart, arteries, or other organs or systems, or they may use some of the drawings and illustrations in this book to form a picture in their minds. Imagine the universal flow of electromagnetic energy spiraling in from the far-distant galaxies, the Milky Way, the solar system, the sun and planets, and the moon, as well as the upward-ascending energy of the Earth as it spins on its axis, entering your body and charging your heart, blood, and other vital organs and functions. If you have atherosclerotic blockages, hardened arteries, swollen tissues, diseased valves, or other disorders, imagine this infinite energy streaming in and circulating through the meridians of the body and gradually dissolving the obstructions or healing diseased areas. Imagine, too, this same energy ripening the grains, beans, and vegetables in the field and the seaweeds in the ocean, as well as a harmonious balance of yin and yang forces in your daily diet contributing to the restoration of your energy and vitality. Various visualizations such as this can be performed and will contribute to harmonizing one's physical, mental, and spiritual conditions.

LITERARY EXERCISE

In his plays and sonnets, William Shakespeare portrays the human heart as the measure of all things. Below is a list of some of the qualities he uses to describe the heart:

Afflicted	Laboring
Angry	Light
Big-swollen	Loyal
Bleeding	Malicious
Broken	Marble
Bruised	Melting
Cleft	Merry
Cold	Mighty
Compassionate	Musing
Constant	Noble
Corrupted	Obdurate
Dear-doting	O'er-fraught
Drumming	Pale
Empty	Penitent
Envious	Pitious
Faint and milky	Poor
Faithful	Rancorous
False	Rapt
Fearful	Sad
Firm	Savage
Flawed	Serpent
Flinty	Sickly
Foul adulterous	Sound
Furnace-burning	Stony
Gentle	Stubborn
Good	Sweet
Great	Tender
Hardened	Throbbing
Heavy	True-divining
Hollow	Tyrannous
Humble	Unrelenting
Icy	Unspotted
Innocent	Valiant
Kind	Warm

Waxen   Worthy
Well-disposed   Wounded
Wild   Wrathful

From what you've learned in this book, see if you can arrange these qualities according to yin and yang tendencies. Of course, all thoughts, emotions, and activities are a combination of yin and yang, but usually one quality predominates.

One way to proceed is to divide these qualities into two categories: (1) more balanced or centered qualities; and (2) more excessive or extreme qualities. Then divide each column into yin (more expansive) and yang (more contractive), according to which tendency predominates. A centrally balanced yang quality may be indicated with an upraised triangle and a centrally balanced yin quality with a downward triangle. Excessive qualities may be indicated with two or three triangles placed next to each other. For example:

$$\triangle \quad \text{firm}$$
$$\triangledown \quad \text{gentle}$$
$$\triangle\triangle \quad \text{angry}$$
$$\triangledown\triangledown\triangledown \quad \text{sad}$$

As a further exercise, try to figure out which daily foods or combinations of foods give rise to each quality and which organ or organs are primarily affected. This is a good exercise to develop your understanding. Of course, there are no absolute right or wrong responses; much depends on context, and our interpretations may differ widely. If you have difficulty at first, you are not alone. This is the type of literary and philosophical material we study together at the Kushi Institute.

Finally, if you have time, consult a concordance to Shakespeare's works in a library and go back to the original plays and verse to see whether the speech, actions, and motives of the different characters are in accord with the dietary and medical information presented. Great poets and writers intuitively understand and express this connection, and that is one of the reasons their work remains timeless.

In addition to Shakespeare, other authors who express a deep understanding of the order of the universe include Homer, Dante,

Lady Murasaki *(The Tale of Genji)*, Wu Chen-en *(Monkey*, or *The Journey to the West)*, Kabir, Basho, Walter Scott, Tolstoy, George Eliot, Lewis Carroll, and Samuel Butler. Reciting from their poetry or novels out loud a few minutes each day is very beneficial for both the mind and heart.

37

Dō-In Exercises

Dō-in is a very simple set of exercises that can be practiced every day for a few minutes to stimulate the electromagnetic activity of the body and contribute to the smooth functioning of the various organs and systems.

A complete introduction to Dō-in including photographs and a discussion of the meridian systems, is provided in my book on the subject. Dō-in is extremely flexible and may be adjusted to meet personal needs and the amount of time available. Usually, it begins with self-massage of the head, face, neck, and shoulders, followed by massage of the arms and hands; the front, back, and sides of the torso; and finally the waist, legs, feet, and toes. For overall health, all these regions should be massaged. However, here we have room to describe only a few techniques that are especially beneficial to the heart and circulation. To begin Dō-in, assume the Seiza posture, sitting on the ground or floor with legs drawn up under the buttocks and hands resting gently on the thighs, as described in Chapter 35.

THE EARS

This exercise will harmonize all circulatory functions and the coordination among the various systems of the entire body. It is also good for kidney and excretory functions and to improve hearing.

Step 1: With the index, middle, and ring fingers, press around the ear several times to release any stagnation in the circulation around the ear. This also helps to give clearer thinking, especially improving the sense of balance.

Step 2: Massage the ears, using the thumb and index finger (and the middle finger, if desired). First, rub the peripheral ridge of the ear to activate the circulation of blood and lymph throughout the body. Second, rub the middle ridge, with the thumb behind the ear and the other finger(s) in front, stimulating the nervous system. Then rub the inner ridges and indentations, helping to activate the digestive functions. During all these processes, the earlobe may be squeezed hard, as may all other areas along the ridges, to release stagnation in this area as well as indirectly throughout the body.

THE CHEEKS

This exercise generates active blood circulation throughout the body, strengthens the respiratory and breathing functions, and regulates active heart beating. It also serves to raise the body temperature.

Step 1: Apply both palms to the cheeks—the right palm to the right cheek, the left palm to the left cheek—and breathe deeply at least three times.

Step 2: Rub the cheeks in an up-and-down motion with the palms until the skin becomes warm (see Figure 36).

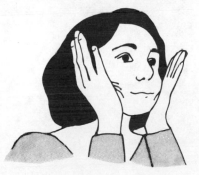

Figure 36. Cheek Massage

THE SHOULDERS

This set of exercises will improve the circulatory and digestive functions by releasing physical and mental stagnation, and will stimulate respiratory activity. It will also help to release fatigue by dissolving general tension in the shoulder region.

Step 1: Raise the shoulders, contracting the shoulder muscles as much as possible. Then, quickly release the contraction, completely relaxing these muscles as much as possible. Repeat five times. Then, tilting the shoulders, contract the upper shoulder and relax the lower shoulder. Repeat three to five times, alternating shoulders.

Step 2: Using the four fingers of one hand, press down upon and massage the opposite shoulder, tilting the head to the other side. Repeat upon the other shoulder. Wherever hardness or stiffness is felt, massage with a circular motion (see Figure 37).

Step 3: Making a fist with one hand, pound the opposite shoulder about ten to twenty times. Repeat on the other shoulder. Wherever pain is felt, pound a little longer and harder. Also pound the top of the spine as well as the back of the neck about ten to twenty times, using the stronger fist.

Step 4: Apply the palms upon the opposite shoulders and breathe in and out three times, slowly but deeply. If desired, the palms may be applied to the shoulders on the same side instead.

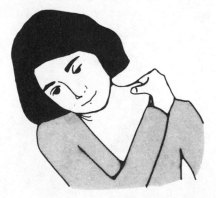

Figure 37. Shoulder Massage

FRONT CHEST AND ABDOMEN

This set of exercises will activate the functioning of all major organs and glands in the torso region, including blood circulation, and generate energy flow through all the meridians related to these organs and systems.

Step 1: Apply both palms to the upper chest and breathe deeply two to three times. Then, apply the palms to the lower chest, and breathe deeply two to three times. Next, apply the palms to the middle or stomach region, and then to the abdominal region, in each case breathing two to three times. On the sides of the torso, apply the same technique to the upper chest, then the stomach, and then to the waist. On the back, apply the palms on the middle region over the kidneys and again breathe deeply two to three times.

Step 2: Begin a light banging or bouncing motion on the entire chest region with the fist, including the sides of the rib cage (see Figure 38). Using the same gentle pounding motion, proceed farther down toward the stomach and continue down to the region of the large and small intestines and the bladder. Also pound the sides of the waist and pelvic region. On the back, bang as high up as possible. You may sit up on your knees and bend your body forward at this time. Then, bang down the back to the hips, including the middle and lower vertebral areas, the back muscles along

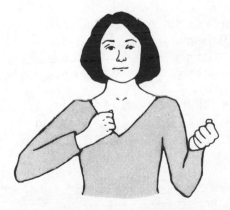

Figure 38. Chest Massage

the vertebrae, the bladder meridians running vertically on the back, and the muscles of the buttocks.

Step 3: Using the four fingers of both hands, press certain points and meridians on the front of the body including (1) underneath the collarbones on both sides, two to three times; (2) along the breastbone, pressing in a vertical line two to three times; (3) from the top of the collarbone vertically down to the pelvic region along the kidney meridian; (4) from the collarbone downward along the stomach meridian to the pelvic region; (5) using either four fingers or the thumb, press down from the indented place near the inside of the shoulder joint, along the spleen meridian, to the pelvic region; (6) on the sides of the body, press from the front of the armpit down along the gallbladder meridian to the sides of the lower hips (to do this, it would be more practical to use the thumb rather than the fingers); (7) using the four fingers of both hands, press in and up under the edge of the rib cage, as if pushing the rib cage up. Press all along the length of the rib cage slowly and deeply. Two points should be pressed especially hard: Ki-Mon (liver meridian no. 14 on the front of the rib cage) and Shō-Mon (liver meridian no. 13 at the bottom edges of the rib cage). See Figures 39 and 40 for the location of these meridians and points.

Step 4: With the palms, press and rub down the whole front of the body, covering the meridians from the top of the collarbone to the bottom of the pelvis.

Step 5: On the back, press the indented area under the rib cage, slightly arching the back to allow an easier grip. Then, suddenly release. Repeat at least five times. Then apply the hands on the region of the kidneys and adrenal glands, stretching backward to make the area softer and relaxed, and breathe deeply three times.

Step 6: Using all four fingers of both hands, press deeply into the abdominal region, bending forward, and then suddenly release and straighten up. While pressing breathe out, and when releasing breathe in. Then massage the abdominal area, first the center, then each side. Then holding the left hand over the right hand, massage the entire abdominal region in a circular motion at least five times, in a clockwise direction. Finally, apply both hands on the abdominal region and breathe deeply in the lower abdomen. During inhalation the abdomen should expand, and during exhalation it should contract. Repeat at least five times.

Figure 39. Front Chest Region

Lines for massaging and pressing in Dō-In exercises. The two liver points, LV 14 and LV 13, should be especially pressed.

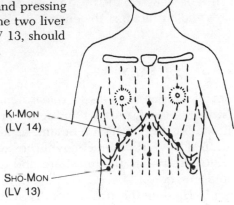

KI-MON
(LV 14)

SHO-MON
(LV 13)

Figure 40. Meridians on the Front of the Torso

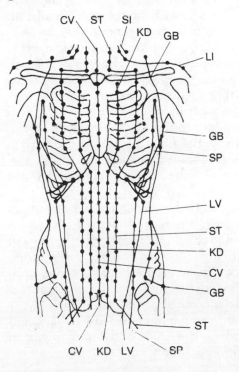

CV ST SI
KD GB
LI
GB
SP
LV
ST
KD
CV
GB
ST
CV KD LV SP

CV = Conception vessel
ST = Stomach
SI = Small intestine
KD = Kidney
GB = Gallbladder
LI = Large intestine
SP = Spleen
LV = Liver

Step 7: Twist the body left and right as far as possible, swinging the arms and keeping the head facing to the front. This exercise activates and harmonizes the energy flow along all the meridians.

ARMS AND HANDS

This set of exercises serves to release stagnation arising in the bloodstream, tissues, muscles and joints and to stimulate the energy flow along the related meridians, resulting in the harmonious activation of the various functions of the heart and circulation, the lungs and respiration, the intestines and digestion, and other organs and functions.

Step 1: Holding the arms naturally at the sides, turn and twist them, stretching them as far as you can, with the fingers spread open. Repeat several times, twisting to the back and to the front. Then lift up the arms to shoulder level and repeat the twisting motion, again as far as possible, several times. Lifting the arms further at about a 45-degree angle, twist them again. Finally, lift the arms far over the head and twist them several times.

Step 2: Gripping the shoulder joint, thoroughly massage that area to release any muscular tension. Then massage down the arm toward the elbow, pressing all indented places around the elbow to release tension there. Further proceed down to the wrist, moving gradually and releasing tension in all areas.

Step 3: Press from the shoulder to the wrist along each meridian running on the arm, namely, the lung, heart governor, triple heater, heart, and small intestine meridians (see Figure 41). You may use four fingers to press these meridians or the thumb if it is more convenient.

Step 4: When the wrist is reached, thoroughly massage all indentations in the area of the wrist. Then press along the bones on the back of the hand. Proceed to the fingers, using the thumb and index finger to massage each finger toward the tip, on the sides, and then on the top and back. This massage should proceed from one finger to another, slowly and carefully (see Figure 42). It is especially important to press and massage the tip of each finger strongly, using the thumb and index finger to twist it back and forth. The heart meridian ends on the inside of the little finger, so concentrating here stimulates circulation.

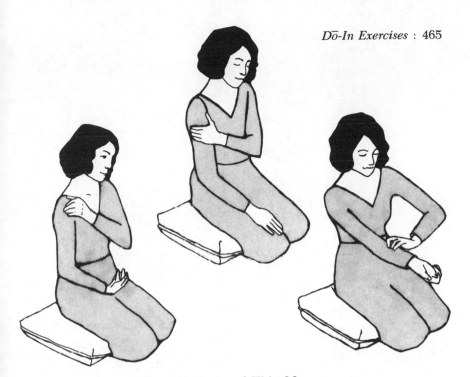

Figure 41. Arm and Wrist Massage

Step 5: Pull and snap each finger to discharge stagnant energy. Then, using the thumb, push down between the fingers. Or press between the fingers by interlacing them and pushing down. Holding the palms together, bend the fingers and try to rest the palms on the ground or floor. This is good for testing the flexibility of the arteries. Ideally, fingers can be bent almost 90 degrees, indicating completely flexible arteries.

Step 6: Press the palms very thoroughly, first along the three major lines on the palm. Then, thoroughly press all areas of the palm in a vertical direction. During this process, press deeply with a circular motion. Two points especially should be strongly pressed: the center of the palm and the point at the junction between the thumb and index finger. After completing the steps 1 through 6, repeat the same exercises on the other arm.

Step 7: Shake the hands loosely and briskly. Release any tension in the joints of the shoulders, elbows, and wrists as well as each joint of the fingers by strong shaking of the arms and hands.

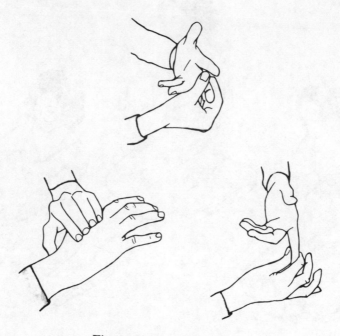

Figure 42. Hand Massage

Leg and foot massage is also part of the usual Dō-in practice and may be done daily. Those with periperal arterial disease, affecting the feet and toes, should emphasize these areas, especially the meridians and key points.

38

Stretching and Walking Exercises

THE THIGHS

This exercise helps prevent hardening of the arteries and arthritis. It extends the thighs, contributing to flexibility in the condition of the muscles and blood circulation. It also harmonizes digestive functions, excretory functions, and breathing by activating the related meridians.

Lying on the back in a relaxed posture, bend the right leg under and extend the right arm upward relaxedly beyond the head (see Figure 43). The left hand is out to the left side about 2 feet, palm up. In this posture, the right leg tends to be slightly off the floor. Now exhale and push the right knee down, touching it to the floor as much as possible and extending the right arm upward as much as possible. At the same time, extend the left arm

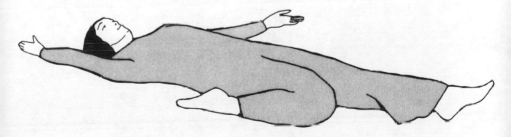

Figure 43. Extension of the Thigh

and left leg downward as much as possible. Then relax. Repeat three times. Then change sides and repeat three times. Then extend the legs, return to the original position, and completely relax.

EXERCISE FOR THE HEART MERIDIAN

Sit with the legs open wide, the knees bent toward the floor, and the soles of the feet together (see Figure 44). Hold the hands around the toes, and bring the feet in toward the body as much as possible. Then slowly bend forward, trying to touch the forehead to the thumbs. In this posture, with all joints relaxed, breathe slowly and deeply two times. During this breathing, energy and blood will stream actively toward the heart and small intestine.

If either knee is higher than the other, tension and disorderly symptoms may appear in that side.

WALKING ON THE GROUND

When we walk, we usually rely on our experience of intuitive balance—left and right, front and back. However, in most cases, we do not fully utilize the energies coming from Heaven and Earth, as well as from the surrounding environment, to make our walking very smooth and effective. Physical imbalances, together with internal disorders and sicknesses, cause most of our walking to be out of harmony with the environment. Individual physical and mental habits also characterize each person's way of walking.

The human body does not grow from the ground; it extends

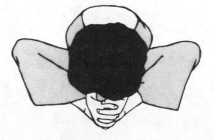

Figure 44. Exercise for the Heart Meridian

vertically in both directions from the region of the mouth cavity and *medulla oblongata*—upward, forming the head, and downward, forming the body, arms, and legs. In other words, the center of the body is floating in space and the lower periphery, the legs and feet, attach lightly to the ground. In Walking on the Ground, therefore, we should hold our body, especially its lower region, including the waist, thighs, legs, and feet, as lightly as possible. Basically, we should walk not with our legs and feet, but with our minds.

To familiarize ourselves with the real way of walking, we can practice the following exercises every day, for as little as ten minutes. Both exercises are beneficial for the heart and circulatory system, though persons with existing heart conditions should be careful about performing the second exercise until their condition has improved.

Ordinary Walking

Keeping the posture straight, receive the forces of Heaven and Earth in their maximum possible power, charging the body, then discharging through the arms and legs. Standing up, keep the sight straight forward as far as you can see, as if you are looking into the infinite distance. Then begin to breathe through the nose very naturally, with the exhalation three to five times longer than the inhalation. This longer exhalation is one of the important factors in walking and running in any circumstance. In fact, a longer exhalation in comparison with the length of the inhalation produces a smoother movement of the body and a more peaceful mind.

As you walk, keep the stomach region as the center of the body, always pushing it forward as if walking from that place. Both arms, if you are not carrying anything, should be held lightly and should move naturally front and back. Don't pay any attention to the legs and feet, allowing them to move as freely as possible.

You will find that with this way of walking you can walk twice as fast as usual, while feeling both lighter and more peaceful. At the same time, you are able to respond instantaneously when you need to change direction, stop walking, or change physical posture to meet new surroundings.

Faster Walking

When you wish to walk faster or almost run for long distances, maintain the posture described in Ordinary Walking to utilize effectively the forces of Heaven and Earth and the environment. Breathing should be done through the nose and the slightly opened mouth, with the exhalation four to seven times longer than the inhalation. Breathing is to be mainly exhaling, with the inhalation merely a reaction to the result of exhaling. Keep the center of the body farther up than in the previous exercise, at the region of the heart, with all lower parts of the body completely relaxed, allowing them to respond freely.

When you walk with the shoulders, which move slightly forward and back, the arms and hands will swing naturally, responding to the movement of the shoulders (see Figure 45). While walking, first put your body weight toward one side, either left or right, and use that foot to support the body, using the foot of the other side to roll or move forward. After about 50 to 100 steps, shift your body weight to the other side and use the opposite side to roll or move. Alternate this way of using the legs every 50 to 100 steps. If you wish to walk more slowly, alternate every 150 to 200 steps, and if you wish to walk faster, alternate every 30 to 50 steps.

The important point in this exercise is that although during the learning period conscious attention is needed to keep the proper posture and movement, eventually the posture is maintained unconsciously, allowing the mind to remain empty and the body to stay strong and untiring while traveling long distances.

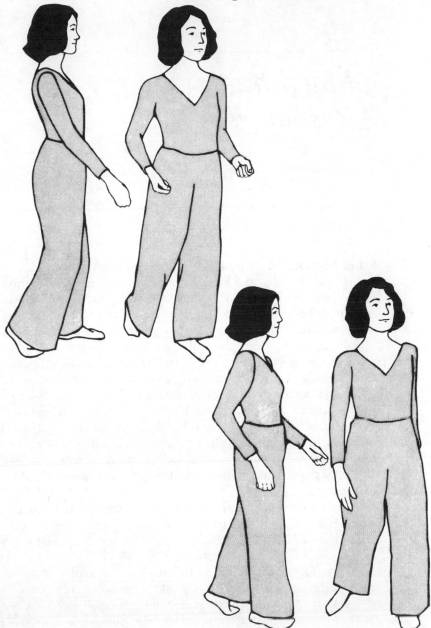

Figure 45. Faster Walking Exercise

39

Macrobiotic
Resources

The Kushi Foundation in Boston and its major educational centers in the United States and Canada offer ongoing classes for the general public in macrobiotic cooking and traditional food preparation and natural processing. They also offer instruction in Oriental medicine, shiatsu massage, pregnancy and natural child care, yoga, meditation, science, culture and the arts, and world peace and world government activities. These educational centers also provide dietary counseling services with trained and certified consultants, referrals to professional health care associates, and cooperate in research and food programs in hospitals, medical schools, prisons, drug rehabilitation clinics, nursing homes, and other institutions. In scores of other cities and communities, there are smaller macrobiotic learning centers, residential centers, and information centers offering some classes and services.

There are also several hundred macrobiotic centers in Central and Latin America, Europe, the Middle East, Africa, Asia, and Australia. There are also friendship and professional associations such as the United Nations Macrobiotics Society.

Most of the foods mentioned in this book are available at natural foods stores, health food stores, and a growing number of supermarkets around the world. Macrobiotic specialty items are also available by mail order from various distributors and retailers.

Please contact the Boston headquarters or one of the selected regional centers listed below for further information on any of the above services or whole foods outlets in your area.

National Headquarters

The Kushi Foundation
Box 1100
Brookline, Massachusetts 02147
(617) 738–0045

Massachusetts

Kushi Marcrobiotic Center of the Berkshires
Box 7
Becket, Massachusetts 01223
(413) 623–5742

New York

Macrobiotic Center of New York
611 Broadway
New York, New York 10012
(212) 877–1110

Washington, D.C.

Macrobiotic Educational Association of Greater Washington
4905 Del Ray Ave. Suite 400
Bethesda, MD 20814
(301) 656–6545

Pennsylvania

The Marcobiotic Assoc. of Pennsylvania
1321 West Wynnewood Rd.
Ardemore, Pa. 19002
(215) 642–4336

Maryland

East West Macrobiotic Foundation
604 East Joppa Road
Towson, Maryland 21204
(301) 321–4474

Florida

Macrobiotic Foundation of Florida
3291 Franklin Avenue
Coconut Grove (Miami), Florida 33133
(305) 448–6625

Ohio

East West Center of Cleveland
1797 Radnor Rd.
Cleveland Heights, OH 44118
(216) 371–3222

Illinois

Midwest Macrobiotic Institute
828 Davis Street
Evanston, Illinois 60201
(312) 328–6632

East West Center
5044 North Western Avenue
Chicago, Illinois 60625
(312) 561–8023

South

Macrobiotic Center of South Carolina
105 Harden St.,
Columbia, S.C. 29205
(803) 765–1400

Rockies

East West Community Center
1931 Mapleton Avenue
Boulder, Colorado 80302
(303) 449-6754

Western Canada

Still Mountain Society
R.R. #1
Fermie, British Columbia, Canada VOB 1MO
(604) 423-6406

Northern California

East West Center for Macrobiotics
1122 M Street
Eureka, California 95501
(707) 445-2290

Southern California

East West Center
11215 Hannum Ave.
Culver City, Calif. 90230
(213) 398-2228

For those who wish to study further, the Kushi Institute, an educational institution founded in Boston in 1979 and with affiliates in London, Amsterdam, Antwerp, Florence, Barcelona, Lisbon, and Tokyo offers full- and part-time instruction for individuals who wish to become certified macrobiotic cooking instructors, teachers, and counselors. The Kushi Institute publishes a *Macrobiotic Teachers and Counselors Directory* every year and makes referrals to graduates who are qualified to give cooking instruction and offer guidance in the macrobiotic way of life.

Kushi Institute
Box 1100
Brookline, Massachusetts 02147
(617) 738-0045

Ongoing developments are reported in the Kushi Foundation's periodicals, including the *East West Journal,* a monthly magazine begun in 1971 and now with an international readership of 200,000. The *East West Journal* features regular articles on the macrobiotic approach to health and nutrition, as well as ecology, science, psychology, and the arts. In each issue there is a macrobiotic cooking column and articles on traditional food cultivation and natural foods processing.

East West Journal
17 Station Street
Brookline, Massachusetts 02146
(617) 232-1000

Notes

Chapter 1: The Heart Disease Epidemic

1. *Dietary Goals for the United States* (Washington, D.C.: Select Committee on Nutrition and Human Needs, U.S. Senate, U.S. Government Printing Office, 1977), 10.

2. All statistics in this paragraph are from *Heart Facts 1984*, (Dallas: American Heart Association, 1984).

3. Michael P. Stern, M.D., "The Recent Decline in Ischemic Heart Disease Mortality," *Annals of Internal Medicine* 91 (1979): 630–40.

4. Patricia Crawford et al., "Serum Cholesterol of Six-Year Olds in Relation to Environmental Factors," *Journal of the American Dietetic Association* 78 (1981): 41–46.

5. Vandie Redaskie, "Coronary Heart Disease in China," *South African Medical Journal* 47 (1973): 1485.

6. J. Judson McNamara et al., "Coronary Artery Disease in Combat Casualties in Vietnam," *Journal of the American Medical Association* 216 (1971): 1185–87; and W. F. Enos et al., "Coronary Disease among U.S. Soldiers Killed in Action in Korea: Preliminary Report," Ibid. 152 (1953): 1090–93.

7. Campbell Moses, M.D., *Atherosclerosis: Mechanisms as a Guide to Prevention* (Philadelphia: Lea and Febiger, 1963), 15.

8. M. S. Seelig, M.D., "Early Nutritional Roots of Cardiovascular Disease," in Herbert K. Naito, ed., *Nutrition and Heart Disease* (New York: SP Medical and Scientific Books, 1982), 31–59.

9. Moses, *Atherosclerosis*, 22.

10. Richard Cooper, M.D., "Rising Death Rates in the Soviet Union: The Impact of Coronary Heart Disease," *New England Medical Journal* 304 (1979): 1259–65.

11. Noboru Kimura, "Changing Patterns of Coronary Heart Disease, Stroke, and Nutrient Intake in Japan," *Preventive Medicine* 12 (1983): 222–27; and Keiko Chiba et al., "Nationwide Survey of HDL Cholesterol among Farmers in Japan," *Preventive Medicine* 12 (1983): 508–22.

12. Michael Gilford, M.D., "Zimbabwe," in H. C. Trowell and D. P. Burkitt, *Western Diseases: Their Emergence and Prevention* (Cambridge, Mass.: Harvard University Press, 1981), 195–96.

13. Genesis 18:1–6 and 19:1–3.

14. Henry C. Lu, trans., *The Yellow Emperor's Classic of Internal Medicine and the Difficult Classic* (Vancouver: Academy of Oriental Heritage, 1978), Book III:8 (p. 58).

15. Ibid., III:10 (p. 70).

16. *Interpreter's Dictionary of the Bible*, Vol. 4, s.v., "Sacrifices and Offerings, Old Testament" (Nashville: Abingdon Press, 1962), 151.

17. Numbers 11:4–5.

18. T. L. Cleave, M.R.C.P., *The Saccharine Disease* (Bristol, England: John Wright & Sons, 1974), 6–7.

19. Ibid., 7.

20. Peter Barry Chowka, "Probing the Medical Pharmaceutical Complex," *East West Journal* (March 1977): 26.

21. William S. Osler, M.D., *Lectures on Angina Pectoris and Allied States* (New York: D. Appleton & Co., 1897), 20.

22. Moses, *Atherosclerosis*, 15.

23. Letitia Brewster and Michael F. Jacobson, *The Changing American Diet* (Washington, D.C.: Center for Science in the Public Interest), 46.

24. Osler, *Lectures*, 145.

25. U.S. Bureau of the Census, *Mortality Statistics*, 1920; 1930; 1940; *Statistical Abstract of the United States*, 1950; 1960.

26. Rob Allanson, "Cutting through the Cream Cheese," *East West Journal* (June 1980): 53.

27. Niles Newton, "Psychologic Differences between Breast and Bottle Feeding," *American Journal of Clinical Nutrition* 24 (1971): 994; and D. B. Jeliffe and E. F. P. Jeliffe, eds., "Symposium—The Uniqueness of Human Milk," *American Journal of Clinical Nutrition* 24 (1971): 968–1024.

28. Quoted in Paul Cressman, "Reproduction Under Seige," *Chino* (December 1981); and "Infertility Increases in Young Women," *New York Times*, February 10, 1983.

29. Rudolph Marx, M.D., *The Health of the Presidents* (New York: G. P. Putnam's Sons, 1960), 316.

30. *Heart Facts*, 3.

31. "Problems Abound in Picking Brink's Jury," *New York Times*, July 19, 1983.

32. Psalms 104:15.

Chapter 2: The Macrobiotic Approach to Heart Disease

1. Clim Yoshimi, "Sagen Ishizuka—The Master's Teacher," *The Macrobiotic*, Oroville, Calif., undated copy of an article published circa 1980.

2. George Ohsawa, *Zen Macrobiotics* (Los Angeles: Ohsawa Foundation, 1965), 33.

3. Ibid., 63.

4. Owsei Temkin and C. Lilian Temkin, eds., "The Hippocratic Oath," *Ancient Medicine: Selected Papers of Ludwig Edelstein* (Baltimore: Johns Hopkins Press, 1967), 6.

5. Hippocrates, "On the Localities of Man," cited in Alfred B. Fishman and D. W. Richards, eds., *Circulation of the Blood* (New York: Oxford University Press, 1964), 130.

6. Christolph W. Hufeland, M.D., *Macrobiotics or the Art of Prolonging Life*, 1797 (English translation, London: John Churchill, 1853), 81, 185.

7. Ibid., 184–85.

8. Peter Pringle and James Spigelman, *The Nuclear Barons* (New York: Avon, 1981), 122.

9. *Dietary Goals for the United States* (Washington, D.C.: Select Committee on Nutrition and Human Needs, U.S. Senate, U.S. Government Printing Office, 1977), 9.

10. *Healthy People: The Surgeon General's Report on Health Promotion and Disease Prevention* (Washington, D.C.: Government Printing Office, 1979).

11. "Quackery: A $10 Billion Scandal," A Report by the Chairman of the Subcommittee on Health and Long-Term Care of the Select Committee on Aging, House of Representatives, May 31, 1984, 67.

12. Stephen S. Schoenthaler, Ph.D., "The Effect of Sugar on the Treatment and Control of Antisocial Behavior," *International Journal of Biosocial Research* 3, no. 1 (1982): 1–9.

Chapter 3: How the Heart Beats

1. *Yellow Emperor's Classic,* quoted in C. R. S. Harris, *The Heart and the Vascular System in Ancient Greek Medicine* (London: Oxford University Press, 1973), 1.

2. William Harvey, quoted in Henry J. Speedby, M.D., *The 20th Century and Your Heart* (London: Centaur Press, 1960), frontispiece.

3. "Heart Diseases in India," *Journal of the Indian Medical Association* 65 (1975): 156–58.

4. "The Gospel According to Thomas," *The Nag Hammadi Library,* James M. Robinson, editor (New York: Harper & Row, 1977), Saying 50, 123.

Chapter 4: Diet, Ecology, and the Heart

1. Jane E. Brody, "Research Yields Surprises About Early Human Diets," *New York Times,* Science Section, May 15, 1979.

2. H. C. Trowell and D. P. Burkitt, *Western Diseases: Their Emergence and Prevention* (Cambridge, Mass.: Harvard University Press, 1981), 15.

Chapter 5: Making Balance Naturally

1. Alexsandr Miasnikov, *Atherosclerosis* (Washington, D.C.: National Institutes of Health, 1962), 71; I. K. Shkhvatsabaya, *Ischemic Heart Disease* (London: C. V. Mosby Co., 1979), 24; and Richard Cooper, M.D., "Rising Death Rates in the Soviet Union: The Impact of Coronary Heart Disease," *New England Medical Journal* 304 (1979): 1259–65.

2. "Primitive Life Keeps Tribesmen's Hearts Strong," *Journal of the American Medical Association* 210 (1969): 1687–88.

3. Henry C. McGill, M.D., "The Relationship of Dietary Cholesterol to Serum Cholesterol Concentration and to Atherosclerosis in Man," *American Journal of Clinical Nutrition* 32 (1979): 2664–2702.

4. Alex Jack, "Passport to Heaven," *East West Journal* (March 1981): 50–57.

5. H. C. Trowell and D. P. Burkitt, *Western Diseases: Their Emergence and Prevention* (Cambridge, Mass: Harvard University Press, 1981), 352–58.

6. Ibid.

7. Ibid., 337–51.

8. T. L. Cleave, M.R.C.P., *The Saccharine Disease* (Bristol, England: John Wright & Sons, 1974), 111–12.

9. "Heart Diseases in India," *Journal of the Indian Medical Association* 65 (1975): 156–58.

10. Trowell and Burkitt, *Western Diseases*, 154–67.

11. J. D. Hunter, "Diet, Body Build, Blood Pressure and Serum Cholesterol Levels in Coconut-Eating Polynesians," *Federal Proceedings* 21, supplement 2 (1962): 36.

12. Trowell and Burkitt, *Western Diseases*, 3–32.

13. A. M. Cohen et al., "Changes of Diet of Yemenite Jews in Relation to Diabetes and Ischemic Heart Disease," *Lancet* 2 (1961): 1399–1401.

14. Jane E. Brody, "New Research on the Vegetarian Diet," *New York Times*, Science Section, October 12, 1983.

15. Ludwig Aschoff, M.D., *Lectures on Pathology* (New York: Paul B. Hoeber, 1924), 139–43.

16. Axel Strom and R. Adelson Jenson, "Mortality from Circulatory Diseases in Norway, 1940–45," *Lancet* 1 (1951): 126–29.

17. Trowell and Burkitt, *Western Diseases*, 113–28.

18. William E. Connor et al., "The Plasma Lipids, Lipoproteins, and Diet of the Tarahumara Indians of Mexico," *American Journal of Clinical Nutrition* 31 (1978): 1131–42.

19. Hugh S. Fulmer et al., "Coronary Heart Disease among the Navajo Indians," *Annals of Internal Medicine* 59 (1963): 740–64.

20. Roland L. Phillips et al., "Coronary Heart Disease Mortality among Seventh Day Adventists with Differing Dietary Habits: A Preliminary Report," *American Journal of Clinical Nutrition* 31 (1978): S191–94.

21. Brody, "New Research on the Vegetarian Diet."

22. H. Kato et al., "Epidemiologic Studies of Coronary Heart Disease and Stroke in Japanese Men Living in Japan, Hawaii, and California: Serum Lipids and Diet," *American Journal of Epidemiology* 97 (1973): 372–85.

23. Trowell and Burkitt, *Western Diseases*, 138–53.

Chapter 7: Nutritional Studies and the Heart

1. P. T. Brown and J. G. Bergan, "Dietary Status of 'New' Vegetarians," *Journal of the American Dietetic Association* 67 (1975): 455–59; and J. G. Bergan and P. T. Brown, "Nutritional Status of 'New Vegetarians,' " *Journal of the American Dietetic Association* 76 (1980): 151–55.

2. J. T. Knuiman and C. E. West, "The Concentration of Cholesterol in Serum and in Various Lipoproteins in Macrobiotic, Vegetarian, and Non-Vegetarian Men and Boys," *Atherosclerosis* 43 (1982): 71–82.

3. *The American Heart Association Heartbook* (New York: Dutton, 1980), 65–66.

4. *Diet, Nutrition, and Cancer* (Washington, D.C.: National Academy of Sciences, 1982), 1–15.

5. Michio Kushi, *The Book of Macrobiotics* (Tokyo: Japan Publications, 1977), 34–48.

6. Jeremiah Stamler, M.D., "Epidemiology as an Investigative Method for the Study of Human Atherosclerosis," *Journal of the National Medical Association* 50 (1958): 161–200.

7. *British Medical Journal* 2 (1977b): 80–81.

8. T. Hirayama, "Relationship of Soybean Paste Soup Intake to Gastric Cancer Risk," *Nutrition and Cancer* 3 (1981): 223–33.

9. *Diet, Nutrition, and Cancer* 15: 1–9.

10. William E. Connor, M.D. et al., "The Plasma Lipids, Lipoproteins, and Diet of the Tarahumara Indians of Mexico," *American Journal of Clinical Nutrition* 31 (1978): 1131–42.

11. G. Chihara et al., "Fractionation and Purification of the Polysaccharides with Marked Antitumor Activity, Especially Lentinan, from *lentinus edodes* (Berk.) Sing. (An Edible Mushroom)," *Cancer Research* 30 (1970): 2776–81.

12. D. R. Meeker and H. D. Kesten, "Experimental Atherosclerosis and High Protein Diets," *Proceedings of the Society for Social Experimentation in Biological Medicine* 45 (1940): 543–45.

13. G. Noseda and Claudia Fragiacomo, "Effects of Soybean Protein Diet on Serum Lipids, Plasma Glucagon, and Insulin," in *Diet and Drugs in Atherosclerosis,* Giorgio Noseda et al., eds. (New York: Raven Press, 1980), 61–65.

14. *Journal of the American Medical Association* 247 (1982): 3045–46.

15. Seibin and Teruko Arasaki, "Dietary and Medical Applications," *Vegetables from the Sea* (Tokyo: Japan Publications, 1983), 32–60.

16. I. Yamamoto et al., "Antitumor Effect of Seaweeds," *Japanese Journal of Experimental Medicine* 44 (1974): 543–46; and N. Iritani and S. Nagi, "Effects of Spinach and Wakame on Cholesterol Turnover in the Rat," *Atherosclerosis* 15 (1972): 87–92.

17. Arasaki, *Vegetables,* 35.

18. Ibid., 60.

19. Ibid.

20. Y. Tanaka et al., "Studies on Inhibition of Intestinal Absorption of Radio-Active Strontium," *Canadian Medical Association Journal* 99 (1968): 169–75.

21. Arasaki, *Vegetables,* 59.

22. H. C. Trowell and D. P. Burkitt, *Western Diseases: Their Emergence and Prevention* (Cambridge, Mass.: Harvard University Press, 1981), 10–11.

23. Thom Leonard et al., "Choosing the Best Sea Salt," *East West Journal* (November 1983): 16–23.

24. Phil Cunby, "It's Not Fishy: Fruit of the Sea May Foil Cardiovascular Disease," *Journal of the American Medical Association* 247 (1982): 729–31.

25. Satoru Kobayashi et al., "Reduction in Blood Viscosity by Eicosapentaenoic Acid," [letter], *Lancet* 2 (1981): 197.

26. B. Armstrong and R. Doll, "Environmental Factors and Cancer Incidence and Mortality in Different Countries with Special Reference to Dietary Practice," *International Journal of Cancer* 15 (1975): 617–31.

27. W. Troll, "Blocking of Tumor Promotion by Protease Inhibitors," in J. H. Burchenal and H. F. Orttgen, eds., *Cancer: Achievements, Challenges, and Prospects for the 1980s, Vol. 1* (New York: Grune and Stratton, 1980), 549–55.

28. William Dufty, *Sugar Blues* (New York: Warner Books, 1975); and Michio Kushi and Alex Jack, *The Cancer-Prevention Diet* (New York: St. Martin's Press, 1983).

29. John Yudkin, M.D., "Diet and Coronary Thrombosis," *Lancet* 2 (1957): 155–62.

30. *Dietary Goals for the United States* (Washington, D.C.: Select Committee on Nutrition and Human Needs, U.S. Senate, U.S. Government Printing Office, 1977), 26.

Chapter 8: Cholesterol and the Heart

1. J. O. Leibowitz, *The History of Coronary Heart Disease* (Berkeley: University of California Press, 1970), 22.

2. "Heart Diseases in India" *Journal of the Indian Medical Association* 65 (1975): 156–58.

3. Leibowitz, *History*, 50–51.

4. Alex Jack and Bill Tims, "A Portrait of Leonardo," *East West Journal* (July 1980): 48–57.

5. Leonardo da Vinci, *Codex Atlanticus, 78v.*

6. Henry Kennedy, *Observations on Fatty Heart* (Dublin: Fannin & Co., 1880), 48–57.

7. Sir William H. Broadbent, M.D., *Heart Disease* (New York: William Wood & Co., 1898), 97.

8. Aleksandr L. Miasnikov, *Atherosclerosis* (Washington, D.C.: National Institutes of Health, 1962).

9. Ludwig Aschoff, M.D., *Lectures on Pathology* (New York: Paul B. Hoeber, 1924), 139–50.

10. Ibid.

11. Unless otherwise noted, all statistics on the Framingham Heart Study in this chapter are from Thomas Royle Dawber, M.D., *The Framingham Study: The Epidemiology of Atherosclerotic Disease* (Cambridge, Mass.: Harvard University Press, 1980.)

12. Ancel Keyes, *Seven Countries: A Multivariate Analysis of Death and Coronary Heart Disease* (Cambridge, Mass.: Harvard University Press, 1980.)

13. H. S. Singman et al., "The Anti-Coronary Club: 1957 to 1972," *American Journal of Clinical Nutrition* 33 (1980): 1183–91.

14. Ingram Hjermains, "A Randomized Primary Prevention Trial in Coronary Heart Disease: The Oslo Study," *Preventive Medicine* 12 (1983): 181–84.

15. P. Leren, "The Oslo Diet-Heart Study: Eleven-Year Report," *Circulation* 42 (1970): 935–42; and M. Miettinen et al., "Effect of Cholesterol Lowering Diet on Mortality from Coronary Heart Disease and Other Causes: A 12-Year Clinical Trial in Men and Women," *Lancet* 2 (1972): 835–38.

16. Dawber, *Framingham Study*, 141.

17. "Hold the Eggs and Butter," *Time* (March 26, 1984): 58.

18. Jane E. Brody, "Panel Urges Cholesterol Cuts to Stem U.S. Heart Disease," *New York Times*, December 13, 1984.

19. Daniel Q. Haney, "Study Says Lifestyle Changes Led Decline in Heart Disease," *Boston Globe*, December 26, 1984.

Chapter 9: The Macrobiotic Studies at Harvard

1. T. M. Dawber, M.D. *The Framingham Study: The Epidemiology of Atherosclerotic Disease* (Cambridge, Mass: Harvard University Press, 1980), 91–120.

2. F. M. Sacks, B. Rosner, and E. H. Kass, "Blood Pressure in Vegetarians," *American Journal of Epidemiology* 100 (1974): 390–98.

3. Dawber, *Framingham Study*, 98.

4. Ibid.

5. Sacks, "Blood Pressure in Vegetarians," 390–98.

6. Ibid.

7. Frank M. Sacks, Sc.B., W. P. Castelli, M.D., Allen Donner, Ph.D., and Edward H. Kass, M.D., Ph.D., "Plasma Lipids and Lipoproteins in Vegetarians and Controls," *New England Journal of Medicine* 292 (1975): 1148–51.

8. William P. Castelli, M.D., "Lessons from the Framingham Heart Study," in Michio Kushi, *Cancer and Heart Disease* (Tokyo: Japan Publications, 1982), 101–05.

9. Ibid., 105.

10. Sacks, "Plasma Lipids," 1148–51.

11. Ibid.

12. J. T. Knuiman and C. E. West, "The Concentration of Cholesterol in Serum and in Various Serum Lipoproteins in Macrobiotic, Vegetarian, and Non-Vegetarian Men and Boys," *Atherosclerosis* 43 (1983): 71–82.

13. F. M. Sacks et al., "Effect of Ingestion of Meat on Plasma Cholesterol in Vegetarians," *Journal of the American Medical Association* 246 (1981): 640–44.

14. Ibid.

15. Telephone interview with Alex Jack, November 2, 1984.

16. Telephone interview with Alex Jack, November 2, 1984.

17. Quoted in a report by Rik Vermuyten, chairman of the medical committee for the European Macrobiotic Congress, *MacroMuse* (Fall/Metal 1984): 39.

18. Mark Mead, "In Search of the Sweet Life: A Dietary Approach to Diabetes Mellitus," Reed College Biology Thesis, in cooperation with the Oregon Health Sciences University, 1984.

19. P. T. Brown and J. G. Bergan, "Dietary Status of 'New' Vegetarians," *Journal of the American Dietetic Association* 76 (1980): 151–55.

Chapter 10: Diet and the Development of Heart Disease

1. John T. Shepherd, M.D., "How the Heart Functions," *American Heart Association Heartbook*, (New York: Dutton, 1980), 129.

2. Lawrence H. Kushi et al., "Diet and Mortality from Coronary Heart Disease in the Ireland-Boston Heart Study," American Heart Association Scientific Sessions, Anaheim, California, November 15, 1983.

3. A. Wright et al., "Dietary Fibre and Blood Pressure," *British Medical Journal,* 2 (1979): 1541–43 and A. M. Fehily et al., "Dietary Determinants of Lipoproteins, Total Cholesterol, Viscosity, Fibrinogen, and Blood Pressure," *American Journal of Clinical Nutrition* 36 (1982): 890–96.

4. A. C. Arutzenius et al., "Effect of Diet on Total Cholesterol/HDL-Cholesterol Ratio in Patients of Leiden Regression Trial," American Heart Association Scientific Sessions, November 16, 1983.

5. Donald H. Heistad et al., "Mechanisms of Altered Vasoconstrictor Responses in Atherosclerosis," American Heart Association Scientific Sessions, November 16, 1983.

6. Henry C. McGill, Jr., "Persistent Questions in the Pathogenesis of Human Atherosclerosis," American Heart Association Scientific Sessions, November 16, 1983; R. L. Kinlough-Rathbone and J. F. Mustard, "Atherosclerosis: Current Concepts," *American Journal of Surgery* 141 (1981): 638–43; and Robert W. Wissler and Henry C. McGill, chairpersons, "Conference on Blood Lipids in Children: Optimal Levels for Early Prevention of Coronary Artery Disease," *Preventive Medicine* 12 (1983): 868–902.

7. *Diet, Nutrition, and Cancer* (Washington, D.C.: National Academy of Sciences, 1982), 5: 1–33.

8. William P. Castelli, M.D., "Lessons from the Framingham Heart Study," in Michio Kushi, *Cancer and Heart Disease* (Tokyo: Japan Publications, 1982), 101–05.

9. Ibid.

10. "Development and Possible Regression of Atherosclerosis: A Symposium," American Heart Association Scientific Sessions, November 13, 1983; and David H. Blankerhorn, "Will Atheroma Regress with Diet and Exercise?" *American Journal of Surgery* 141 (1981): 644–45.

11. L. H. Newburgh and S. Clarkson, "The Production of Atherosclerosis in Rabbits by Feeding Diets Rich in Meat," *Archives of Internal Medicine* 31 (1923): 653–76.

12. D. R. Meeker and H. D. Kesten, *Proceedings in Social Experimental Biological Medicine* 45 (1940): 543–45.

13. Frank M. Sacks et al., "Lack of an Effect of Dairy Protein (Casein) and Soy Protein on Plasma Cholesterol of Strict Vegetarians: An Experiment and a Critical Review," *Journal of Lipid Research* 24 (1983): 1012–20.

14. Ibid.

15. K. K. Carroll, "Dietary Protein in Relation to Plasma Cholesterol Levels and Atherosclerosis," *Nutrition Reviews* 36 (1978): 1–5.

16. Michio Kushi and Alex Jack, "The Myth of Carcinogens," *The Cancer-Prevention Diet* (New York: St. Martin's Press, 1983), 98–114.

17. Martha P. McMurry et al., "Dietary Cholesterol and the Plasma Lipids and Lipoproteins in the Tarahumara Indians: A People Habituated to a Low Cholesterol Diet after Weaning," *American Journal of Clinical Nutrition* 35 (1982): 741–44 and William E. Connor, "Cross-Cultural Studies of Diet and Plasma Lipids and Lipoproteins," in *Childhood Prevention of Atherosclerosis and Hypertension*, R. M. Lauer and R. B. Shekelle, eds. (New York: Raven Press, 1980), 99–111.

18. Kushi, *Ireland-Boston Heart Study.*

19. Murray W. Huff, Ph.D., et al., "Turnover of Very Low-Density Lipoprotein: Apoprotein B Is Increased by Substitution of Soybean Protein for Meat and Dairy Protein in the Diet of Hypercholesterolemic Men," *American Journal of Clinical Nutrition* 39 (1984): 888–97.

Chapter 11: Evaluating the Heart Naturally

1. Lawrence K. Altman, M.D., "Decline in Autopsies Raises Concern," *New York Times*, September 18, 1983.

2. "Effects of Blood-Pressure Measurement by the Doctor on Patient's Blood Pressure and Heart Rate," *Lancet* 2 (1983): 695–698.

3. "Nosebleeds May Prolong Clark's Hospitalization," undated Associated Press clipping.

4. *Boston Globe*, December 10, 1983.

5. Loretta McLaughlin, "New Operation Cures Snoring, Removing Threats to Heartbeat and Blood Pressure," *Boston Globe*, January 13, 1983.

6. Bill Tims, "How Strong Is Your Heart?" *East West Journal* (February 1982): 65.

Chapter 12: Sex, Race, Genetics, and Smoking

1. Elliot Rapaport, M.D., "Coronary Artery Disease," in the *American Heart Association Heartbook* (New York: Dutton, 1980), 178.

2. Ibid.

3. Patricia Wahl et al., "Effect of Estrogen/Progestin Potency in Lipid/ Lipoprotein Cholesterol," *New England Journal of Medicine* 308 (1983): 862–67.

4. *Heart Facts 1984* (Dallas: 1984), 4.

5. Ibid.

6. Peter Barry Chowka, "Up from Soul Food: Dick Gregory's Journey from Night Club to Juice Bar," *East West Journal* (July 1981): 30–37.

7. Duneya Matumbi, "Diet of the African Homeland," *East West Journal* (July 1981): 38–41.

8. H. C. Trowell and D. P. Burkitt, *Western Diseases: Their Emergence and Prevention* (Cambridge, Mass.: Harvard University Press, 1981), 341–42.

9. Ancel Keys, "The Diet and the Development of Coronary Heart Disease," *Journal of Chronic Diseases* 4 (1956): 364–80.

10. T. R. Dawber, M.D., *The Framingham Study: The Epidemiology of Atherosclerotic Disease* (Cambridge, Mass.: Harvard University Press, 1980), 172–80.

11. Revel A. Stallones, "The Rise and Fall of Ischemic Heart Disease," *Scientific American* 243 (1980): 56.

12. Michio Kushi and Alex Jack, *The Cancer-Prevention Diet* (New York: St. Martin's Press, 1983), 238–46.

13. Richard J. Evans et al., "Hazards of Smoking," in *American Heart Association Heartbook*, 22–40.

14. Gary Glober and Grant Stemmermann, "Hawaii Ethnic Groups," in Trowell and Burkitt, *Western Diseases*, 323.

15. Stallones, "Rise and Fall," 58.

Chapter 13: Diet, Emotions, and the Heart

1. J. O. Leibowitz, *The History of Coronary Heart Disease* (Berkeley: University of California Press, 1970), 44.

2. Henry C. Lu, trans., *The Yellow Emperor's Classic of Internal Medicine and the Difficult Classic* (Vancouver: Academy of Oriental Heritage, 1978), 57–58.

3. Ibid.

4. Richard Burton, *The Anatomy of Melancholy*, 1621, revised 1651.

5. *Richard III*, 1.1.135–40.

6. Larry Dossey, M.D., *Space, Time, and Medicine* (Boulder: Shambhala Publications, 1982).

7. "Emotions Found to Influence Nearly Every Human Ailment," *New York Times*, May 24, 1983.

8. *Love's Labour's Lost*, 4.3.301–04.

9. "Stress: Can We Cope," *Time* (June 6, 1983): 50.

10. Dean Ornish, M.D., *Stress, Diet, and Your Heart* (New York: Holt, Rinehart, and Winston, 1982), 59.

11. Norman Cousins, *The Healing Heart* (New York: Norton, 1983).

12. "Stress," *Time*, 54.

13. Jean Marx, "Coronary Artery Spasms and Heart Disease," *Science* 208 (1980): 1127–30.

14. See an article by John Mann based on my lectures, "The Tao of Music," *East West Journal* (May 1979): 49–55.

15. *Hamlet*, 4.7.180.

16. Eric Partridge, *Origins: A Short Etymological Dictionary of Modern English* (New York: Macmillan, 1958), 671–72.

Chapter 14: Diet, Exercise, and the Heart

1. Michael Dehn and Jere H. Mitchell, "Exercise," *American Heart Association Heartbook* (New York: Dutton, 1980), 67–84.

2. Bryan W. Smith et al., "Serum Lipids and Lipoprotein Profiles in Elite Age-Group Endurance Runners," American Heart Association Scientific Sessions, Anaheim, California, November 15, 1983.

3. Henry Blackburn, M.D., "Risk Factors and Cardiovascular Disease," *American Heart Association Heartbook*, 12.

4. John T. Shepherd, M.D., "How the Heart Functions," *American Heart Association Heartbook*, 137.

5. T. R. Dawber, M.D., *The Framingham Study: The Epidemiology of Atherosclerotic Disease* (Cambridge, Mass: Harvard University Press, 1980), 160.

6. Patricia Houseman, *Jack Sprat's Legacy: The Science and Politics of Fat and Cholesterol,* (New York: Richard Marek, 1981), 80.

7. P. D. Thompson et al., "Incidence of Death During Jogging in Rhode Island from 1975 through 1980," *Journal of the American Medical Association* 247 (1982): 2535–38.

8. David S. Siscovick et. al., "The Incidence of Primary Cardiac Arrest During Vigorous Exercise," *New England Journal of Medicine* 311 (1984): 874.

9. Tom Monte, "Sports Doctor's Advice: Interview with T. J. Maggs," *East West Journal* (July 1982): 16–24.

10. Beverly Brough, "America's Native Runners: Interview with Peter Nabokov," *East West Journal* (June 1982): 32–38.

11. Peter Nabakov, *Indian Running* (Santa Barbara, Calif.: Capra Press, 1981), 185.

12. Irving Wallace et al., "The Veggie Baseball Team," *Parade Magazine,* April 15, 1984.

Chapter 15: The Artificial Heart and the Future of Humanity

1. Harry Schwartz, "Toward the Conquest of Heart Disease," *New York Times Magazine,* March 27, 1983, 59.

2. J. R. Crouse and S. M. Grundy, "Effects of Sucrose Polyester on Cholesterol Metabolism in Man," *Metabolism* 28 (1979): 994.

3. Schwartz, "Conquest," 58.

4. "Meet HERO, JR.: The Home and Personal Robot with an Entertaining Personality," Heathkit® Mail Order Catalog No. 867 (Benton Harbor, Mich.: 1984), 2.

5. "Who Should Play God?: Jeremy Rifkin on Genetic Engineering," *East West Journal* (December 1984): 39–46.

6. Thomas Hobbes, *Leviathan,* introduction, 1651.

Chapter 16: Getting Well

1. Norman M. Kaplan, M.D., "Therapy for Mild Hypertension: Toward a More Balanced View," *Journal of the American Medical Association* 249 (1983): 365–67.

2. Jeremy N. Ruskin et al., "Antiarrhythmic Drugs: A Possible Cause of Out-of-Hospital Cardiac Arrest," *New England Journal of Medicine,* 309 (1983): 1302–06.

3. S. H. Taylor et al., "A Long-Term Prevention Study with Oxprenolol in Coronary Heart Disease," *New England Journal of Medicine* 307 (1982): 1293–1301.

4. Robert Mendelsohn, M.D., "Inderal," in *The People's Doctor,* 5, no. 3. (1981), 1–8.

5. Harold M. Schmeck, Jr., "Heart Stimulant Linked to Acidity," *New York Times,* January 14, 1983.

6. Richard A. Knox, "New Treatment for Heart Attacks," *Boston Globe,* November 28, 1983.

7. Richard S. Blacher, M.D., "The Hidden Psychosis of Open-Heart Surgery," *Journal of the American Medical Association* 222 (1972): 305–08.

8. Richard A. Knox, "Study: Some Bypass Surgery Can Be Delayed," *Boston Globe,* October 27, 1983.

9. Frank C. Spencer, M.D., "Emergency Coronary Bypass for Acute Infarction: An Improved Clinical Experiment," *Circulation* 68, supplement II, (1983): 17–19.

10. Marcus A. DeWood et al, "Acute Myocardial Infarction: A Decade of Experiments with Surgical Reperfusion in 701 Patients," *Circulation* 68, supplement II (1983): 8–16.

11. Brenden Phibbs, M.D., *The Human Heart* (New York: New American Library, 1982), 72.

12. H. V. Schaft, "Survival Functional Status After Coronary Artery Bypass Grafting Results 10 to 12 Years after Surgery in 500 Patients," *Circulation* 68, supplement II (1983): 200–04.

13. Phibbs, *Human Heart,* 153.

14. *The Yellow Emperor's Classic of Internal Medicine and the Difficult Classic,* translated by Dr. Henry C. Lu, Ph.D. (Vancouver: The Academy of Oriental Heritage, 1978), 14.

Chapter 17: Dietary Recommendations

1. Some of the material in this section is derived from an article on visual diagnosis by Bill Tims edited by Alex Jack and based on my lectures at the East West Foundation. See Bill Tims, "How Healthy Is Your Heart?," *East West Journal* (November 1980): 48–49.

Chapter 26: Diseases of the Veins

1. H. C. Trowell and D. P. Burkitt, *Western Diseases: Their Emergence and Prevention* (Cambridge, Mass.: Harvard University Press, 1981), 38.

2. Ibid.

3. Ibid.

4. Ibid.

Chapter 27: Congenital Heart Disease

1. "Birth Defects Reported Doubled," *Boston Globe*, July 19, 1983.

Chapter 29: The Tragical Case History of Prince Hamlet

1. All quotations from *Hamlet* in this chapter are from *The Arden Shakespeare: Hamlet*, Harold Jenkins, ed. (London and New York: Methuen, 1982). 5.2.208–09.

2. 3.1.47–49.

3. 1.2.180–81.

4. 1.2.146.

5. 3.4.72–73.

6. 3.2.356–57.

7. 2.2.524–25.

8. 2.2.435–36.

9. 2.2.440–41.

10. 4.3.16–21.

11. Shree Purohit Swami and W. B. Yeats, *The Ten Principal Upanishads* (London: Faber and Faber, 1937), 69, 78.

12. 1.4.81–83.

13. 1.5.93–95.

14. 3.4.64.

15. 1.5.66–70.

16. 3.4.184.

17. 3.3.89.

18. 3.3.70–71.

19. 2.2.573–74.

20. 1.4.40.

21. 3.2.68–73.

22. 3.2.381–86.

23. 5.2.77–78.

24. 1.2.79.

25. 3.1.84–85.

26. 5.2.170–71.

27. 5.2.290.

28. 2.2.374–75.

29. Timothy Bright, *A Treatise of Melancholy,* 1586.

30. 1.4.27–29.

31. 3.2.291–99.

32. 1.2.129–30.

33. 2.2.303–08.

34. 2.2.300–303.

35. 2.2.569–70.

36. 2.2.243.

37. Cyrus Hoy, *Hamlet* (New York: Norton, 1963), 107.

38. 5.2.351–54.

39. 5.2.364–65.

40. Giorgio de Santillana and Hertha von Dechend, *Hamlet's Mill* (Boston: David Godine, 1977).

41. 4.3.9–11.

42. 4.3.68–70.

43. 4.7.122–23.

44. 1.5.85.

45. 5.2.60–62.

46. 5.2.4–5.

47. 1.4.17–20.

48. 3.4.91–93.

49. 3.4.154–56.

50. 5.2.218–220.

51. 5.2.215–216.

52. 5.2.10–11.

53. 3.4.48–49.

54. John Russell, "The Image of the Buddha Continues to Enthrall," *New York Times*, December 2, 1984.

55. 5.2.386–90.

Glossary

Amasake A sweet, creamy beverage made from fermented sweet rice.

Aneurysm A ballooning-out of the wall of the heart or a blood vessel.

Angina pectoris A chronic pain in the chest caused by coronary heart disease, usually relieved when the level of activity is reduced.

Aorta The great artery receiving blood from the left ventricle and distributing it to the rest of the body.

Arame A thin, wiry black sea vegetable similar to hiziki.

Arepa An oval-shaped corn ball or cake made from whole corn dough and baked or fried.

Arrhythmia Any abnormal heartbeat.

Arrowroot A starch flour processed from the root of an American plant used as a thickening agent in cooking.

Arteriole A small arterial blood vessel connecting an artery to the capillaries.

Arteriosclerosis Generalized hardening of the arteries.

Artery Blood vessel transporting blood away from the heart.

Atheroma A fatty deposit on the inside walls of artery; also called *plaque;* plural *atheromata.*

Atherosclerosis A form of arteriosclerosis in which hardened plaque from fat and cholesterol builds up on the inner walls of arteries, narrowing them and reducing the flow of blood; the underlying cause of most heart attacks and strokes.

Atrioventricular node A small mass of special muscle fibers connecting the upper and lower chambers of the heart; also called AV node.

Atrium One of the two top chambers of the heart; plural *atria.*

Autonomic nervous system The system regulating largely involuntary functions such as heartbeat, blood pressure, etc.

Azuki bean   A small, dark, red bean originally from Japan but now also grown in the West.

Bancha tea   The twigs, stems, and leaves from mature Japanese tea bushes; bancha twig tea also known as *kukicha tea.*
Barley malt   A natural sweetener made from malted barley.
Blood pressure   The force that flowing blood exerts against artery walls.
Boiled salad   Salad whose ingredients are lightly boiled or dipped in hot water before serving.
Bradycardia   Abnormally slow heartbeat, usually under 60 beats per minute.
Brown rice   Whole unpolished rice, containing an ideal balance of nutrients.
Buckwheat   A hardy cereal grass eaten in the form of kasha (whole groats) or soba noodles.
Burdock   A wild hardy plant whose long, dark root is valued in cooking for its strengthening qualities.

Capillary   The smallest blood vessel, in which nutrients and gases are exchanged to the cells and tissues.
Cardiomyopathy   A degenerative weakening of the heart muscle.
Carotid artery   One of the two major arteries supplying blood to the head and neck.
Cholesterol   A waxy constituent of all animal fats and oils, which can contribute to heart disease, cancer, and other diseases. Vegetable-quality foods do not contain cholesterol. The liver naturally produces all the serum cholesterol needed by the body.
Claudication   Pain, soreness, or lameness in the limbs resulting from faulty circulation.
Congestive heart failure   Progressive loss of the heart's pumping function, leading to fluid accumulation in the lungs, legs, or abdomen.
Coronary bypass   Surgical operation in which usually a vein from the leg is inserted into the heart to detour around the obstructed part of an artery.
Coronary heart disease   Degeneration of the coronary arteries or other vessels of the heart; the most common form of modern heart disease.

Daikon   A long, white radish used in many types of dishes and for medicinal purposes.
Dashi   Traditional Japanese soup stock made from kombu broth.
Diastole   The relaxing period of the heartbeat where incoming blood fills up the atria or ventricles.

Dry-roast   To toast a grain, seed, or flour in an unoiled skillet, stirring gently until brown or golden and a nutty aroma is released.

Dulse   A red-purple sea vegetable used in soups, salads, and vegetable dishes or as a garnish.

Electrocardiogram   A graph recording the electrical impulses produced by the heart; called an *ECG* or *EKG*.

Embolism   The obstruction of a blood vessel by a clot or other substance transported in the bloodstream.

Embolus   A blood clot or other substance that drifts in the bloodstream and becomes lodged in a small vessel, impeding or obstructing circulation.

Epinephrine   A hormonal secretion of the adrenals, which constricts the arterioles, increases heart rate, and raises blood pressure; also called *adrenalin*.

Fiber   The part of whole grains, vegetables, and fruits that is not broken down in digestion and gives bulk to wastes.

Fibrillation   Chaotic heart rhythm characterized by rapid, irregular contractions.

Fu   Dried wheat gluten cakes or sheets.

Ginger   A spicy, pungent, golden-colored root used in cooking and for medicinal purposes.

Ginger compress   A compress made from grated gingerroot and water. Applied hot to an affected area of the body, it serves to stimulate circulation and dissolve stagnation.

Gomashio   Sesame seed salt made from dry-roasting and grinding sea salt and sesame seeds and crushing them in a suribachi.

Hara   Energy center located in the intestinal area.

Heart attack   The death of a portion of the heart muscle resulting from an obstruction in one of the coronary arteries, preventing an adequate supply of oxygen to the heart; also called a *myocardial infarction*.

Heart failure   Inability of the heart to pump sufficient blood to maintain normal circulation; a condition resulting from many disorders, including high blood pressure and coronary disease.

Hemorrhage   Loss of blood from a blood vessel.

High blood pressure   A state of chronic abnormal elevation of blood pressure; also known as *hypertension*.

Hiziki   A dark brown sea vegetable that when dried turns black; also spelled *hijiki*.

Hypertension   High blood pressure.
Hypotension   Low blood pressure.

Ischemia   A temporary deficiency of oxygen in some localized part of the body.
Ischemic heart disease   General term for coronary heart disease or degeneration of the heart as a result of atherosclerosis.

Jinenjo   A light brown Japanese mountain potato that grows to be several feet long and two to three inches wide.

Kanten   A jelled fruit dessert made from agar-agar.
Kasha   Roasted buckwheat groats.
Kelp   A large family of sea vegetables similar to kombu.
Kinpura   A style of cooking root vegetables by first sautéing, then adding a little water, and seasoning with tamari soy sauce at the end of cooking.
Koi koku   A rich, thick soup made from carp, burdock, bancha tea, and miso.
Kombu   A wide, thick, dark green sea vegetable that grows in deep ocean water. Used in making soup stocks and condiments, and cooked as a separate dish or with vegetables, beans, or grains.
Kuzu   A white starch made from the root of a prolific wild vine. Used in thickening soups, gravies, sauces, desserts, and for medicinal beverages; also known as *kudzu.*

Lipid   A fat, oil, or fatlike substance such as cholesterol; also called *lipoid.*
Lipoprotein   A substance combining lipid and protein molecules, allowing substances that are insoluble in the blood to circulate through the body.
Lotus root   Root of the water lily, brown-skinned with a hollow, chambered, off-white inside, used in many dishes and for medicinal preparations.

Macrobiotics   From the traditional Greek words for "Great Life" or "Long Life." The way of life according to the largest possible view, the infinite order of the universe. The practice of macrobiotics includes the understanding and practical application of this order to daily life, including the selection, preparation, and manner of cooking and eating, as well as the orientation of consciousness.
Masa   Dough made from whole corn, used in making arepas, tortillas, and other traditional dishes.

Meridian   One of the channels of electromagnetic energy circulation in the body in traditional Oriental medicine.

Millet   A small, yellow grain that can be prepared whole and added to soups, salads, and vegetable dishes.

Mirin   A sweet cooking wine made from sweet rice.

Miso   A fermented paste made from soybeans, sea salt, and usually rice or barley. Used in soups, stews, spreads, baking, and as a seasoning. Miso gives a nice sweet taste and salty flavor.

Mitral valve   The valve connecting the upper and lower chambers of the left side of the heart.

Mochi   A cake or dumpling made from cooked, pounded sweet rice.

Mu tea   A tea made from a variety of herbs that warms the body, strengthens the female organs, and has other medicinal properties.

Murmur   Any abnormal heart sound.

Myocardial infarction   The death of an area of heart muscle; also known as *heart attack*.

Myocardium   The muscular wall of the heart.

Natto   A lightly fermented soybean dish with sticky, long strands and a strong odor.

Natural foods   Whole foods that are unrefined and untreated with artificial additives or preservatives.

Nishime   Long, slow style of boiling in which vegetables or other ingredients cook primarily in their own juices, giving strong, peaceful energy.

Norepinephrine   A hormonal secretion that raises the blood pressure.

Nori   Thin sheets of dried sea vegetable, black or dark purple in color, that turn green when roasted; used as a garnish, to wrap rice balls, in making sushi, or cooked with tamari soy sauce as a condiment.

Occlusion   Obstruction of a blood vessel.

Open-pollinated   Type of traditional Indian corn that is pollinated by the wind as opposed to hybrid corn; also known as *standard corn*.

Organic foods   Foods grown without the use of chemical fertilizers, herbicides, pesticides, or other artificial sprays.

Pacemaker   The sinoatrial node that activates the heartbeat; an artificial pacemaker is often inserted when the heart's natural pacemaker fails to perform properly.

Pan-fry   To sauté with a little oil over a low to medium heat, stirring occasionally but not so often as stir-frying.

Peripheral artery disease   Disorders of the arteries in the limbs or vessels outside of the heart.

Phlebitis   Inflammation of a vein, usually in a leg, subject to clotting.

Plaque   An atherosclerotic deposit of fatty substances in the inner lining of an artery.

Platelets   One of the formed elements in the blood.

Polyunsaturated fats   Essential fatty acids found in high concentration in whole grains, beans, seeds, and to a lesser extent in fish.

Pressed salad   Salad prepared by pressing sliced vegetables and sea salt in a small pickle press or an improvised weight on a plate.

Pressure-cooker   An airtight metal pot that cooks food quickly by steaming under pressure at high temperature. Used primarily in macrobiotic cooking for whole grains and occasionally for beans and vegetables.

Pulmonary artery   The large artery conveying unoxygenated blood from the right ventricle to the lungs.

Pulmonary vein   The large vein conveying oxygenated blood from the lungs to the left atrium.

Pulse   The rhythmic expansion and contraction of an artery.

Refined oil   Cooking oil that has been chemically processed to alter or remove its natural color, taste, and aroma.

Regurgitation   The flow of blood backward through a diseased valve.

Rheumatic fever   A disease growing out of a streptococcal infection, often affecting children and often weakening the heart.

Rice cake   A light, round cake made of puffed brown rice enjoyed as a snack.

Rice syrup   A natural sweetener made from malted brown rice.

Saturated fats   Fats found primarily in meats, poultry, eggs, dairy food, and a few vegetable oils such as coconut and palm tree oil; these fats elevate serum cholesterol and contribute to atherosclerosis.

Sea salt   Salt obtained from the ocean; unrefined sea salt is high in trace minerals and contains no chemicals, sugar, or added iodine.

Sea vegetable   An edible seaweed such as kombu, wakame, arame, hiziki, nori, or dulse.

Seitan   A whole wheat product cooked in tamari soy sauce, kombu, and water; used for stews, croquettes, grainburgers, and many other dishes; high in protein and gives a strong, dynamic taste; also called *wheat gluten* or *wheat meat.*

Septum   A wall dividing the left and right chambers of the heart and the upper and lower chambers.

Serum cholesterol   Cholesterol measured or produced in the body as distinct from dietary cholesterol, measured or found in animal foods.

Shiitake   A mushroom used, fresh or dried, for soups and stews and for medicinal purposes.

Shio kombu Salty kombu; pieces of kombu cooked for a long time in tamari soy sauce and used as a condiment.

Shiso Leaves usually pickled with umeboshi plums; also known as *beefsteak leaves.*

Sinoatrial node The heart's natural pacemaker located in the right atrium, generating electrical activity to keep the heart beating.

Soba Noodles made from buckwheat flour or buckwheat combined with whole wheat.

Stenosis A narrowing or contraction, especially of a valve.

Stoneground Unrefined flour that has been ground in a stone mill that preserves the germ, bran, and other nutrients.

Stroke An obstruction of blood to some part of the brain, resulting from a blood clot, a hemorrhage, an embolus, or pressure on a blood vessel; also called a *cerebral vascular accident.*

Stroke volume The amount of blood pumped out of the heart during each contraction.

Suribachi A serrated, glazed clay bowl or mortar, used with a pestle for grinding and pureeing foods.

Sweet rice A glutinous type of rice that is slightly sweeter to the taste and used in making mochi, amasake, and various dishes.

Systole The period of contraction of the heartbeat.

Tachycardia Abnormally rapid heartbeat, usually over 100 beats per minute.

Tamari soy sauce Traditional, naturally made soy sauce, distinguished from refined, chemically processed soy sauce; also known as *organic* or *natural shoyu.* A stronger, wheat-free soy sauce called *real* or *genuine tamari,* a by-product of making miso, is used for special dishes. Tamari soy sauce is used for daily cooking in macrobiotic food preparation.

Tekka Condiment made from soy miso, sesame oil, burdock, lotus root, carrot, and gingerroot, cooked down to a black powder.

Tempeh A traditional Indonesian soyfood made from split soybeans, water, and a special bacteria; high in protein with a rich, dynamic taste, tempeh is used in soups, stews, sandwiches, casseroles, and other dishes.

Thrombosis The formation or presence of a blood clot inside a blood vessel or the heart itself.

Thrombus A blood clot that forms inside a blood vessel and may impede or obstruct the flow of blood.

Tofu Soybean curd made from soybeans and nigari; high in protein and prepared in cakes, it is used in soups, vegetable dishes, salads, sauces, dressings, and other dishes.

Triglyceride   A fatty acid, high levels of which are associated with atherosclerosis.

Udon   Japanese whole wheat noodles.
Umeboshi   A salted pickled plum that has aged usually for several years. Its nice zesty sour taste and salty flavor go well with many foods, and it is used as a seasoning, in sauces, as a condiment, in beverages, and in many medicinal preparations.
Umeboshi vinegar   The liquid that umeboshi plums are aged in; used for sauces, dressings, and seasoning and making pickles; also known as *ume-su*.
Unrefined oil   Vegetable oil that has been naturally processed to retain its natural color, taste, aroma, and nutrients.

Varicose vein   Swollen vein in the leg.
Vascular   Pertaining to the blood vessels or circulatory system as a whole.
Vein   A blood vessel conveying blood from various parts of the body back toward the heart.
Vena cava   One of two large veins that return unoxygenated blood back to the right atrium.
Ventricle   One of the two pumping chambers of the heart.

Wakame   A long thin, green sea vegetable used in making daily miso soup, as well as salads and other dishes.
Whole foods   Foods in their natural form that have not been refined or processed, such as brown rice or whole wheat berries.
Whole grains   Unrefined cereal grains to which nothing has been added or subtracted in milling except for the inedible outer hull. Whole grains include brown rice, millet, barley, whole wheat, oats, rye, buckwheat, and corn.
Whole wheat   A whole cereal grain that may be prepared in whole form or made into flour. Whole wheat products such as noodles, seitan, fu, bulghur, couscous, and cracked wheat make a variety of dishes.

Yang   One of the two fundamental energies of the universe. Yang refers to the relative tendency of contraction, centripetality, density, heat, light, and other qualities. Yang energy tends to go down and inward. Its complementary and antagonistic force is yin.
Yin   One of the two fundamental energies of the universe. Yin refers to the relative tendency of expansion, growth, centrifugality, diffusion, cold, darkness, and other qualities. Yin energy tends to go up and outward. Its complementary and antagonistic force is yang.

Recommended Reading

Books

Aihara, Cornellia. *Macrobiotic Kitchen*. Tokyo: Japan Publications, 1983.

Aihara, Herman. *Basic Macrobiotics*. New York: Japan Publications, 1985.

Brewster, Letitia, and Michael F. Jacobson, Ph.D. *The Changing American Diet*. Washington, D.C.: Center for Science in the Public Interest, 1979.

Brown, Virginia, with Susan Stayman. *Macrobiotic Miracle: How a Vermont Family Overcame Cancer*. New York: Japan Publications, 1985.

Dietary Goals for the United States. Washington, D.C.: Select Committee on Nutrition and Human Needs, U.S. Senate, 1977.

Diet, Nutrition, and Cancer. Washington, D.C.: National Academy of Sciences, 1982.

Dufty, William. *Sugar Blues*. New York: Warner Books, 1975.

Esko, Edward, and Wendy Esko. *Macrobiotic Cooking for Everyone*. Tokyo: Japan Publications, 1980.

Esko, Wendy. *Introducing Macrobiotic Cooking*. Tokyo: Japan Publications, 1978.

Fukuoaka, Masanobu. *The One-Straw Revolution*. Emmaus, Pa.: Rodale Press, 1978.

Healthy People: The Surgeon General's Report on Health Promotion and Disease Prevention. Washington, D.C., 1979.

Heidenry, Carolyn. *An Introduction to Macrobiotics.* Brookline, Mass.: Aladdin Press, 1984.

Hippocrates. *Hippocratic Writings.* G. E. R. Lloyd. Translated by J. Chadwick and W. N. Mann. New York: Penguin Books, 1978.

I Ching or *The Book of Changes.* Translated by Richard Wilhelm and Cary F. Baynes. Princeton: Bollingen Foundation, 1950.

Kohler, Jean, and Mary Alice Kohler. *Healing Miracles from Macrobiotics.* West Nyack, N.Y.: Parker, 1979.

Kotzsch, Ronald E., Ph.D. *Macrobiotics: Yesterday and Today.* Tokyo: Japan Publications, 1985.

Kushi, Aveline. *How to Cook with Miso.* Tokyo: Japan Publications, 1978.

———. *Cooking for Health: Allergies.* Edited by Lillian Kushi. Tokyo: Japan Publications, 1985.

———. *Cooking for Health: Diabetes and Hypoglycemia.* Edited by Veronique Kushi. Tokyo: Japan Publications, 1985.

Kushi, Aveline, with Wendy Esko. *Changing Seasons Macrobiotic Cookbook.* Wayne, N.J.: Avery Publishing Group, 1985.

Kushi, Aveline, with Alex Jack. *Aveline Kushi's Complete Guide to Macrobiotic Cooking for Health, Harmony, and Peace.* New York: Warner Books, 1985.

Kushi, Michio. *The Book of Dō-In: Exercise for Physical and Spiritual Development.* Tokyo: Japan Publications, 1979.

———. *The Book of Macrobiotics.* Tokyo: Japan Publications, 1977.

———. *The Era of Humanity.* Edited by Sherman Goldman. Brookline, Mass.: East West Journal, 1980.

———. *How to See Your Health: The Book of Oriental Diagnosis.* Tokyo: Japan Publications, 1980.

———. *Macrobiotic Home Remedies.* Edited by Marc Van Cauwenberge, M.D. Tokyo: Japan Publications, 1985.

———. *Natural Approach: Allergies.* Edited by Mark Mead. Tokyo: Japan Publications, 1985.

———. *Natural Approach: Diabetes and Hypoglycemia.* Edited by John David Mann. Tokyo: Japan Publications, 1985.

———. *Natural Healing through Macrobiotics.* Tokyo: Japan Publications, 1978.

Kushi, Michio, with Alex Jack. *The Cancer-Prevention Diet.* New York: St. Martin's Press, 1983.

Kushi, Michio, and Aveline Kushi. *Macrobiotic Pregnancy and Care of the Newborn.* Edited by Edward and Wendy Esko. Tokyo: Japan Publications, 1984.

———. *Macrobiotic Childcare and Family Health.* Edited by Edward and Wendy Esko. Tokyo: Japan Publications, 1985.

———. *Macrobiotic Diet.* Edited by Alex Jack. Tokyo: Japan Publications, 1985.

Mendelsohn, Robert S., M.D. *Confessions of a Medical Heretic.* Chicago: Contemporary Books, 1979.

———. *Male Practice.* Chicago: Contemporary Books, 1980.

Miller, Saul, with Joanne Miller. *Food for Thought: A New Look at Food and Behavior.* Englewood Cliffs, N.J.: Prentice-Hall, 1979.

Ohsawa, George. *Cancer and the Philosophy of the Far East.* Oroville, Calif.: George Ohsawa Macrobiotic Foundation, 1971.

———. *You Are All Sanpaku.* Edited by William Dufty. New York: University Books, 1965.

Ohsawa, Lima. *Macrobiotic Cuisine.* Tokyo: Japan Publications, 1984.

Price, Weston A., D.D.S. *Nutrition and Physical Degeneration.* Santa Monica, Calif.: Price-Pottenger Nutritional Foundation, 1945.

Sattilaro, Anthony, M.D., with Tom Monte. *Recalled by Life: The Story of My Recovery from Cancer.* Boston: Houghton-Mifflin, 1982.

Yamamoto, Shizuko. *Barefoot Shiatsu.* Tokyo: Japan Publications, 1979.

Tara, William. *Macrobiotics and Human Behavior.* Tokyo: Japan Publications, 1985.

The Yellow Emperor's Classic of Internal Medicine. Translated by Ilza Veith. Berkeley: University of California Press, 1949.

Periodicals

East West Journal, Brookline, Massachusetts

MacroMuse, Rockville, Maryland

Nutrition Action, Washington, D.C.

The People's Doctor, Evanston, Illinois

Index

abortion, 226
Abraham, 7–8, 18, 34
Academic Hospital of Ghent
  University, 131–132
aches, 242
acid/alkaline quality of blood,
  141–142
acid/alkaline ratio of nutrients, 21
acrocynanosis, 294–295
acupuncture, 42, 192, 217
acute thrombosis, *see* embolism
adrenal glands, 47, 145, 203, 262
adrenalin (epinephrine), 203, 239, 262
aerobic exercise, 215–216
Afghanistan, diet in, 51
Africa, diet and diseases in, 64, 69
age, smoking and, 191
agriculture:
  chemicalized, 11, 22
  self-sufficiency in, 22
AIDS, 14, 31
alcohol, 9
  atherosclerosis and, 249
  blood quality and, 139, 142
  cancer and, 27
  cardiovascular disease and, 27, 60,
    138, 265, 272, 275, 279, 281, 288
  dietary guidelines for, 95
  hypertension and, 249, 261, 263
  hypotension and, 250

liver disease and, 27
  in modern diets, 13, 59
  in patient's diet, 249, 260
  in traditional diets, 51
Algeny (Rifkin), 230
alveoli, 190
American Cancer Society, 31
American Heart Association, xii, 3, 17,
  28, 98, 106, 109, 119, 146, 171, 242
*American Journal of Clinical
  Nutrition*, 103, 160
American Journal of Epidemiology,
  29, 125
American Type Culture Collection, 411
amniocentesis, 227
Anatomy of Melancholy, The
  (Burton), 195–196
anemia, 250
aneurysms, 4, 136, 292–293
  home cares for, 293
angina:
  diet and, 11, 62, 131
  in heart surgery patients, 240
  in traditional cultures, 62
angina pectoris, 135, 203
  cholesterol and, 120
  description of, 10, 267–268
  diagnosis of, 162
  drug treatments for, 268
  smoking and, 188

507

Recipe Index

Note on the Authors

Michio Kushi, leader of the international macrobiotic, natural health movement, has guided thousands of people with cancer and heart disease toward physical, psychological, and spiritual health and lectured on Oriental medicine and philosophy to medical professionals across North and South America, Europe, and the Far East. He has inspired macrobiotic research projects at the Harvard School of Public Health, Tulane University Medical School, University Hospital and Shattuck Hospital in Boston, and other hospitals, medical schools, and prisons around the country. He is the president of the Kushi Foundation, Kushi Institute, and East West Foundation in Boston with 500 affiliate centers worldwide. He has also spoken at numerous international seminars, governmental conferences, universities, medical schools, civic organizations, and the United Nations.

Born in Kokawa, Wakayama-ken, Japan, in 1926, Michio Kushi devoted his early years to the study of international law at Tokyo University. Following World War II, he became interested in world peace through world government and met Yukikazu Sakurazawa (known in the West as George Ohsawa), who had revised and reintroduced the principles of Oriental medicine and philosophy under the traditional name *macrobiotics*. Inspired by Ohsawa's teaching, he began his lifelong study of the application of traditional understanding to solving the problems of the modern world.

In 1949 Michio Kushi came to the United States to pursue graduate studies at Columbia University. Since that time he has resided in this country and lectured on diet, philosophy, and culture and given personal counseling to individuals and families. In 1972 he founded the East West Foundation, a nonprofit cultural and educational organization, with headquarters in Boston, to help develop and spread the macrobiotic way of life through seminars, publications, research, and other means. He is also the founder of Erewhon, a leading distributor of natural and macrobiotic foods in North America, and of the *East West Journal*, a monthly magazine unifying traditional Oriental philosophy and medicine with Western science. In 1978 he founded the Kushi Institute, an educational organization for the training of macrobiotic teachers, counselors, and cooks, with affiliates in London, Amsterdam, Florence, and Antwerp. As a further means toward addressing problems of world health and world peace, he established the Macrobiotic Congresses of North America, the Caribbean, and Western Europe, which meet annually and draw delegates from many states and nations.

Michio Kushi has published a dozen books including *The Book of Macrobiotics, How to See Your Health: Book of Oriental Diagnosis, The Macrobiotic Way of Natural Healing, The Cancer-Prevention Diet,* and *Macrobiotic Pregnancy and Care of the Newborn.* He currently resides in Brookline, Massachusetts, with his wife Aveline, several of his five children, and their families.

Alex Jack was born in Chicago in 1945 and grew up in Evanston, Illinois and Scarsdale, New York. His interest in the Far East developed at age eleven when he accompanied his father, a Unitarian minister, to an international peace conference in Japan. During the mid-1960s, he served as a civil rights organizer in Mississippi, helped set up an arts festival with atomic bomb survivors in Hiroshima, and reported on the war in Southeast Asia for a syndicate of university, small-town, and peace publications. He adopted a natural foods diet while studying philosophy and religion at Banaras Hindu University in India in 1965.

After graduating from Oberlin College in 1967 with a degree in philosophy, he pursued graduate studies, traveled, and edited several newspapers and periodicals. In 1973 he founded Kanthaka Press, a small publishing company named after the Buddha's horse. In 1975 Alex joined the staff of the *East West Journal,* serving as editor from 1979 to 1982 and writing extensively on diet, nutrition, heart disease, cancer, and various historical and literary subjects.

Alex's books include *The Adamantine Sherlock Holmes: The Adventures in Tibet and India, The New Age Dictionary,* and *Dragon Brood: An Epic Poem of Vietnam and America.* With Michio Kushi, he is the co-author of *The Cancer-Prevention Diet* and with Aveline Kushi the co-author of *Aveline Kushi's Complete Guide to Macrobiotic Cooking for Health, Harmony, and Peace.* He lives in Brookline, Massachusetts.